CONTEMPORARY MANAGEMENT IN CRITICAL CARE

MARTIN J. TOBIN, MD, Editor-in-Chief

Professor of Medicine
Division of Pulmonary and Critical Care Medicine
Stritch School of Medicine
Loyola University of Chicago
Chicago, Illinois

AKE GRENVIK, MD, PhD, Editor-in-Chief

Professor of Anesthesiology, Medicine & Surgery
Director, Multidisciplinary CCM Training Program
University of Pittsburgh Medical Center
Pittsburgh, Pennsylvania

D1537954

■:■ CHURCHILL LIVINGSTONE
New York, Edinburgh, London, Melbourne, Tokyo 1991

FORTHCOMING ISSUES

CRITICAL CARE TOXICOLOGY

ROBERT S. HOFFMAN, MD, ABMT, Editor

Director, Medical Toxicology Fellowship Training
  Program
Associate Medical Director
New York City Poison Control Center
Instructor Clinical Surgery/Emergency Medicine
New York University School of Medicine
New York, New York

LEWIS R. GOLDFRANK, MD, ABMT, Editor

Director, Emergency Services
Bellevue and New York University Hospital
Medical Director
New York City Poison Control Center
New York, New York

CHURCHILL LIVINGSTONE
New York, Edinburgh, London, Melbourne, Tokyo 1991

Copyright © 1991 by Churchill Livingstone Inc.
Contemporary Management in Critical Care is published quarterly.
Annual subscription rates (1991): U.S., $65 individual, $85 institution; foreign, add $30 for airmail or $15 for surface mail; single copy, $32.50.

ISSN 1050-9623
ISBN 0-443-08830-6

Direct subscription orders, changes of address, and claims for missing issues (within five months of publication) to Churchill Livingstone Inc. (650 Avenue of the Americas, New York, NY 10011). In Japan, contact Nankodo Co., Ltd., 42-6, Hongo 3-chome, Bunkyo-ku, Tokyo 113, Japan.

The authors, editors, and publisher have exerted every effort to ensure that drug selection and dosage and descriptions of instruments and recommendations for their use set forth in all articles appearing in *Contemporary Management in Critical Care* are in accord with current recommendations and practice at the time of publication. However, many considerations necessitate caution in applying in practice any information appearing in *Contemporary Management in Critical Care*. The reader is advised to check package inserts for each drug for indications and dosages and the descriptions provided by instrument manufacturers for warnings and precautions.

The publishers have made every effort to trace the copyright holders for borrowed material. If they have inadvertently overlooked any, they will be pleased to make the necessary arrangements at the first opportunity.

Printed in the United States of America

Volume 1 Number 3
First published in 1991

CONTRIBUTING AUTHORS

LEAH BALSAM, MD
Attending Nephrologist
Nassau County Medical Center
East Meadow, New York
Instructor of Medicine
State University of New York at Stony Brook
Health Sciences Center
Stony Brook, New York

THEODORE C. BANIA, MD
Chief Resident
Department of Emergency Medicine
Metropolitan Hospital Center
New York, New York

GEORGE N. CORITSIDIS, MD
Attending Nephrologist
Nassau County Medical Center
East Meadow, New York
Instructor of Medicine
State University of New York at Stony Brook
Health Sciences Center
Stony Brook, New York

KATHLEEN A. DELANEY, MD, ABMT
Assistant Professor
Division of Emergency Medicine
University of Texas Southwestern Medical School
Dallas, Texas

DONALD A. FEINFELD, MD, FACP
Co-Director of Nephrology
Nassau County Medical Center
East Meadow, New York
Associate Professor of Medicine
State University of New York at Stony Brook
Stony Brook, New York
Consultant in Nephrology
New York City Poison Control Center
New York, New York

MARSHA FORD, MD, FACEP, ABMT
Director
Division of Toxicology
Assistant Chairman
Department of Emergency Medicine
Carolinas Medical Center
Charlotte, North Carolina

LEWIS R. GOLDFRANK, MD, ABMT
Director, Emergency Services
Bellevue and New York University Hospital
Medical Director
New York City Poison Control Center
New York, New York

ROBERT S. HOFFMAN, MD, ABMT
Director, Medical Toxicology Fellowship Training
    Program
Associate Medical Director
New York City Poison Control Center
Instructor Clinical Surgery/Emergency Medicine
New York University of Medicine
New York, New York

MARY ANN HOWLAND, PharmD, ABAT
Clinical Professor of Pharmacy
St. John's University College of Pharmacy
Consultant
New York City Poison Control Center
New York, New York

MARK A. KIRK, MD, ABMT
Assistant Director
Division of Toxicology
Department of Emergency Medicine
Carolinas Medical Center
Charlotte, North Carolina

DAVID C. LEE, MD
Division of Toxicology
Department of Emergency Medicine
Mercy Catholic Medical Center and The Medical
    College of Pennsylvania
Philadelphia, Pennsylvania

DIANE LIU, MD, MPH
San Francisco Bay Area Regional Poison Control
    Center
San Francisco General Hospital
Center for Municipal Occupational Safety and
    Health
San Francisco, California

KENT R. OLSON, MD, FACEP, ABMT
Medical Director
San Francisco Bay Area Regional Poison Control
    Center
Associate Clinical Professor of Medicine
Lecturer in Pharmacy
University of California, San Francisco
San Francisco General Hospital
San Francisco, California

JAMES R. ROBERTS, MD, FACEP, ABMT
Division of Toxicology
Department of Emergency Medicine
Mercy Catholic Medical Center and The Medical
    College of Pennsylvania
Philadelphia, Pennsylvania

MARTIN J. SMILKSTEIN, MD, ABMT
Assistant Professor
Emergency Medicine and Trauma
University of Colorado Health Sciences Center
Denver, Colorado

CANDICE SMITH, PharmD
Assistant Clinical Professor
St. John's University
Jamaica, New York

DIANE SAUTER, MD, FACEP, ABMT
Director
Emergency Medicine Residency Training Program
Metropolitan Hospital Center
New York, New York

PAUL M. WAX, MD
Senior Fellow
New York City Poison Control Center
Instructor Clinical Surgery/Emergency Medicine
New York University School of Medicine
New York, New York

RICHARD S. WEISMAN, PharmD, ABAT
Director
New York City Poison Control Center
New York City Department of Health
Bellevue Department of Emergency Services
New York, New York

INTRODUCTION

In today's world of medicine, the amount of new research and new concepts is growing at an exponential rate. This makes it extremely difficult for the busy physician to keep pace with new advances. Due to its multidisciplinary nature and high technology base, the field of Critical Care Medicine may be affected more than any other subspecialty. Accordingly, the availability of timely and pertinent reviews in a convenient form becomes an essential tool for the achievement of excellence in the practice of Critical Care Medicine.

The aim of *Contemporary Management in Critical Care* is to provide the practitioner with concise surveys of major topics in Critical Care Medicine. The Guest Editors and authors are leaders in their respective fields, and the orientation is clinical and practical. The *contemporary* nature of the series is emphasized, as we strive to cover the most current topics and keep the reader abreast of the latest issues and advances in Critical Care Medicine.

As Editors of the series, we look forward to suggestions and comments from our readers.

Martin J. Tobin, MD
Ake Grenvik, MD, PhD

CRITICAL CARE TOXICOLOGY

CONTENTS

CRITICAL CARE TOXICOLOGY

PREFACE

The poisoned or overdosed patient provides a unique challenge for physicians in virtually every medical specialty. Mortality for this patient, much like those with other disease states, can usually be prevented, and morbidity can be reduced when the diagnosis is rapidly established and consequential therapeutic interventions are initiated early in the clinical course. Unlike most other disease states, however, poisoning is often a completely reversible process. The physician practicing in a critical care environment is most likely to encounter poisoned patients in extremus. Thus, a fundamental knowledge of intensive care toxicology is essential.

While common poisonings and their manifestations are familiar to most clinicians, one must realize that any chemical or drug is a potential toxin. Hence, a thorough understanding of the assessment and management of the myriad of toxicologic emergencies requires specialty training. To that end, the American Academy Board of Clinical Toxicology (AACT) established two sister organizations: The American Board of Medical Toxicology (ABMT) in 1974 and the American Board of Applied Toxicology (ABAT) in 1985. Diplomates of the ABMT (who are MDs) and the ABAT (who are PhDs and PharmDs) have devoted their careers specifically to the diagnosis and management of poisoning and overdose.

Most chapters in this volume are authored by ABMT or ABAT diplomates. Many of the coauthors are currently completing requirements for board certification. The aim of this issue of *Contemorary Management in Critical Care* is to integrate Intensive Care Medicine with Medical Toxicology; that is, to allow the intensivist to approach the poisoned patient through the eyes of a clinical toxicologist. Early chapters focus on general principles: utilization of the intensive care unit toxicokinetics, utilization of activated charcoal, extracorporeal drug removal, the special role of bicarbonate, and immunotoxicology. The latter chapters deal with specific issues that we have found problematic: the approach to the agitated delirious patient, hemodynamic assessment and management of the poisoned patient, smoke inhalation, and alkali acid injuries.

In addition to general principles, the reader will find specific, practical management strategies for assessment and treatment of poisonings. These strategies reflect the authors' and editors' critical interpretation of the literature and their extensive clinical experience. Because of the explosive nature of pharmacologic and toxicologic research, the unending creation of new chemicals and pharmaceuticals, and the remarkable range of legitimate and illegitimate use and misuse of available drugs and toxins, toxicology is a continually evolving science. Many of our recommendations, therefore, are only meant to serve as guidelines. The individual patient must always be assessed in the context of his or her individual circumstances and general medical condition. The editors strongly encourage regular contact with Certified Regional Poison Centers for contemporary recommendations regarding individual cases. In addition, we request that you become actively involved with your poison center so that they may use your knowledge of Intensive Care Medicine to assist with their management of severely poisoned or overdosed patients. We hope that you find this volume useful and interesting, and that it stimulates further reading in Medical Toxicology.

Robert S. Hoffman, MD, ABMT
Lewis R. Goldfrank, MD, ABMT

RATIONAL UTILIZATION OF THE INTENSIVE CARE UNIT IN MANAGING THE POISONED PATIENT

MARK A. KIRK, MD, ABMT[†]

Toxicologic emergencies challenge many components of the health care system. Poisoned patients frequently enter the health care system through the prehospital emergency medical services and the emergency department and may then require many specialized hospital services such as intensive care, laboratory, and psychiatric care. The majority of patients with acute poisoning will be assessed, treated, and discharged from the emergency department.[1] A critically ill, poisoned patient will require the unique benefits of the intensive care unit (ICU). In modern times, the ICU has dramatically increased survival from many serious conditions due to continuous monitoring, supportive care, and the most modern medical technology and treatment. While the ICU allows patients the best opportunity to minimize morbidity and decrease mortality, it is also a major source of expensive health care that has contributed significantly to the escalation of health care costs. Every physician must address the appropriate use of the ICU and consider the rationing of health care as an ethical issue. Few poisoned patients will become critically ill, defining those who will need intensive care is the purpose of this paper.

A critically ill, poisoned patient will require the unique benefits of the intensive care unit.

UNIQUE ASPECTS OF TOXICOLOGIC EMERGENCIES

Knowledge of many factors contributes to the adequate evaluation and treatment of a poisoned patient. Unfortu-

[†] Assistant Director, Division of Toxicology, Department of Emergency Medicine, Carolinas Medical Center, Charlotte, North Carolina

nately, this information is frequently unavailable or unreliable. Specifically, historical information is likely to be unreliable. Understanding the pharmacology, toxicokinetics, and natural history of a toxin will assist in determining both risks of developing toxicity and a treatment plan. Toxic emergencies may require treatment modalities unfamiliar to the health care providers. In addition to medical issues, the psychiatric component of a patient's illness must be addressed.

The uncertainties of overdosed patients prevent more than an educated guess at the true risk of developing toxicity. The accuracy of the history is always suspect. The toxin and the amount are frequently determined by indirect evidence. In the intentionally overdosed patient, ingesting more than one drug is common and the interactions of multiple toxins must be considered.[2]

Many diseases managed in the ICU have a well-recognized, predictable course and expected complications. This is not necessarily the case with poisoning. Our environment contains a multitude of chemicals and pharmaceuticals that may have little or no human exposure data available with regard to toxic amounts and effects. The information that is available may be derived solely from animal studies. The clinician must therefore make therapeutic decisions and anticipate potential toxicity with little or no reliable data related to toxicity of a substance. In this case, expectant observation may be the only rational approach. Early recognition of serious toxicity could prevent an adverse outcome.

As an example, a worker presented to a hospital after working in a poorly ventilated area with a resin coating containing 2–nitropropane. Toxicologic information about the substance was not immediately available. The patient developed nonspecific symptoms and mild elevations of liver aminotransferases. Two days after discharge he returned in fulminant hepatic failure and died.[3] A similar example involved a child exposed to methylene iodide. No information was available concerning potential human toxicity. A rapidly progressive hepatocellular necrosis evolved and the child died.[4] If literature had been available that identified the toxic nature of these substances, aggressive monitoring and intervention would have likely occurred once toxicity was recognized.

The natural history of acute poisoning is unique because it is a dynamic disease. An asymptomatic patient may be a "timebomb" with the potential to rapidly deteriorate. Failure to appreciate the potential for serious toxicity is a major concern in the management of the poisoned patient. In an acute toxic exposure, one can expect a variable amount of time before symptoms of toxicity occur. As

The natural history of acute poisoning is unique because it is a dynamic disease. An asymptomatic patient may be a "timebomb" with the potential to rapidly deteriorate. Failure to appreciate the potential for serious toxicity is a major concern in the management of the poisoned patient.

symptoms develop and are treated, the underlying cellular or metabolic injury may continue as long as toxin absorption occurs, toxic metabolites are present, or end-organ toxicity develops. An important goal of therapy in this asymptomatic period is to reduce or prevent toxicity by gastrointestinal decontamination.[5]

Certain toxins will prolong gastrointestinal absorption, thereby delaying onset of toxicity. Opioids and the anticholinergic effects of drugs, such as cyclic antidepressants and antihistamines, will delay gastric emptying and potentially prolong drug absorption.[6] In children, Lomotil (atropine and diphenoxylate) can produce delayed and prolonged coma from slowed gastrointestinal motility. Salicylates produce pylorospasm that will delay gastric emptying.[7] Bromides, meprobamate, and salicylates may form gastric bezoars, thus producing prolonged gastrointestinal absorption. Recently, the act of smuggling (body-packer) or hiding (body-stuffer) contraband drugs in the gastrointestinal tract has resulted in delayed onset of serious toxicity from ruptured bags.[8,9]

Certain toxins will prolong gastrointestinal absorption, thereby delaying onset of toxicity.

Sustained release preparations have been developed to enhance patient compliance by increasing dosing intervals. In overdoses, sustained release and enteric-coated preparations may delay absorption and, in turn, the onset of toxicity.[10] A patient with an overdose of a sustained-release theophylline preparation did not attain a peak level until 26 hours after ingestion.[11,12] Reported overdoses of enteric-coated aspirin reached peak levels at 24–36 hours after ingestion.[7,13] Cardiac arrhythmias developed as late as 16 hours following ingestion of sustained-release verapamil in two cases.[14] Sustained release preparations of toxicologic importance include theophylline, phenylpropanolamine, potassium, calcium channel blockers, beta-adrenergic blockers, and lithium. Serial levels (when available) are necessary to verify peaks and ensure that levels are decreasing. Some of these drugs do not have readily obtainable serum levels that can be monitored. In such cases, admission and observation are required.

In overdoses, sustained release and enteric-coated preparations may delay absorption and, in turn, the onset of toxicity.

Some toxins may have a delayed onset or an unpredictable course. Clinical effects may be delayed when toxicity requires alteration of enzyme functions, cellular reproduction, or metabolic function. Toxicity of monoamine oxidase inhibitors (MAOI) may appear more than 12 hours after an overdose and may progress rapidly to cardiovascular collapse.[15] Because of delay in onset of severe toxicity, even if asymptomatic, a history of MAOI ingestion mandates ICU monitoring for 24 hours. Colchicine's gastrointestinal toxicity may resolve within hours of ingestion with apparent recovery, only to have multisystem organ failure occur 24–72 hours later.[16] Another example is the "inter-

Clinical effects may be delayed when toxicity requires alteration of enzyme functions, cellular reproduction, or metabolic function.

mediate syndrome" of organophosphate insecticide poisoning. Marked respiratory and proximal muscle weakness develop 1–4 days following a cholinergic crisis in a patient with apparent resolution of toxicity.[17] The syndrome may simply be a manifestation of inadequate treatment with pralidoxime.[18] Where there is potential for serious delayed toxicity, the patient may need close monitoring for a prolonged period after resolution of toxicity.

Anticipated complications of certain toxins may require close observation. Possible complications or delayed effects can include noncardiogenic pulmonary edema, rhabdomyolysis, hepatotoxicity, renal failure, or bone marrow toxicity. Several toxins may produce noncardiogenic pulmonary edema (salicylates, opioids, cyclic antidepressants, carbon monoxide, sedative-hypnotics).[19–23] Overdose of barbiturates, amphetamines, and cocaine are examples of toxins associated with a high incidence of rhabdomyolysis.[24] Aspiration pneumonitis is a frequent complication in comatose or seizing patients.[19,25] ICU observation may be necessary until the risk of complications is lessened.

Predictors of outcome in cardiac arrest, such as coma, do not apply to poisoning.[26,27] Severe poisoning may clinically mimic brain death.[28,29] As an example, a barbiturate overdose resulted in a Glasgow Coma Scale of 3 and an isoelectric EEG. Treated with only supportive care, the patient had complete neurologic recovery.[28] In addition, many toxic emergencies occur in young patients who are relatively free of underlying cardiac disease. This increases the likelihood of surviving significant insults such as prolonged hypotension or hypoxia. Prolonged, aggressive resuscitation efforts may be warranted in this case. Case studies have reported a good neurologic outcome with prolonged external cardiac massage during asystole from tricyclic antidepressant overdoses.[30,31] Cardiopulmonary bypass was reportedly successful in resuscitating a patient from a massive toxic ingestion and is currently being evaluated in animal studies.[32,33]

Treatment of the poisoned patient is unique in that antidotes and specific treatments may be unfamiliar to the physicians and the ICU staff. Similarly, familiar medications, such as atropine or glucagon, may be used as antidotes in doses that far exceed conventional doses. These antidotes and specific treatments, while they may be lifesaving, also carry their own inherent risks. For example, antivenin for rattlesnake envenomations may result in anaphylaxis and rapid intravenous infusion of deferoxamine for iron poisoning may result in hypotension. Because these treatments may be unfamiliar, complicated, and have their own inherent risks, the ICU is the most prudent environment in which to monitor such treatments.

Many toxic emergencies occur in young patients who are relatively free of underlying cardiac disease. This increases the likelihood of surviving significant insults such as prolonged hypotension or hypoxia. Prolonged, aggressive resuscitation efforts may be warranted in this case.

Eighty percent of recognized suicide attempts are due to an overdose of medications.[34] Complications of poisoning make it difficult to adequately assess the suicidal risks of such patients. Until these are resolved, it should be assumed that the patient remains a suicidal risk. Outside of the psychiatric ward, policies concerning monitoring for suicidal behavior may differ among institutions. Providing a safe environment may include admitting all patients with suicidal risks to the ICU, physically restraining a ward patient, or providing a ward patient with one-to-one observation. In many hospitals, the ICU is the safest place to observe a patient with suicidal risks until that patient is medically clear of toxicity. Nevertheless, every suicide attempt should be taken seriously, as it has been demonstrated that patients have an increased rate of suicide following discharge from an ICU for drug overdose.[35]

ADVANTAGES OF ICU CARE FOR THE POISONED PATIENT

The ICU offers the most highly skilled staff, aided by modern technologic advances, to manage many complex diseases. The treatment of poisoned patients involves routine supportive care measures that ICUs are most skilled in providing. In the 1930s, barbiturate overdoses were common and mortality was greater than 20%. At that time, treatment consisted of gastric lavage and administration of "central analeptics." In the 1950s, the mortality of barbiturate overdoses decreased to less than 2%.[36] This significant decrease was attributed to the awareness that maintaining a patent airway, preventing hypoxia with the administration of oxygen, and treatment of shock resulted in improved patient outcome. Elk et al. reported a good outcome in the majority of 103 critically ill, overdosed patients with only supportive care (ie, in the form of ventilator support, vasopressor support, and close monitoring).[27] In a pediatric study, only 2 of 105 pediatric patients admitted to the ICU required aggressive treatment in addition to general, nonspecific (supportive) care.[37] In most instances, antidotes and specific treatments do not take the place of supportive care.

Early detection of toxicity and prevention of complications are fundamental to management. The ICU provides a ratio of nursing care to each patient that allows close monitoring of basic physiologic parameters. Noninvasive measurements of vital signs, neurologic status, and intake/output measurements, along with continuous cardiac monitoring, will provide important clues to the early development of serious toxicity or complications.

The treatment of poisoned patients involves routine supportive care measures that ICUs are most skilled in providing.

In most instances, antidotes and specific treatments do not take the place of supportive care.

Bedside monitoring can detect the need for active intervention or guide the discontinuation of present treatment. Overdosed patients with alterations in mental status may be unable to protect their airways and are ideally monitored by continuous techniques in order to recognize the need for airway protection. Routine clinical assessment, appropriate use of arterial blood gas analysis, pulse oximetry, bedside pulmonary function parameters (vital capacity, PEFV) and inductance plethysmography are valuable aids in clinical decision making. Sedated or paralyzed patients may need continuous EEG monitoring to identify occult seizures.

Invasive monitoring is routinely used in the ICU and may be indicated in some poisoned patients. Hemodynamic parameters are valuable for the patient with hypotension, intravascular volume depletion, or noncardiogenic pulmonary edema. Intraarterial monitoring will provide a more accurate and continuous record of actual blood pressure in a patient with cardiovascular compromise. Fluid therapy may be best managed by using a pulmonary artery catheter. Certain toxins may require specific invasive procedures. Extracorporeal methods of elimination, such as hemodialysis or hemoperfusion, are best performed in the ICU.

The ICU plays a role in advancements in the field of clinical toxicology.[38] For many toxins, little data has been published regarding human toxicity. The ICU is an essential source of physiologic parameters gathered from critically ill patients exposed to toxins. Publications of detailed analyses of poisoned patients, including this physiologic information, are necessary to advance the science of clinical toxicology.

DEVELOPING RATIONAL GUIDELINES

The poisoned patient is admitted to the ICU either for intervention or for observation. Patients with acute reversible conditions that require intervention, such as mechanical ventilation, vasopressor support, arrhythmia management, or hemodialysis, clearly benefit from intensive care.[39]

A large number of patients are admitted to the ICU not for intervention, but for observation. In a clinical series from New Zealand, 50% of the patients admitted to the ICU for observation and monitoring had a diagnosis of poisoning.[40] Of all ICU admissions, including poisonings, Henning found that only 10–15% required aggressive management and invasive monitoring.[41] The decision to admit

The poisoned patient is admitted to the ICU either for intervention or for observation. Patients with acute reversible conditions that require intervention, such as mechanical ventilation, vasopressor support, arrhythmia management, or hemodialysis, clearly benefit from intensive care.

a poisoned patient to the ICU for observation may be based only on a history of exposure to a potentially life-threatening toxin. With limited historical information, physicians may be justified in admitting and closely monitoring a patient since toxicity can develop rapidly and remain unrecognized to the point of life-threatening complications. If a mildly toxic salicylate-poisoned patient, for example, is placed on the ward for intravenous hydration and urinary alkalinization, continued gastrointestinal absorption can produce a gradual increase in toxicity with a resultant poor outcome from severe pulmonary and cerebral edema. To the contrary, retrospective data of 209 hospitalized poisoned patients does not support the fear of delayed deterioration once a patient is stabilized.[42] The ICU provides necessary monitoring and individual nursing care that can assist in early recognition of developing toxicity.

Overcrowded ICUs and escalating health care costs have been the incentives to develop indices that predict the benefits of ICU care. Numerous indices have been developed to select those patients who would benefit from ICU admission, the goal being to deter excessive use of resources. One index, the Acute Physiology and Chronic Health Evaluation (APACHE II), assesses and scores certain physiologic parameters at admission.[43]

Clinical studies to validate such a scoring system have evaluated patients with a variety of conditions, but none have looked solely at overdosed patients or have included large numbers of these patients.[40] Such scoring systems are less useful for the poisoned patient because parameters that would define patients as unlikely to benefit from ICU intervention by predicting clinical outcome, such as coma following cardiac arrest, are not reliable in the poisoned patient.[26,27]

Brett et al. developed a set of criteria to determine whether initial clinical assessment could identify those poisoned patients at risk of complications.[42] Criteria defining high-risk patients were: need for intubation; unresponsiveness to verbal stimuli; seizures; P_aCO_2 >45 mmHg; systolic blood pressure <80 mmHg; any cardiac rhythm except normal sinus, sinus tachycardia, or sinus bradycardia; second- or third-degree AV block; and QRS duration >120 ms. Patients were classified as low-risk when none of the above criteria were present in the emergency department. Retrospectively, 209 cases were analyzed using the above parameters obtained in the emergency department. The most commonly ingested drugs in both the high- and low-risk groups were alcohol, cyclic antidepressants, benzodiazepines, barbiturates, phenothiazines, opioids, and salicylates. Of the 151 patients considered low-risk, none developed complications or required ICU interventions after

The ICU provides necessary monitoring and individual nursing care that can assist in early recognition of developing toxicity.

admission. Of the 58 patients deemed high-risk, 35 required ICU interventions such as intubation, treatment of arrhythmias, treatment of seizures, intravenous vasopressors, or hemodialysis/hemoperfusion. Seven patients developed high-risk complications, such as need for intubation, hypotension, and seizures after admission, but all had other high-risk criteria in the emergency department. The authors concluded that the clinical course of poisoned patients can be predicted during the first hours of observation.

In this series, 70% of the low-risk patients were admitted to the ICU for observation. Since none of these low-risk patients developed complications or required ICU intervention, the authors contend that using their criteria would have eliminated 50% of the ICU days without compromising care.

This study is a retrospective collection of a small number of patients with a limited diversity in the type of toxin exposures and does not allow generalization of these criteria to all poisoned patients. However, it does suggest that, with some clinical judgment, not all poisoned patients require ICU admission.

Nothing is more useful than experience and good clinical judgment in predicting those likely to die, even with ICU intervention, and those likely to survive, even if deprived of ICU intervention.[44] Between these extremes is a large group of patients in whom a distinction is not always possible. Withholding ICU care from poisoned patients based solely on a "score" will not result in significant cost savings in the ICU but will create risks in increased morbidity and mortality.[45]

Optimally, clinical indicators of toxicity must be defined for each toxin. Few toxins have been studied in order to determine indicators of toxicity and safe disposition to the extent that cyclic antidepressants have. Most patients who have overdosed on cyclic antidepressants and have abnormal vital signs or ECGs are admitted to the ICU, due to the inability to predict outcome. Several studies to define predictive criteria for serious toxic reactions with cyclic antidepressants have been generated by (1) unnecessary admissions for trivial overdoses, and (2) the fact that cyclic antidepressants are the most common life-threatening prescribed drug ingested in the United States, accounting for more than 25% of all serious drug overdoses admitted to adult ICUs.[46]

Studies concerning cyclic antidepressant overdoses suggest that patients who remain asymptomatic for a 6-hour observation period after presentation may be safely discharged.[30,47-49] Otherwise, only patients with a normal mental status and sinus tachycardia that resolves within

Seventy percent of the patients who were classified by study criteria as low-risk were admitted to the ICU for observation. Since none of these low-risk patients developed complications or required ICU intervention, the authors contend that using their criteria would have eliminated 50% of the ICU days without compromising care.

the 6-hour observation period should be considered safe for discharge. It has been reported that prolonged QRS duration, seen on a 12-lead ECG, is predictive of serious complications such as seizures and arrhythmias.[50–52] Any case manifesting a persistent tachycardia, ECG abnormalities (including QRS ≥ 0.10 s), anticholinergic signs, or neurologic symptoms needs ICU monitoring.[30,49] Tokarski prospectively validated these recommendations in 45 overdosed patients.[48]

SPECIFIC REASONS TO CONSIDER ADMISSION TO THE ICU

Guidelines to help the clinician make decisions regarding ICU admission are presented in Table 1. The presence of certain signs or symptoms requires ICU observation or intervention, regardless of the toxic exposure. Indications for ICU admission based on end-organ toxicity are presented in Table 2. Using end-organ toxicity as the basis for admission to the ICU requires no knowledge of the toxin. This approach may prove most helpful for polydrug ingestions.

Central nervous system manifestations are common to many poisonings. Alteration of mental status in the form of acute delirium or coma needs immediate intervention. In most cases, ICU admission will be necessary because the alteration of mental status will not be quickly corrected. Any comatose patient without an identifiable cause requires continued investigation in the ICU. Toxin-induced seizures are best managed in the ICU.

Respiratory compromise must not be overlooked. Several mechanisms may produce respiratory compromise. As an example, organophosphate poisoning produces respiratory compromise by central nervous system depression, respiratory muscle weakness, and copious pulmonary secretions. Upper-airway edema may develop secondary to a caustic ingestion. Liberal admission to the ICU for any patient, even with mild symptoms, after an inhalation exposure should be considered because certain inhaled toxins, such as chlorine, nitrogen oxides, and phosgene, may produce noncardiogenic pulmonary edema many hours after exposure.

Any evidence of cardiac toxicity, such as conduction disturbances (QRS prolongation and QT segment prolongation), bradyarrhythmias, supraventricular arrhythmias, or ventricular arrhythmias, requires ICU admission. The mechanism of toxin-induced hypotension may be any combination of decreased myocardial contractility, arrhythmias, peripheral vasodilation, or hypovolemia. Chest pain

TABLE 1   Specific Reasons to Consider ICU Admission—With Examples

Patients requiring intervention to maintain normal physiological parameters
    intubation
    mechanical ventilation
    vasopressors
Patients with signs of severe poisoning
    salicylates: CNS alteration, metabolic acidosis, pulmonary edema
    theophylline: persistent GI symptoms, CV toxicity
    cardiac drugs (digitalis, beta-adrenergic blockers, calcium channel blockers, antiarrhythm-
      ics): arrhythmias or hypotension
    cyclic antidepressants: persistent tachycardia >6 h, QRS duration >0.10 s, lethargy, and
      seizures
    cocaine: persistent arrhythmias, hypertension, chest pain, status epilepticus, focal neuro-
      logic deficits
    carbon monoxide: altered mental status, chest pain, arrhythmias
Patients with worsening signs of toxicity
Patients with laboratory evidence of a significant ingestion that is likely to result in serious toxicity
    elevated serum drug levels of some drugs (eg, salicylates, theophylline, iron, digoxin)
    prolonged coagulation factors after Crotalid envenomation
    large number of radiopaque pills or substance on KUB (eg, iron tablets or heavy metals)
    CXR findings of pulmonary edema (eg, inhalation exposures, salicylates, or opioids)
    ECG changes (eg, QRS prolongation with cyclic antidepressants, ischemic changes with
      cocaine or carbon monoxide)
Patients with underlying medical conditions that increase the risk of developing serious toxicity
    extremes of age
    cardiovascular pulmonary, renal, or hepatic disease
    pregnancy
Patients exposed to potentially serious toxins with insufficient literature on human exposure
Patients exposed to toxins with a potential for prolonged absorption
    enteric-coated or sustained release preparations (eg, salicylate, theophylline, lithium, β-
      adrenergic blockers, and calcium channel blockers)
Patients exposed to toxins with a delayed onset of toxicity
    monoamine oxidase inhibitors
    Lomotil
    colchicine
    inhalation of chlorine or phosgene
    oral hypoglycemic agents/insulin overdose
    cocaine body stuffers
    ergotamines
    Amanita phalloides mushroom poisoning
Patients needing invasive procedures or invasive monitoring
    arterial blood pressure monitoring
    arterial infusion of calcium gluconate for hydrofluoric acid burns
    CVP monitoring
    hemoperfusion/hemodialysis
Patients requiring administration of an antidote with the potential for serious side effects
    Crotalid, Elapidae, or black widow spider antivenin
    deferoxamine for iron poisoning
    ethanol for methanol and ethylene glycol poisoning
    cyanide antidote kit
    glucagon for beta-adrenergic blockers
Patients receiving an antidote with a shorter duration of action than the toxin
    naloxone for long-acting opioids
    glucose for oral hypoglycemic agents
    flumazenil for benzodiazepines
    atropine for organophosphates
    physostigmine for anticholinergics
Patients with evidence of consequential drug withdrawal
Actively suicidal patients needing close monitoring

TABLE 2   End-organ Toxicity as Criteria for ICU Admission

Neurologic	**Thermoregulation**
coma	hyperthermia
delerium	hypothermia
seizures	**Gastrointestinal**
Respiratory	corrosive upper GI burns
respiratory depression	severe vomiting/diarrhea
hypoxia	**Hepatic**
airway obstruction	hepatic necrosis
pulmonary edema	hepatic encephalopathy
bronchospasm	**Renal**
Cardiovascular	acute renal failure
arrhythmias	**Metabolic**
hypotension	unexplained metabolic acidosis
persistent hypertension	hypoglycemia
ischemic chest pain	**Dermal**
Hematologic	large body surface area chemical burns
decreased oxygen carrying capacity	potential systemic toxicity from dermal exposure
coagulopathy	
hemolysis	

from myocardial ischemia can be induced by exposure to toxins such as cocaine or carbon monoxide. Persistent, toxin-induced hypertension, especially with associated headache or chest pain, requires ICU admission.

Arsine gas may produce a serious hemolytic anemia, while cyanide, carbon monoxide, and methemoglobin inducers will impair oxygen utilization or oxygen-carrying capacity, thus producing tissue hypoxia. Life-threatening coagulopathy may result from rattlesnake envenomation.

Core body temperature is vitally important to monitor in the poisoned patient. Temperature regulation is altered by various mechanisms and needs rapid intervention.

Gastrointestinal symptoms, particularly vomiting and diarrhea, are an early manifestation of many toxins. In cases of severe persistent symptoms, significant fluid and electrolyte losses may occur. A serious iron ingestion will cause caustic gastrointestinal mucosal effects that lead to vomiting and diarrhea so severe that profound volume losses will produce hypotension. A patient ingesting an acid or alkaline caustic needs ICU admission because serious complications include esophageal perforation, airway compromise, and shock.

Hepatotoxicity usually occurs days after toxin exposure. If hepatotoxicity, especially with hepatic encephalopathy, is evident at admission, ICU observation is suggested.

Renal toxicity may be a direct toxic effect or the result of other toxic manifestations, such as hypotension or rhabdomyolysis. Impaired renal function is a serious problem in poisoning because an important route of toxin elimination may be limited.

Metabolic acidosis is an important clue to the presence of toxins such as ethylene glycol, methanol, and salicylates. Toxin-induced metabolic acidosis needs ICU intervention. Investigation into the cause of an unexplained acidosis needs to continue in the ICU. Unexplained, persistent, or refractory hypoglycemia resulting from an oral hypoglycemic, insulin overdose, or other toxins, necessitates ICU admission.

Chemical burns of the skin have similar complications to thermal burns. The injured dermis may produce significant fluid losses, alter core body temperature regulation, and increase the risk of infection. In addition to these complications, systemic toxic effects may occur through dermal absorption. A 2.5% body surface area exposure to concentrated hydrofluoric acid has produced systemic hypocalcemia and death.[53]

SAFE DISPOSITION FROM THE ICU

Once toxicity has resolved, most patients may be safely transferred to a hospital ward. Cyclic antidepressants have been extensively studied in order to determine a safe period at which to discontinue monitoring. Concern arose from case reports of patients developing sudden death up to several days following a cyclic antidepressant overdose.[6,54,55] Continued toxicity, such as lethargy or sinus tachycardia, was evident when delayed complications developed in the majority of these cases. More recently, studies have demonstrated that arrhythmias do not occur after signs of toxicity have resolved (ie, central nervous system and cardiac manifestations).[49,56,57] Current recommendations based on these studies suggest the use of cardiac monitoring for an additional 24 hours after normalization of the ECG and when no other signs of continued toxicity are present.[58] This additional period of monitoring should occur after discontinuation of specific therapy such as serum alkalinization. Unfortunately, most toxins have not received the extensive attention given to cyclic antidepressants. Until further research and experience are obtained, clinical judgment with the assistance of an experienced clinical toxicologist will be the only way to determine safe disposition from the ICU.

Until further research and experience are obtained, clinical judgment with the assistance of an experienced clinical toxicologist will be the only way to determine safe disposition from the ICU.

When antidotes are administered, recurrence of potentially serious toxic effects can result. The duration of action of the toxin may be longer than the duration of action of the specific treatment or antidote. The half-life of naloxone, for example, is shorter than certain opioids such as heroin.

Another example is that the cholinergic effects of organophosphate poisoning may reoccur after the administration of atropine.[59] A further precaution is that one must ensure that gastrointestinal absorption is not continuing and that the risk of delayed toxicity has diminished prior to ICU transfer. Continued absorption is not likely to be clinically significant when serum drug concentrations are decreasing.

OBSERVING PATIENTS ON THE WARD

Until further clinical studies are available to define those patients at risk, the majority of seriously poisoned patients will be admitted to the ICU. However, not all poisoned patients admitted to the hospital require ICU intervention. Many factors such as the amount of toxin and its inherent toxicity, the type of coingestants, and underlying medical conditions of the patient will help determine the need for ICU admission. An informed decision can be made with the assistance of a clinical toxicologist or Certified Regional Poison Center.

Accidental chronic toxicity of certain drugs may be observed on a hospital ward. For example, mild to moderate chronic phenytoin toxicity, with verification of diminishing serum levels, may be managed effectively on a ward. This is not an all-inclusive recommendation, as phenytoin toxicity can produce central nervous system depression that may require intervention or ICU monitoring.

An overdose of acetaminophen has a well-defined clinical course and an effective antidote. Toxicity develops slowly and will not be clinically evident until several days after ingestion. Administering the antidote, N-acetylcysteine, within 8 hours, will minimize the risk of hepatotoxicity.[60] The efficacy of this antidote diminishes with time when administration begins after 8 hours. High-risk patients are those treated more than 16 hours after ingestion, with hepatotoxicity developing in as many as 41%.[60] Liver function tests should be followed closely. Early elevation of liver function tests will alert the need to watch closely for hepatotoxicity and subsequent hepatic encephalopathy. Once toxicity is evident, the ICU may be the appropriate place to continue therapy. Antidote administration does not require ICU care, and the ICU can offer little to prevent hepatotoxicity. From this perspective, the majority of acetaminophen overdoses can be treated on a hospital ward, providing suicidal risks can be monitored and regular administration of the antidote is assured.

SUMMARY

Acute poisoning is a dynamic disease with an unpredictable clinical course and therapy that is unfamiliar to many medical and nursing staff. Lacking both historical data on individuals and literature on toxic amounts and effects of toxins on humans creates many uncertainties in management. Since many uncertainties exist and the ICU offers the highest level of skilled staff and modern technology, most potentially seriously poisoned patients will be admitted to the ICU. The question remains whether or not this is clinically justified or is an effective use of resources. Admission of the poisoned patient continues to be a clinical judgment based on the best available information. Consultation with a Certified Regional Poison Control Center or a clinical toxicologist is encouraged.

References

1. Litovitz TL, Schmitz BF, Bailey KM: 1989 annual report of the American Association of Poison Control Centers National Data Collection System. Am J Emerg Med 8:394, 1990

2. Stern TA, Mulley AG, Thibault GE: Life-threatening drug overdose: precipitants and prognosis. JAMA 251:1983, 1984

3. Harrison R, Letz G, Pasternak G, Blanc P: Fulminant hepatic failure after occupational exposure to 2-nitropropane. Ann Intern Med 107:466, 1987

4. Weimerskirch PJ, Burkhart KK, Bono MJ et al: Methylene iodide poisoning. Ann Emerg Med 19:1171, 1990

5. Spyker DA, Minocha A: Toxicodynamic approach to management of the poisoned patient. J Emerg Med 6:117, 1988

6. Callaham M: Admission criteria for tricyclic antidepressant ingestion. West J Med 137:425, 1982

7. Bogacz K, Caldron P: Enteric-coated aspirin bezoar: elevation of serum salicylate level by barium study. Am J Med 83:733, 1987

8. McCarron MM, Wood JD: The cocaine body packer syndrome. JAMA 250:1417, 1983

9. Roberts JR, Price D, Goldfrank L et al: The body stuffer syndrome: a clandestine form of drug overdose. Am J Emerg Med 4:22, 1986

10. Minocha A, Spyker DA: Acute overdose with sustained release drug formulations. Med Toxicol 1:300, 1986

11. Dederich RA, Szefler SJ, Green ER: Intrasubject variation in sustained release theophylline absorption. J Allerg Clin Immunol 67:465, 1981

12. Robertson NJ: Fatal overdose from a sustained-release theophylline preparation. Ann Emerg Med 14:154, 1985

13. Wortzman DJ, Grunfeld A: Delayed absorption following enteric-coated aspirin overdose. Ann Emerg Med 16:434, 1987

14. Spiller HA, Meyers A, Ziemba T, Riley M: Delayed onset of cardiac arrhythmias from sustained-release verapamil. Ann Emerg Med 20:201, 1991

15. Linden CH, Rumack BH, Strehlke C: Monoamine oxidase inhibitor overdose. Ann Emerg Med 13:1137, 1984

16. Boehnort M, McGuigan MA: Colchicine. Clin Toxicol Rev 5:1, 1983

17. Senanayake N, Karalliedde L: Neurotoxic effects of organophosphorus insecticides: an intermediate syndrome. N Engl J Med 316:761, 1987

18. Aaron CK, Smilkstein MJ: Organophosphate poisoning: intermediate syndrome or inadequate therapy? (Abstr) Vet Hum Toxicol 30:370, 1988

19. Shannon M, Lovejoy FH: Pulmonary-complications of severe tricyclic antidepressant ingestion. J Toxicol Clin Toxicol 25:443, 1987

20. Duberstein JL, Kaufman DM: A clinical study of an epidemic of heroin intoxication and heroin-induced pulmonary edema. Am J Med 51:704, 1971

21. Frand UI, Shim CS, Williams MH: Heroin-induced pulmonary edema. Ann Intern Med 77:29, 1972

22. Heffner JE, Sahn SA: Salicylate-induced pulmonary edema. Ann Intern Med 95:405, 1981

23. Fisher CJ, Albertson TE, Foulke GE: Salicylate-induced pulmonary edema: clinical characteristics in children. Am J Emerg Med 3:33, 1985

24. Curry SC, Change D, Connor D: Drug- and toxin-induced rhabdomyolysis. Ann Emerg Med 18:1068, 1989

25. Allen J: Aspiration pneumonitis. Clin Toxicol Rev 7:1, 1984

26. Rinaldo JE, Snyder JV: Survival data base: central nervous system injury. Am Rev Respir Dis 140:S25, 1989

27. Elk JR, Linton DM, Potgieter PD: Treatment of acute self-poisoning in a respiratory intensive care unit. S Afr Med J 72:532, 1987

28. Bird TD, Plum F: Recovery from barbiturate overdose coma with a prolonged isoelectric electroencephalogram. Neurology 18:456, 1968

29. Powner DJ: Drug-associated isoelectric EEGs: a hazard in brain death certification. JAMA 236:1123, 1976

30. Frommer DA, Kulig KW, Marx JA, Rumack B: Tricyclic antidepressant overdose. JAMA 257:521, 1987

31. Orr DA, Bramble MG: Tricyclic antidepressant poisoning and prolonged external cardiac massage during asystole. Br Med J 283:1107, 1981

32. Noble J, Kennedy DJ, Latimer RD et al: Massive lignocaine overdose during cardiopulmonary bypass. Br J Anaesth 56:1439, 1984

33. Martin TG, Klain MM, Molner RL et al: Extracorporeal life support vs thumper after lethal desipramine OD. (Abstr) Vet Hum Toxicol 4:349, 1990

34. Murphy GE, Wetzel RD: Family history of suicidal behavior among suicide attempters. J Nerv Ment Dis 170:86, 1982

35. Strom J, Thisted B, Krantz T, Bredgaard Sorensen M: Self-poisoning treated in an ICU: drug pattern, acute mortality and short-term survival. Acta Anaesthesiol Scand 30:148, 1986

36. Clemmesen C, Nilsson E: Therapeutic trends in the treatment of barbiturate poisoning: the Scandinavian method. Clin Pharmacol Ther 2:220, 1961

37. Lacroix J, Gaudreault P, Gauthier M: Admission to a pediatric intensive care unit for poisoning: a review of 105 cases. Crit Care Med 17:748, 1989

38. Kulling P, Persson H: Role of the intensive care unit in the management of the poisoned patient. Med Toxicol Adverse Drug Exp 1:375, 1986

39. Ron A, Aronne LJ, Kalb PE et al: The therapeutic efficacy of critical care units. Arch Intern Med 149:338, 1989

40. Zimmerman JE, Knaus WA, Judson JA et al: Patient selection for intensive care: a comparison of New Zealand and United States hospitals. Crit Care Med 16:318, 1988

41. Henning RJ, McClish D, Daly B et al: Clinical characteristics and resource utilization of ICU patients: implications for organization of intensive care. Crit Care Med 15:264, 1987

42. Brett AS, Rothchild N, Gray R, Perry M: Predicting the clinical course in intentional drug overdose. Arch Intern Med 147:133, 1987

43. Knaus WA, Draper EA, Wagner DP, Zimmerman JE: APACHE II: a severity of disease classification system. Crit Care Med 13:818, 1985

44. Kruse JA, Thill-Baharozian MC, Carlson RW: Comparison of clinical assessment with APACHE II for predicting mortality risk in patients admitted to a medical intensive care unit. JAMA 260:1739, 1988

45. Civetta JM: Setting objectives: perspectives for care. p. 5. In Civetta JM, Taylor RW, Kirby RR (eds): Critical care. JB Lippincott, Philadelphia, 1988

46. Dec WG: Tricyclic antidepressants in the intensive care unit. J Intensive Care Med 5:69, 1990

47. Pentel PR, Benowitz NL: Tricyclic antidepressant poisoning: management of arrhythmias. Med Toxicol 1:101, 1986

48. Tokarski GF, Young MJ: Criteria for admitting patients with tricyclic antidepressant overdose. J Emerg Med 6:121, 1988

49. Callaham M, Kassel D: Epidemiology of fatal tricyclic antidepressant ingestion: implications for management. Ann Emerg Med 14:1, 1985

50. Boehnert MT, Lovejoy FH: Value of the QRS duration vs the serum drug level in predicting seizures and ventricular arrhythmias after an acute overdose of tricyclic antidepressants. N Engl J Med 313:474, 1985

51. Niemann JT, Bessen HA, Rothstein RJ, Laks MM: Electrocardiographic criteria for tricyclic antidepressant cardiotoxicity. Am J Cardiol 57:1154, 1986

52. Wolfe TR, Caravati EM, Rollins DE: Terminal 40-ms frontal plane QRS axis as a marker for tricyclic antidepressant overdose. Ann Emerg Med 18:348, 1989

53. Tepperman PB: Fatality due to acute systemic fluoride poisoning following a hydrofluoric acid skin burn. J Occup Med 22:691, 1980

54. Sedal L, Korman MG, Williams PO et al: Overdosage of tricyclic antidepressants: a report of two deaths and a prospective study of 24 patients. Med J Aust 2:74, 1972

55. McAlpine SB, Calabro JJ, Robinson MD, Burkle FM: Late death in tricyclic antidepressant overdose revisited. Ann Emerg Med 15:1349, 1986

56. Goldberg RJ, Capone RJ, Hunt JD: Cardiac complications following tricyclic antidepressant overdose. JAMA 254:1772, 1985

57. Pentel P, Sioris L: Incidence of late arrhythmias following tricyclic antidepressant overdose. J Toxicol Clin Toxicol 18:543, 1981

58. Smilkstein MJ: Reviewing cyclic antidepressant cardiotoxicity: wheat and chaff. J Emerg Med 8:645, 1990

59. Tafuri J, Roberts J: Organophosphate poisoning. Ann Emerg Med 16:193, 1987

60. Smilkstein MJ, Knapp GL, Kulig KW, Rumack BH: Efficacy of oral N-Acetylcysteine in the treatment of acetaminophen overdose. N Engl J Med 319:1557, 1988

TOXICOKINETICS

APPLYING PHARMACOKINETIC PRINCIPLES TO THE POISONED PATIENT

RICHARD S. WEISMAN, PharmD, ABAT[†]
CANDICE SMITH, PharmD[††]
LEWIS R. GOLDFRANK, MD, ABMT[†††]

Toxicokinetics enables the clinician to mathematically predict the onset and duration of toxic effects and to monitor the efficacy of therapeutic procedures and antidotes intended to prevent absorption, block metabolism, or hasten elimination. The critically ill poisoned patient, by nature of the intricacy of pharmacologic interactions, therapeutic interventions, and the rapid rate at which organ function changes, is an excellent candidate for the use of kinetic calculations. Unfortunately, the very indications for making these calculations dramatically complicate the accuracy of the mathematical predictions. In order for the clinician and the patient to benefit from these attempts at mathematical modeling, calculations will have to be performed frequently and timely therapeutic drug monitoring will be needed to enhance the accuracy and value of the predictions.

Pharmacokinetics has long been the unwanted stepchild of clinical pharmacology. Clinicians have avoided the use of pharmacokinetics believing that it requires advanced mathematics and complex engineering equations that can only be solved with the aid of a computer. Even when simple applications were used, the accuracy of the predictions nearly always made the exercise more time-consuming than clinically relevant.

One of the benefits that has grown from the frustration of pharmacokinetics is an understanding of numerous physiologic and pathologic events that will modify ab-

The critically ill poisoned patient, by nature of the intricacy of pharmacologic interactions, therapeutic interventions, and the rapid rate at which organ function changes, is an excellent candidate for the use of kinetic calculations. Unfortunately, the very indications for making these calculations dramatically complicate the accuracy of the mathematical predictions.

[†] Director, New York City Poison Control Center, New York City Department of Health, Bellevue Department of Emergency Services, New York, New York
[††] Assistant Clinical Professor, St. John's University, Jamaica, New York
[†††] Director, Emergency Services, Bellevue & New York University Hospitals, Medical Director, New York City Poison Center, New York, New York

sorption, tissue and protein binding, volumes of distribution, metabolism, elimination, and clearance.

This chapter will address some of the situations that modify pharmacokinetics and combine this knowledge with some basic toxicologic principles, thus defining our present understanding of toxicokinetics in the poisoned or intoxicated patient.

ABSORPTION

Absorption is defined as the extent and rate of substance movement from outside the body to the intravascular (blood) compartment. The route of substance administration (ie, oral, intravenous, cutaneous, subcutaneous, inhaled, intranasal, intramuscular, rectal) is a major determinant of both the fraction of substance reaching the systemic circulation (bioavailability) and the rate of absorption.[1] Following the ingestion of 200 mg of cocaine hydrochloride, the onset of action is 20 minutes with peak levels of 200 ng/ml.[2] This compares with smoking 250 mg of cocaine freebase with an onset of action of 8 seconds and a peak level of 800 ng/ml or intravenous administration of 200 mg of cocaine hydrochloride with an onset of action of 30 seconds and peak levels of 1,000 ng/ml.[2]

When a substance is ingested, many factors will modify the bioavailability, the time to achieve a peak concentration, and when the onset of pharmacologic activity can be anticipated. The absorption of acetaminophen from the gastrointestinal tract can be accelerated with metoclopramide or delayed with the administration of propantheline.[3] Factors that must be considered when a substance is ingested include physical characteristics such as solubility, molecular weight, dissolution rate, and the presence of adsorbent substances such as activated charcoal, as well as physiologic variables, including gastric emptying time, intestinal motility, tissue perfusion, and first-pass metabolism. Most substances are absorbed from the gastrointestinal tract by passive diffusion. The rate of diffusion across the lipophilic gastrointestinal membrane is described by Fick's first law, which states that the rate of diffusion across a membrane (dC/dt) is equal to the product of the difference in concentration on each side of the membrane ($C_1 - C_2$) and the diffusion constant of the drug or toxin (ka).

$$dC/dt = ka \times (C_1 - C_2)$$

In order for a substance to be passively absorbed into the systemic circulation, it must be soluble in the gastrointestinal fluid yet both lipophilic enough and of low enough

The rate of diffusion across the lipophilic gastrointestinal membrane is described by Fick's first law, which states that the rate of diffusion across a membrane (dC/dt) is equal to the product of the difference in concentration on each side of the membrane ($C_1 - C_2$) and the diffusion constant of the drug or toxin (ka).

molecular weight to diffuse across the phospholipid membranes of the gut.[4] Attempts to alter the solubility of ingested substances have not been successful *in vivo*. One clinical model that has been studied extensively is the patient with an iron overdose. The administration of oral sodium bicarbonate or phosphate solutions has been unable to convert iron to the less well absorbed carbonate or phosphate salt in the animal overdose model.[5]

Passive absorption of alkaline substances is more rapid in the alkaline small intestine, while passive absorption of acidic substances is more efficient in the acid environment of the stomach. Most pharmacologically active substances are primarily absorbed in the proximal small intestine. This is due to the small intestine's large surface area, high permeability to substances, and extensive blood flow.[6] Clinical situations that increase the rate of physiologic gastric emptying may increase the rate of absorption and hasten the onset of toxicity of basic drugs. Increasing the rate of absorption does not necessarily mean that there will be a corresponding increase in the amount of drug or toxin absorbed.[6] Factors that hasten transport of a substance to the primary site of absorption may continue to rapidly move the substances past the absorptive surface, thus resulting in an overall decrease in bioavailability. This hypothesis serves as the justification for the use of cathartics[7] and whole bowel irrigation.[8] Active transport systems for absorption are located in specific regions of the gastrointestinal tract. Iron is absorbed predominantly in the intestines proximal to the mid-jejunum.[9] Drugs that require bile salts to enhance their absorption such as L-amino acids, monosaccharides, and certain pyrimidines will only be absorbed in the ileum.[10]

The amount of a substance absorbed through the epithelial layer of the gut membrane is usually diminished with the presence of a toxin or gastrointestinal disease that decreases gastrointestinal transit times. The absorption of sustained release theophylline preparations is reduced to a greater extent when a cathartic is added to activated charcoal than when activated charcoal is given alone.[11] The absorption of both vitamin K and the oral anticoagulants has been proposed to be decreased in patients with laxative-induced decreased gastrointestinal transit times[12] and in patients with sprue, regional enteritis, enterocolitis, ulcerative colitis, and dysentery.[13] Although increased gastrointestinal motility may increase bioavailability if rapid absorption saturates hepatic metabolism,[14] cathartic-induced increases in gastrointestinal motility would be likely to speed the ingested substance past the sites of rapid absorption, leading to a decrease in overall absorption.

Disease states such as congestive heart failure, nephrotic

Most pharmacologically active substances are primarily absorbed in the proximal small intestine. This is due to the small intestine's large surface area, high permeability to substances, and extensive blood flow.

syndrome, or concurrent ingestions of alcohol, opioids, or substances with anticholinergic effects can prolong gastric emptying and gastrointestinal transit time, decrease the rate of absorption, and delay the onset of action.[15] Any substance that lowers either blood pressure or cardiac output will not only decrease perfusion of the vital organs of elimination (kidney and liver) but will also decrease blood flow to the gastrointestinal tract. As a result of diminishing the blood flow to the small intestines, unpredictable absorption will occur.[6] In overdose, a delay in absorption may be observed due to the formation of bezoars, concretions, or an agglutinated mass. This absorptive delay is well described in the literature for iron, bromides, and meprobamate.[16-18] Plasma drug concentrations performed soon after ingestion may not be representative of the peak plasma drug concentration. For example, when acetaminophen levels were compared to pharmacokinetically derived predictions based on the history, a coefficient of correlation of 0.98 was obtained if the level was obtained at least 4 hours after the ingestion. Acetaminophen levels obtained sooner after the ingestion at 0–2 hours and 2–4 hours had correlations of 0.59 and 0.85, respectively.[19]

If a chelating agent is to be administered orally, it is important to establish that the chelated substance does not have greater bioavailability than the drug or toxin alone. When deferoxamine is administered orally following iron in the dog overdose model, the absorption of the iron is increased rather than prevented because the iron chelate (ferrioxamine) is rapidly absorbed.[20] Conversely, the oral administration of 2,3-dimercaptosuccinic acid results in a beneficial decrease in gastrointestinal lead absorption.[21]

The administration of activated charcoal to the poisoned patient will significantly reduce the gastrointestinal absorption of many substances. The few notable exceptions are iron, lithium, alcohols, and caustics.

The administration of activated charcoal to the poisoned patient will significantly reduce the gastrointestinal absorption of many substances. The few notable exceptions are iron, lithium, alcohols, and caustics.[22] Binding to activated charcoal is related to specific stereochemical and electrochemical characteristics of binding affinity, the potential for contact, the amount of activated charcoal present in relationship to the substances, and the amount of time that has elapsed since the ingestion.[23] Multiple doses of activated charcoal are also effective in limiting secondary absorption by breaking the entero-hepatic recirculation of drugs such as digoxin and diphenoxylate,[24] and interrupting the entero-gastric recirculation of phencyclidine.[25]

Substances are adsorbed to activated charcoal most readily in their undissociated form. Weak acids bind better in an acid pH, while weak alkalis bind most avidly in an alkaline milieu.[26] The phenomena of drug desorption from activated charcoal has been reported for a weak acid such as salicylate when it is administered prebound to activated charcoal.[27] After administration of the prebound salicylate, an initial delay followed by sustained absorption of the salicylate for 30 hours occurred. The desorption of the salicylate may not have occurred until the salicylate entered the more alkaline pH of the small intestine. Desorption can be overcome by simply administering larger doses of activated charcoal more frequently.

FIRST-PASS METABOLISM

The anatomic relationship between the liver and the gastrointestinal tract plays an important role in the overall bioavailability of ingested substances that have a high hepatic extraction ratio. Before reaching the systemic circulation, an orally ingested drug must pass through the gastrointestinal wall into the liver via the portal circulation. The fraction of drug that is eliminated or metabolized in one pass of blood through the liver is defined as the hepatic extraction ratio.[14] A proportion of the dose may be eliminated by the liver or gut before reaching the systemic circulation. When this occurs it is referred to as first-pass metabolism.[28,29] In overdose, the bioavailability of drugs such as the cyclic antidepressants, phenothiazines, opioids, and many of the beta-blockers is increased because the first-pass metabolic process may become saturated.[30]

In patients with hepatic compromise such as cirrhosis, an increased bioavailability of an ingested substance with a normally high hepatic extraction ratio can be observed due to portosystemic shunting and/or decreased metabolic enzyme activity of the liver.[28,29] Poisoned patients with hepatic compromise who have been exposed to a substance that requires extensive hepatic metabolism are likely to have elevated levels of the substance for a protracted period of time. The reduced clearance of acetaminophen, opioids, diazepam, theophylline, or lidocaine in patients with hepatic failure demonstrates this concept. In untreated acetaminophen overdoses, the half-life of acetaminophen will become greater than 4 hours as hepatic necrosis progresses.[31] Alternatively, if the poisoned patient has been chronically exposed to a hepatic mixed-function oxidase inducer, first-pass hepatic metabolism may be increased, resulting in a decrease in bioavailability. Common inducers of the mixed-function oxidase system include phenobarbital, phenytoin, and cigarette smoking.[32,33]

Drugs such as propranolol that demonstrate significant first-pass metabolism will have lower systemic bioavailability after oral administration than after intravenous administration. In the case of lidocaine, the first-pass hepatic metabolism is so extensive that the use of oral administration to attain a therapeutic blood level is impractical.[34] Fol-

In overdose, the bioavailability of drugs such as the cyclic antidepressants, phenothiazines, opioids, and many of the beta-blockers is increased because the first-pass metabolic process may become saturated.

lowing accidental intravenous bolus administration of 1–2 g doses of lidocaine in a dog, cardiopulmonary bypass intended to maintain cardiac output and hepatic blood flow has been shown to result in rapid lidocaine clearance (40 ml/kg/min) by the liver.[35] In humans only about one-third of the orally administered dose of lidocaine will reach the systemic circulation.

The intramuscular administration of substances, either therapeutically or by the parenteral drug abuser, may also be affected by unexpected kinetic factors altering absorption. These factors include the amount of blood flow to the muscle group into which the injection is made and the rate of diffusion of the substance into the blood stream. The presence of potent vasoconstrictors such as epinephrine or cocaine may retard the absorption of concurrently administered substances.[36] When cocaine and heroin are administered together ("speedball") by the subcutaneous route, it can be postulated that the absorption of the heroin will be delayed. The rate of diffusion of the injected substance will also be affected by volume, pH, the viscosity of the diluent, varied adjuvant materials, and lipid solubility. Toxins that are very lipophilic will tend to move more rapidly into fat than into the aqueous blood compartment.

DISTRIBUTION

The way in which a substance distributes throughout the body is dependent upon several factors, including tissue perfusion, pH, protein and tissue binding, and lipid solubility.

The way in which a substance distributes throughout the body is dependent upon several factors, including tissue perfusion, pH, protein and tissue binding, and lipid solubility. The rate in which a substance distributes will be decreased by factors that decrease blood flow or cardiac output.

Changes in systemic and urinary pH can modify drug distribution. While this approach is most commonly thought of as a means of enhancing elimination, it also changes distribution into the central nervous system. Acidemia increases the proportion of both salicylate and phenobarbital found in the unionized form that is capable of entering the brain.[37,38] Alkalinizing the urine pH to between 7.5 and 8.5 will maximize the renal elimination of ionized salicylate and reduce the distribution of drug into the central nervous system.[37,39] Conversely, the renal elimination of phencyclidine can be increased by acidification of the urine.[40] While acidification is no longer recommended as a therapy because of the complication associated with a metabolic acidosis and the potential of precipitating myoglobin in the urine, this concept of ion entrapment can be utilized by placing the patient on continuous nasogastric suction, which has been shown to remove large amounts of phencyclidine as it distributes into gastric acid.[41]

In general, well-perfused tissues take up and distribute substances more rapidly and efficiently than poorly per-fused tissues.[42] The distribution of a drug to various tissues will take longer and the volume of distribution may be altered in the poisoned patient manifesting congestive heart failure, hypotension, or circulatory collapse.[43] It has been suggested that a smaller loading dose be administered for some substances (ie, lidocaine) in congestive heart fail-ure because of a reduced volume of distribution.[43] In con-trast, in a patient with chronic liver disease, the volume of distribution for lidocaine may increase, thus requiring a larger loading dose.[44] During periods of hypoperfusion, the response of the autonomic nervous system results in more drug being distributed to the central nervous system and myocardium and less to the eliminating organs such as the kidney and liver.[29] This redistribution may tend to exaggerate alterations in central nervous system or cardio-vascular function such as mental status, seizures, cardiac arrhythmias, and cardiac output. This pattern of toxicity is often seen with severe theophylline poisoning. Theoph-ylline causes an increase in circulating epinephrine result-ing in vasodilation and a reduction in peripheral vascular resistance.[45] Under these circumstances, the administra-tion of a beta-blocker has been shown to increase blood pressure by antagonizing this effect.[46]

Once a substance is in the blood compartment, it diffuses into a wide variety of different fluids and tissues: it can enter the highly perfused organs (ie, kidney, liver), become protein- or tissue-bound, enter adipose tissue, or stay in the extracellular compartment. For a variety of reasons, the body does not behave as if it were a single homogenous compartment where substances are uniformly distributed throughout all body fluids and tissues. The body is not a simplistic model in which the concentration of drug throughout the body reflects the same concentration as in the plasma. For most substances, it is more accurate to depict the body as being divided into two or more com-partments. The first compartment (central compartment) in which substances distribute rapidly is made up of blood and highly perfused organs such as the liver, lung, and kidney. From this central compartment, the substance dis-tributes to other body tissues (peripheral compartment) such as muscle and adipose tissue. The time it takes for a substance to distribute and equilibrate is referred to as the alpha distribution phase (Fig. 1). Changes in plasma con-centration during the distribution phase primarily reflect movement within the various body fluids and tissues rather than elimination from the body. This is especially

During periods of hypoperfusion, the response of the autonomic nervous system results in more drug being distributed to the central nervous system and myocardium and less to the eliminating organs such as the kidney and liver.

true if the patient is hypotensive or demonstrates hypo-perfusion states, where elimination may be impaired. Lithium, naloxone, and lidocaine are exceptions to this generalization because a significant loss of drug occurs during the distribution phase. The post-distribution plasma concentration reflects the amount of substance in the body and the extent of distribution throughout the body.[6] The extent to which a substance distributes throughout the body can be determined by relating the plasma concentration after distribution with the amount of substance in the body. The volume of distribution (Vd) represents the volume into which a substance distributes in the body at equilibrium.

$$Vd = \frac{\text{amount of substance in the body}}{\text{plasma concentration}}$$

The volume of distribution is not a real volume, but the size of the single compartment that would be created when one assumes that all of the drug or toxin in the body exists at the same concentration as it does in the plasma.

The volume of distribution is not a real volume, but the size of the single compartment that would be created when one assumes that all of the drug or toxin in the body exists at the same concentration as it does in the plasma. A large volume of distribution (defined as a Vd greater than 1 l/kg) indicates that the substance has distributed outside the plasma compartment into other body tissues or fluids. For some substances, such as digoxin (Vd = 7–8 l/kg) or the cyclic antidepressants (Vd = 10–50 l/kg), the volume of distribution is far larger than the actual volume of the

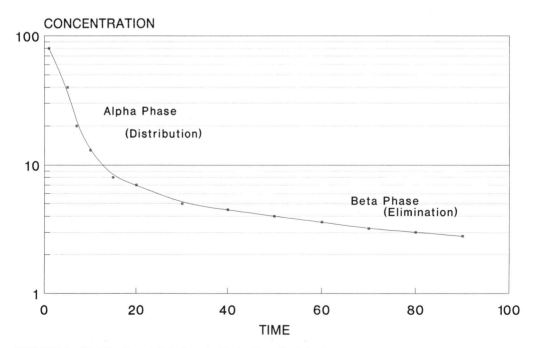

FIGURE 1   Distribution (alpha) and elimination (beta) phases.

body. As these volumes of distribution become larger, the concentration of the drug or toxin in the tissues becomes proportionally greater than the plasma concentration of the substance.[42] Volume of distribution only indicates the extent of substance distribution and not the specific tissue or fluid of distribution or relative concentrations in these tissues.

The volume of distribution can be used to estimate plasma concentrations when a known amount of substance has been ingested. If a 60 kg patient ingests 3,000 mg of theophylline and the volume of distribution of theophylline is 0.45 l/kg, the patient's maximum plasma concentration will be predicted as:

$$\frac{\text{amount of drug in body}}{\text{Vd}} = \text{maximum plasma concentration}$$

$$\frac{3{,}000\,\text{mg}}{0.45\,\text{l/kg} \times 60\,\text{kg}} = 110\,\text{mg/l}$$

This formula is useful for predicting the worst-case scenario. Peak levels will always be lower than this prediction because distribution and elimination occur during the absorption phase.

When an intravenous loading dose is administered, time is required for the drug to distribute into the various body tissues and fluids from the plasma compartment (alpha phase). Toxicity can be seen following rapid administration of a loading dose with some drugs due to a transiently high plasma concentration. Toxicity occurs because receptor sites for these substances are located within the central compartment and sufficient time has not elapsed for either alpha phase distribution to equilibrate with a peripheral compartment or for beta phase elimination to remove the drug from the compartment. Beta phase elimination is defined as the rate of elimination after the completion of both absorption and distribution. Too rapid administration of any of the substances in Table 1 will result in this type of toxicity.

After the ingestion of lithium or digoxin, a substantial amount of time is required for the drug to distribute into the peripheral compartment. The initial high concentration is not associated with toxic effects because the receptor sites responsible for toxicity are located in the peripheral compartment (long alpha phase). However, plasma concentrations taken before completion of distribution (equilibrium) will not reflect the tissue concentrations at the sites of pharmacologic activity. While theoretically it is important to allow for completion of the alpha distribution phase that defines equilibration of the plasma and tissue concentrations, this may not always be possible. Lithium requires

When an intravenous loading dose is administered, time is required for the drug to distribute into the various body tissues and fluids from the plasma compartment (alpha phase). Toxicity can be seen following rapid administration of a loading dose with some drugs due to a transiently high plasma concentration.

TABLE 1   Drugs That Cause Toxicity if Administered Rapidly

Drug	Administration Rate (not to exceed)	Toxicity (if rate exceeded)
Theophylline	20 mg/min	Seizures/arrhythmias
Lidocaine	25–50 mg/min	Seizures
Procainamide	25–50 mg/min	Cardiac
Quinidine	0.5 mg/kg/min	Cardiac
Propylene glycol (phenytoin diluent)	50 mg/min	Cardiac
Deferoxamine	15 mg/kg/h	Hypotension

Blood levels obtained prior to the completion of distribution may cause an apparent disparity between laboratory and clinical findings.

8–10 days for an equilibrium to be achieved between serum, brain, bone, and muscle.[47] Blood levels obtained prior to the completion of distribution may cause an apparent disparity between laboratory and clinical findings. For example, significantly elevated carboxyhemoglobin levels have been reported in patients that are asymptomatic if they are obtained soon after exposure.[48]

The use of Fab fragments of digoxin-specific antibodies demonstrates that an antidote can actually change the volume of distribution of digoxin. Digoxin normally has a large volume of distribution (7–8 l/kg), an indication that most of the drug resides in the tissue compartment with only a small percentage remaining in the intravascular compartment. After the alpha distribution phase, the concentration of digoxin in myocardial tissue is 15 to 30 times the plasma concentration.[49] Following the administration of the Fab fragments, the digoxin is pulled into the plasma where it is strongly bound to the Fab fragment. This results in a dramatic increase in the amount of digoxin in the blood (presumably as the digoxin-antibody complex).[50] If the free and bound digoxin are then used to calculate the volume of distribution, the Vd will be reduced, demonstrating the increased amount of drug in the plasma. The administration of multiple doses of activated charcoal may have the opposite effect on Vd. As a drug moves from the blood stream to the lumen of the gastrointestinal tract, plasma levels will decline. If these values are used to calculate Vd, an apparent increase in the volume of distribution will occur. While multiple dose activated charcoal may rapidly remove phenobarbital from the plasma, if equilibration from the central nervous system is not equally rapid, the patient may not show clinical improvement despite the presence of lower phenobarbital levels.[51]

PROTEIN BINDING

Another factor that influences the distribution of substances is binding to plasma proteins. Many substances are extensively bound to plasma proteins, the most important being albumin, alpha-1-acid glycoprotein, and globulins. Salicylates, disopyramide, and several of the nonsteroidal antiinflammatory drugs saturate their protein-binding sites at therapeutic levels. Most other drugs that are extensively bound to proteins do not reach saturation until toxic levels are attained.[30] Acidic substances are primarily bound to the most abundant plasma protein, albumin, while basic substances are usually bound to alpha-1-acid glycoprotein.

In general, substances that are extensively plasma protein-bound tend to have a small volume of distribution, whereas drugs or toxins with a high affinity for peripheral tissues have larger volumes of distribution. Only free, non-protein-bound substances are able to diffuse through cell membranes and equilibrate with receptor sites in tissues thereby causing pharmacologic and/or toxicologic effects.[52] Most toxicology laboratories primarily measure total drug (plasma protein-bound and unbound) concentrations due to cost and technical difficulties.[53]

Alterations in protein binding due to various disease states can affect a substance's distribution and ultimately its pharmacologic and toxicologic effect. Systemic toxicity results from the exposure to excessive amounts of free or unbound iron. Normally, iron binds to transferrin, a beta-1 globulin carrier protein with two high-affinity iron-binding sites for transfer to storage. Malnutrition, severe infection, rheumatoid arthritis, and the anemia of chronic disease are associated with significantly lower transferrin levels. These chronically ill patients can be predicted to be more susceptible to iron toxicity at lower levels of iron exposure. Once the binding sites on transferrin are overwhelmed, absorbed iron is taken up primarily by hepatocytes with accumulation in the mitochondria and resultant swelling and dysfunction.[54]

Physiologic and pathologic conditions can alter drug protein binding primarily through two mechanisms. These mechanisms are (1) the alteration of affinity of substances for plasma proteins and (2) the alteration of the concentration of plasma proteins available for binding.[55] In patients with normal protein binding, the therapeutic range for phenytoin is 10–20 μg/ml of which 10% (1–2 mg/ml) corresponds to free drug. When alterations in protein binding result in a decrease in the available binding sites, the desired therapeutic range as determined by a measurement of total available drug must be reduced. If a patient with hypoalbuminemia overdoses on phenytoin, nystagmus, ataxia, and central nervous system depression may be found, with phenytoin levels well below 20 mg/l. The consequences of diminished albumin include a comparable decrease in available binding sites with a resultant increase

Alterations in protein binding due to various disease states can affect a substance's distribution and ultimately its pharmacologic and toxicologic effect.

in the availability of free drug for pharmacologic or toxicologic effects.[56]

The tricyclic antidepressants are extensively bound to alpha-1-acid glycoprotein (AAG) in serum. The administration of AAG in the anesthetized rat desipramine overdose model resulted in less QRS complex prolongation 30 minutes after the protein was administered.[57] Although this effect was both limited and transient, the administration of specific binding proteins to poisoned patients may have great promise as an antidote of the future.

TISSUE BINDING

Most pharmacologically active receptor sites are located in highly vascular tissue compartments. The major determinant of toxicity is the amount of drug or toxin that is physically present to bind to these receptor sites.

Most pharmacologically active receptor sites are located in highly vascular tissue compartments. The major determinant of toxicity is the amount of drug or toxin that is physically present to bind to these receptor sites. Pharmacodynamics is the study of the dose response relationship at the level of the receptor site. Little is known about tissue-binding changes in overdose because of our inability to measure drug or toxin concentrations at receptor sites, although clinically we can predict that the changes do occur.[58]

The antidotal use of amyl and sodium nitrite in the treatment of cyanide or hydrogen sulfide poisoning is an example of a toxicologic modification of tissue binding. The formation of a toxic hemoglobin state rapidly removes cyanide from its tissue-binding sites. Since cyanide and hydrogen sulfide bind more avidly to the Fe^{+3} of methemoglobin than to the Fe^{+3} of cytochrome A_3, the addition of nitrites to transform approximately 20% of oxyhemoglobin to methemoglobin will allow methemoglobin to draw cyanide off of the cytochrome oxidase chain and form cyanomethemoglobin. Subsequently, in the presence of sodium thiosulfate, the cyanide is removed from the cyanomethemoglobin, thus regenerating methemoglobin and forming sodium thiocyanate, which can be eliminated by the kidneys.[59] Sodium thiosulfate will not be effective for hydrogen sulfide poisonings.

The use of hyperbaric oxygen to treat carbon monoxide poisoning is another example of a therapeutic intervention that will favorably alter the concentration of a toxin bound to tissue. Hyperbaric oxygen, in addition to displacing carbon monoxide from hemoglobin, also decreases carbon monoxide's binding to myoglobin and the cytochromes.[60]

Disease states such as hypo- or hyperthyroidism, congestive heart failure, and renal failure have all been shown to alter the relationship between the plasma concentration and the pharmacodynamic activity of digoxin. This has been postulated to be due to alterations in tissue binding.[61,62] In order to achieve the desired therapeutic effect with digoxin in the hyperthyroid patient, higher-than-normal doses may be required. Conversely, patients with hypothyroidism may be exquisitely sensitive to lower-than-normal doses of digoxin.[63]

Additional research in the area of tissue binding and pharmacodynamics may result in a better understanding of what happens to the tissue concentration of a cyclic antidepressant as its binding to the sodium channels is altered by serum alkalinization associated with either the use of sodium bicarbonate or hyperventilation.[64]

LIPID SOLUBILITY

The extent that a substance distributes into the peripheral fat compartment depends on the physical-chemical properties of the substance. A substance that is highly lipophilic penetrates most membrane barriers and therefore has a higher volume of distribution. Drugs that are lipophilic tend to have longer duration of effects because they accumulate in fat tissue and then slowly diffuse out as the plasma concentration decreases.

Following an overdose of ethchlorvynol, plasma drug levels begin to decline after 3–5 hours as the lipophilic drug distributes into fatty tissue stores. At about 7–10 hours after ingestion, plasma drug levels remain elevated and central nervous system depression persists as the drug redistributes from tissue stores back into the plasma. A similar pattern of distribution into adipose tissue and then redistribution back into plasma is seen with another sedative-hypnotic of abuse, glutethimide.[65]

Thiopental is a lipophilic anesthetic that is dependent on distribution for its short duration of effect. After intravenous administration, the patient will lose consciousness in 10–20 seconds. Maximum activity is reached at 40 seconds and then decreases progressively until the patient awakens at about 25 minutes. The rapid onset of action reflects the high initial brain concentrations. As the drug rapidly distributes into fat and other tissues, the plasma concentration decreases until no pharmacologic effect is observed. As the thiopental is liberated from body fat, it is eventually metabolized by the liver. If too much thiopental is administered, the fat storage compartment can become "filled" and the duration of anesthesia could become dramatically prolonged (half-life = 9 hours).[66]

ELIMINATION

The accurate characterization of elimination in the poisoned or intoxicated patient is of paramount importance. Many of the treatment strategies involve enhancing the

TABLE 2 Drugs and Toxins That Are Associated With Acute Renal or Hepatic Failure

Renal Failure	Hepatic Failure
Aminoglycosides	Acetaminophen
Mercury	Iron
Hydrocarbons (halogenated)	Cyclopeptide (mushrooms)
Ethylene glycol	Carbon tetrachloride
Arsenic	Arsenic
Cyclosporine	Yellow phosphorus
Chromium	Methotrexate
Cisplatinum	Phosphine
Cyclopeptide (mushrooms)	
Amphotericin	
Orellanine (mushrooms)	

Elimination is affected by changes in vital signs or tissue perfusion and is modified by changes in absorption, binding, and distribution. Elimination also changes with age.

elimination of a substance. Without a mathematical approach to quantitate the impact of an intervention, it is difficult to judge a treatment's benefit or to scientifically compare it to a new or innovative therapy.

Elimination is an extremely complex, dynamic process in the poisoned patient. Acute exposure to the substances in Table 2 may result in the development of renal or hepatic failure with a progressive decline in elimination. Elimination is affected by changes in vital signs or tissue perfusion and is modified by changes in absorption, binding, and distribution.[30] Elimination also changes with age. Although the overall rate of elimination of acetaminophen in the neonate is the same as in the adult, the difference in the amount of drug metabolized by sulfate formation and glucuronidation is significant.[67] Alcoholism may also alter elimination. Chronic ingestion of ethanol has been shown to stimulate the cytochrome P-450 mixed-function oxidase system that may increase the formation of free radicals from the metabolism of carbon tetrachloride or halothane and increase the production of the toxic metabolite of acetaminophen, N-acetyl-p-benzoquinoneimine.[68,69]

CLEARANCE

Clearance is one of the most clinically useful pharmacokinetic techniques for evaluating substance elimination in the overdosed patient. While defining a substance's elimination as being either zero-order, first-order, or Michaelis-Menten may be useful for therapeutic drug monitoring, the concept of clearance has a greater clinical utility for the poisoned patient. Clearance is defined as the measurement of the body's ability to eliminate a substance from blood or plasma over time. One of the major advantages of clearance is that it enables the clinician to easily evaluate the impact of a new treatment intervention. It does not require the knowledge of previously reported elimination parameters for a toxin or previous knowledge of how an individual patient will eliminate a substance. Clearance is expressed as a volume of blood or plasma that is cleared of drug per unit of time. The elimination of a substance may be a result of metabolic processes, renal excretion, chelation, or binding to activated charcoal. Total body clearance is equal to the sum of all of the clearance processes.

Cl total body = Cl renal + Cl hepatic

+ Cl activated charcoal + Cl chelation

Total body clearance is also equal to the product of the rate constant of elimination and the volume of distribution.

Cl = rate of elimination (Ke) × volume of distribution (Vd)

If this equation is to be used, it must be remembered that the clearance derived is only correct for a specific moment in time. Both the rate of drug elimination and the volume of distribution may change continuously. This calculation is valuable for monitoring changes and trends in clearance when both the Ke and Vd reach equilibrium during the beta phase of elimination. When this occurs, projections for the rate of drug elimination or the time it will take to reach a particular level can be made by calculating the half-life.

$$\text{half-life } (t\tfrac{1}{2}) = \frac{0.693Vd}{Cl}$$

Two major organs of elimination are the kidneys and the liver. In the poisoned patient, the gastrointestinal tract can also function as a major pathway of elimination. Many of the therapeutic interventions used to treat poisoned patients are directed at increasing clearance. Clearance can be thought of as the loss of drug across an organ of elimination. By modifying the urine pH, the renal clearance of several drugs can be enhanced by increasing the percentage of drug in the renal tubules that is in the ionized (water-soluble) state. The renal clearance of salicylates and phenobarbital can be enhanced at least four-fold with alkalinization of the urine through use of sodium bicarbonate.[70,71] While the clearance of the amphetamines and phencyclidine can also be enhanced with acidification of the urine, the complications of inducing a metabolic acidosis pose an unacceptable risk to the patient.

Many of the therapeutic interventions used to treat poisoned patients are directed at increasing clearance. Clearance can be thought of as the loss of drug across an organ of elimination.

A patient with preexistant renal failure who has been exposed to excessive amounts of a substance requiring renal clearance may require extracorporeal removal. The renal clearance of active drug or toxins, metabolites, chelated toxins, or drugs bound to Fab fragments is critical when it is the body's major route of elimination.

A patient with preexistant renal failure who has been exposed to excessive amounts of a substance requiring renal clearance may require extracorporeal removal. The renal clearance of active drug or toxins, metabolites, chelated toxins, or drugs bound to Fab fragments is critical when it is the body's major route of elimination. Many substances that are primarily eliminated by the kidney are well-recognized nephrotoxins. Some of the more notable of these are lead, lithium, oxalic acid from the metabolism of ethylene glycol, the aminoglycoside antibiotics, mercury, the cyclopeptide- and orellanine-containing mushrooms, and the nonsteroidal antiinflammatory drugs.[72] The elimination of these substances by the kidneys is proportional to the creatinine clearance. A patient who has been exposed to one of these drugs or toxins should have frequent assessments of his or her BUN and creatinine. The patient's urine should be frequently examined for protein, glucose, red or white blood cells, crystals, tubular elements, casts, and bacteria. The development of worsening renal function may require the use of hemodialysis or hemoperfusion to remove any remaining toxin.[73]

Antidotes that depend on renal elimination include D-penicillamine, calcium disodium edetate, deferoxamine, dimercaptosuccinic acid, digoxin-specific Fab fragments, and the cyanide antidote kit. In a recent report, a functionally anephric patient with digoxin poisoning was treated with digoxin Fab fragments. Although the patient was receiving multiple doses of activated charcoal and hemodialysis three times a week, a biphasic elimination half-life of 43 hours and 330 hours was described.[74] It has not been established if the digoxin-Fab complex was stable over this prolonged period of time. The biphasic elimination half-life may have documented dissociation of the digoxin from the Fab fragment. Future research is needed to determine the stability of the Fab-digoxin complex in patients with renal failure.

When multiple doses of activated charcoal are administered in certain overdoses, the gastrointestinal tract can be considered to be an organ of elimination. Multiple doses of activated charcoal will enhance the clearance of digitoxin, phenobarbital, carbamazepine, phenylbutazone, dapsone, methotrexate, nadolol, theophylline, salicylate, cyclosporin E, propoxyphene, nortriptyline, and amitriptyline.[75] It is proposed that activated charcoal in the lumen of the gut binds drug that is moving across a concentration gradient from the mesenteric blood vessels into the gut.[76]

The intrinsic hepatic clearance (metabolism) of drugs or toxins involves two phases. Phase I includes the oxidation-reduction, hydrolysis, and conjugation with sulfhydryl or amide groups. The cytochrome mixed-function oxidase enzyme system (Phase I) has toxicologic importance because it has been shown to produce hepatotoxic intermediates of both acetaminophen and carbon tetrachloride. The administration of N-acetylcysteine to protect the liver from acetaminophen toxicity may increase the metabolic clearance of acetaminophen by enhancing glutathione stores, thus providing a glutathione substitute for the mixed-function oxidase system, or by providing additional substrate for the nontoxic sulfation pathway.[77]

An increased clearance of theophylline can be seen when the hepatic microsomal enzyme system is stimulated by enzyme-inducing substances such as phenobarbital, ethanol, rifampin, carbamazepine, cigarette smoking, or phenytoin.[15,29]

The Phase II pathways include acetylation, sulfation, and glucuronidation. These enzymatic reactions increase the polarity of the metabolites, which leads to an increased urinary or biliary elimination. Drugs or toxins that are primarily eliminated from the body by oxidation appear to be more affected by diseases of the liver than by being metabolized by conjugation.[78] The benzodiazepines diazepam and lorazepam demonstrate this principle. The clearance of diazepam has been reported to decrease from 1.7 l/h to 0.8 l/h in patients with cirrhosis because an oxidative reaction is required before conjugation. The clearance of lorazepam (low-extraction drug), which only requires conjugation, is not affected by cirrhosis.[58]

The inhibition of selective metabolic pathways is occasionally used in toxicology as a therapeutic intervention. The administration of ethanol or 4-methylpyrazole (investigational) is used to inhibit the enzyme alcohol dehydrogenase.[79,80] The inhibition of alcohol dehydrogenase prevents the metabolism of methanol or ethylene glycol to their first metabolites, formaldehyde and glycoaldehyde, respectively, and allows for removal by hemodialysis of the (less toxic) parent alcohols and any of the metabolites should they have been produced.

Disulfiram, which is a potent inhibitor of the enzyme aldehyde dehydrogenase, is often used as a deterrent for drinking in alcoholics. If ethanol is ingested with aldehyde dehydrogenase blocked, acetaldehyde accumulates, causing the patient to develop nausea, vomiting, a flush, headache, and possibly hypotension. Once the enzyme is blocked, it may require 14 days after exposure to disulfiram for the enzyme to begin to function normally.[81]

Cimetidine is presently being investigated for acetaminophen overdoses because of its ability to inhibit the cytochrome P-450 mixed-function oxidase system. Cimetidine appears to be able to decrease toxicity in animals but not in humans.[82,83]

CONCLUSION

In evaluating the poisoned patient, the ability to predict the situations that will modify absorption, distribution, and elimination of drugs or toxins is essential. An understanding of the toxicokinetic and pharmacodynamic fate of these substances provides the clinician with a better understanding of what interventions will be necessary to limit morbidity.

Our understanding of these principles allows for the development of new and creative strategies to enhance the quality of care of the poisoned patient.

References

1. Benet LZ, Massoud N: Pharmacokinetics. p. 1. In Benet L (ed): Pharmacokinetic basis for drug theapy. Raven Press, New York, 1984

2. Verebey K, Gold MS: From coca leaves to crack: the effect of dose and routes of administration in abuse liability. Psychiatr Ann 18:513, 1988

3. Nimmo J, Heading RC, Tothill P, Prescott LF: Pharmacologic modification of gastric emptying: effects of propantheline and metoclopramide on paracetamol absorption. Br Med J 1:587, 1973

4. Welling PG: Effects of gastrointestinal disease on drug absorption. p. 29. In Benet L (ed): Pharmacokinetic basis for drug therapy. Raven Press, New York, 1984

5. Dean B, Oehme FW, Krenzelok E: A study of iron complexation in a swine model. Vet Hum Toxicol 30:313, 1988

6. Rowland M, Tozer TN: Clinical pharmacokinetics concepts and applications. 2nd ed. Lea & Febiger, Philadelphia, 1989

7. Riegel J, Becker C: Use of cathartics in toxic ingestions. Ann Emerg Med 10:254, 1981

8. Tennenbein M: Whole bowel irrigation as gastrointestinal decontamination procedure after acute poisoning. Med Toxicol Adverse Drug Exp 3:77, 1988

9. Wheby MS: Site of iron absorption in man. Scand J Haematol 7:56, 1970

10. Lack L, Weiner JM: In-vitro absorption of bile salts by small intestines of rats and guinea pigs. Am J Physiol 200:313, 1961

11. Goldberg M, Spector R, Park G: The effect of sorbitol and activated charcoal on serum theophylline concentrations after slow release theophylline. Clin Pharmacol Ther 41:108, 1987

12. Hanston PD: Drug-drug interactions. p. 39. In Hanston PD (ed): Drug interactions. 3rd ed. Lea & Febiger, Philadelphia, 1975

13. Marcus R, Coulson AM: Fat soluble vitamins: vitamins A, K, and E. p. 1553. In Goodman LS, Gilman AG (eds): The pharmacologic basis of therapeutics. 8th ed. Macmillan, New York, 1990

14. Pond SM, Tozer TN: First-pass elimination: basic concepts and clinical consequences. Pharmacokinet 9:1, 1984

15. Shammas FV, Deckstein K: Clinical pharmacokinetics in heart failure: an updated review. Clin Pharmacokinet 15:94, 1988

16. Foxford R, Goldfrank L: Gastrotomy: a surgical approach to iron overdose. Ann Emerg Med 14:1223, 1985

17. Iberti T, Patterson B, Fisher C: Prolonged bromide intoxication resulting from a gastric bezoar. Arch Intern Med 144:402, 1984

18. Jenis EH, Payne RJ, Goldbaum LR: Acute meprobamate poisoning: a fatal case following a lucid interval. JAMA 207:361, 1969

19. Edwards DA, Fish SF, Lamson MJ, Lovejoy FH: Prediction of acetaminophen levels from clinical history of overdose using a pharmacokinetic model. Ann Emerg Med 15:1314, 1986

20. Whitten CF, Chen Y-C, Gibson GW: Studies in acute iron poisoning. II. Further observations on desferrioxamine in the treatment of acute experimental iron poisoning. Pediatrics 38:102, 1966

21. Kapoor SC, Wielopolski L, Graziano JH, LoIacono NJ: Influence of 2,3-dimercaptosuccinic acid on gastrointestinal lead absorption and whole body lead retention. Toxicol Appl Pharmacol 97:525, 1989

22. Neuvonen P, Olkkola K: Oral activated charcoal in the treatment of intoxications. Med Toxicol Adverse Drug Exp 3:33, 1988

23. Olkkola K: Factors affecting the antidotal efficacy of oral activated charcoal. Ph.D. Thesis. University of Helsinki, Helsinki, 1985

24. Baselt R: Disposition of toxics drugs and chemicals in man. Vol. 1. Biomedical Publications, Canton, 1978

25. Picchioni AC, Consroe PF: Activated charcoal: a phencyclidine antidote, or hog in dogs. N Engl J Med 300:202, 1979

26. Anderson H: Experimental studies on the pharmacology of activated charcoal. II. The effect of pH on the adsorption by charcoal from aqueous solutions. Acta Pharmacol 3:199, 1947

27. Filippone GA, Fish SS, Lacouture PG et al: Reversible adsorption (desorption) of aspirin from activated charcoal. Arch Intern Med 147:1390, 1987

28. Blaschke TF, Rubin PC: Hepatic first-pass metabolism in liver disease. Clin Pharmacokinet 4:423, 1979

29. Wilkinson GR: Influence of hepatic disease on pharmacokinetics. p. 116. In Evans WE, Schentag J, Justo W (eds): Applied pharmacokinetics principles of therapeutic drug monitoring. Applied Therapeutics, Spokane, 1986

30. Rosenberg J, Benowitz NL, Pond S: Pharmacokinetics of drug overdose: Clin Pharmacokinet 6:161, 1981

31. Prescott LF, Roscoe P, Wright N: Plasma-paracetamol half-life and hepatic necrosis in patients with paracetamol overdosage. Lancet 1:519, 1971

32. Grygiel JJ, Birkett DJ: Cigarette smoke and theophylline clearance and metabolism. Clin Pharmacol Ther 4:491, 1981

33. Lohmann SM, Miech RP: Theophylline metabolism by the rat microsomal system. J Pharmacol Exp Ther 196:213, 1976

34. Boyes RN, Scott DB, Jebson PJ et al: Pharmacokinetics of lidocaine in man. Clin Pharmacol Ther 12:105, 1971

35. Freedman MD, Gal J, Freed CR: Extracorporeal pump assistance: novel treatment for acute lidocaine poisoning. Eur J Clin Pharmacol 22:129, 1982

36. Weiner N: Norepinephrine, epinephrine, and the sympathomimetic amines. p. 138. In Goodman LS, Gilman AG (eds): The pharmacologic basis of therapeutics. 6th ed. Macmillan, New York, 1980

37. Hill JB: Salicylate intoxication. N Engl J Med 288:1110, 1973

38. Waddell WJ, Butler TC: The distribution and excretion of phenobarbital. J Clin Invest 36:1217, 1956

39. Prescott LF, Balali-Mood M, Critcheley JA et al: Diuresis or urinary alkalinization for salicylate poisoning? Br Med J 285:1383, 1982

40. Aronow R, Done AK: Phencyclidine overdose: an emerging concept of management. JACEP 7:56, 1978

41. Goldfrank LR, Lewin NA, Osborn H: Phencyclidine. p. 517. In Goldfrank LR, Flomenbaum NE, Lewin NA et al (eds): Toxicologic emergencies. 4th ed. Appleton & Lange, Norwalk, 1990

42. Klotz U: Pathophysiological and disease-induced changes in drug distribution volume: pharmacokinetic implications. Clin Pharmacokinet 1:204, 1976

43. Woosley RL: Pharmacokinetics and pharmacodynamics of antiarrhythmic agents in patients with congestive heart failure. Am Heart J 114:1280, 1987

44. Thomson PD, Melmon KL, Richardson JA et al: Lidocaine pharmacokinetics in advanced heart failure, liver disease, and renal failure in humans. Ann Intern Med 78:499, 1973

45. Vestal RE, Eiriksson CE, Musser J: Effect of intravenous aminophylline on plasma levels of catecholamines and related cardiovascular and metabolic responses in man. Circulation 67:162, 1983.

46. Biberstein MP, Ziegler MG, Ward DM: Use of beta-blockade and hemoperfusion for acute theophylline poisoning. West J Med 141:485, 1984

47. Jaeger A, Sander P, Kopferschmitt J et al: Toxicokinetics of lithium intoxication treated by hemodialysis. Clin Toxicol 23:501, 1985

48. Davis SM, Levy RC: High carboxyhemoglobin levels without acute or chronic findings. J Emerg Med 1:539, 1984

49. Hoffman BF, Bigger JT: Digitalis and allied cardiac glycosides. p. 729. In Goodman LS, Gilman AG (eds): The pharmacologic basis of therapeutics. 6th ed. Macmillan, New York, 1980

50. Smith TW, Haber E, Yeatman L, Butler VP Jr: Reversal of advanced digoxin intoxication with Fab fragments of digoxin-specific antibodies. N Engl J Med 294:797, 1976

51. Pond S, Olson K, Osterloh J, Tong T: Randomized study of the treatment of phenobarbital with repeated dose of activated charcoal. JAMA 251:3104, 1984

52. Perucca E, Grimaldi R, Crema A: Interpretation of drug levels in acute and chronic disease states. Clin Pharmacokinet 10:498, 1985

53. Svensson CK, Woodruff MN, Baster JG: Free drug concentration monitoring in clinical practice: rational and current status. Clin Pharmacokinet 11:450, 1986

54. Robotham JL, Lietman PS: Acute iron poisoning: a review. Am J Dis Child 134:875, 1980

55. Baire J, Didey F, Delion F: Problems in therapeutic drug monitoring: free drug levels monitoring. Ther Drug Monit 10:133, 1988

56. Kilpatrick CJ, Wanwimolruk S, Wing LMH: Plasma concentrations of unbound phenytoin in the management of epilepsy. Br J Clin Pharmacol 17:536, 1984

57. Pentel PR, Keyler DE: Effects of high dose alpha-1-acid glycoprotein on desipramine toxicity in rats. J Pharmacol Exp Ther 246:1061, 1988

58. Bodenham A, Shelly MP, Park GR: The altered pharmacokinetics and pharmacodynamics of drugs commonly used in critically ill patients. Clin Pharmacokinet 14:347, 1989

59. Way JL: Cyanide antagonism. Fundam Appl Toxicol 3:383, 1985

60. Davis JC, Dunn JM, Heimbach RD: Indications for hyperbaric oxygen therapy. Tex Med 76:44, 1980

61. Mooradian AD: Digitalis: an update of clinical pharmacokinetics, therapeutic monitoring techniques and treatment recommendations. Clin Pharmacokinet 15:165, 1988

62. Rodin SM, Johnson BF: Pharmacokinetic interaction with digoxin. Clin Pharmacokinet 15:227, 1988

63. Morrow DH: Studies on digitalis-influence of hyper- and hypothyroidism on the myocardial response to ouabain. J Pharmacol Exp Ther 140:324, 1963

64. Sasyniuk BI, Jhamandas V, Valois M: Experimental amitripytyline intoxication: treatment of cardiac toxicity with sodium bicarbonate. Amm Emerg Med 15:1052, 1986

65. Ellenhorn MJ, Barceloux DG: Sedative-hypnotics. p. 573. In Ellenhorn MJ, Barceloux DG (eds): Medical toxicology: diagnosis and treatment of human poisoning. Elsevier, New York, 1988

66. Benet LZ: Effect of route of administration and distribution on drug action. J Pharmacokinet Biopharm 6:559, 1978

67. Miller RP, Roberts RJ, Fischer LJ: Acetaminophen elimination kinetics in neonates, children, and adults. Clin Pharmacol Ther 19:284, 1976

68. Lieber CS, DeCarli LM: Ethanol oxidation by hepatic microsomes: adaptive increases after ethanol feeding. Science 162:917, 1968

69. Sipes GI, Gandolfi AJ: Biotransformation of toxicants. p. 64. In Klaassen CD, Amdur MO, Doull J (eds): Casarett and Doull's toxicology: the basic science of poisons. 3rd ed. Macmillan, New York, 1986

70. Morgan AG, Polak A. The excretion of salicylate in salicylate poisoning. Clin Sci 41:475, 1971

71. Linton AL, Luke AG, Briggs JD: Methods of forced diuresis and its application in barbiturate poisoning. Lancet 2:377, 1967

72. Feinfeld DA: Renal principles. p. 167. In Goldfrank LR, Flomenbaum NE, Lewin NA et al (eds): Goldfrank's toxicologic emergencies. 4th ed. Appleton & Lange, Norwalk, 1990

73. Pond SM, Diuresis, dialysis, and hemoperfusion: indications and benefits. Emerg Med Clin North Am 2:29, 1984

74. Nuwayhid NF, Johnson GF: Digoxin elimination in a functionally anephric patient after digoxin-specific Fab fragment therapy. Ther Drug Monit 11:680, 1989

75. Howland MA: Antidotes in depth: activated charcoal. p. 129. In Goldfrank LR, Flomenbaum NE, Lewin NA et al (eds): Goldfrank's toxicologic emergencies. 4th ed. Appleton & Lange, Norwalk, 1990

76. Levy G: Gastrointestinal clearance of drugs by activated charcoal (editorial) N Engl J Med 307:676, 1982

77. Slattery JT, Wilson JM, Kalhorn TF, Nelson SD: Dose-dependent pharmacokinetics of acetaminophen: evidence of glutathione depletion in humans. Clin Pharmacol Ther 41:413, 1987

78. Kaplowitz N: Drug-induced hepatotoxicity. Ann Intern Med 104:826, 1986

79. Agner K, Hook O, Von Porat B: The treatment of methanol poisoning with ethanol. J Stud Alcohol 9:515, 1949

80. Li TK, Theorell H: Human liver alcohol dehydrogenase: inhibition by pyrazole and pyrazole analogs. Acta Chem Scand 23:892, 1969

81. Eneanya DI, Bianchine JR, Duran DO et al: The actions and metabolic fate of disulfiram. Annu Rev Pharmacol Toxicol 21:575, 1981

82. Mitchell M, Schenker S, Avant G et al: Cimetidine protects against acetaminophen hepatotoxicity in rats. Gastroenterology 81:1052, 1981

83. Ruffalo R, Thompson J: Cimetidine and acetylcysteine as antidotes for acetaminophen overdose. South Med J 75:954, 1982

USE OF ORAL ACTIVATED CHARCOAL IN MEDICAL TOXICOLOGY

DAVID C. LEE, MD[†]
JAMES R. ROBERTS, MD, FACEP, ABMT[†]

The medical treatment of patients with an acute drug overdose usually consists of a four-point approach to management consisting of: (1) general supportive care, (2) inhibition of drug/toxin absorption, (3) specific antidotal treatment (if any is available), and (4) enhancement of drug/toxin elimination from the body. As it is currently applied to medical toxicology, oral activated charcoal (AC) both limits drug/toxin absorption and enhances elimination. Activated charcoal is well recognized as a superlative adsorbent of many substances, and it has assumed a role as the primary intervention to limit gastrointestinal absorption of many drugs and toxins. Activated charcoal is physiologically inert with no inherent toxicity.[1] In addition to its primary adsorptive role, recent studies have indicated that serial pulsed dosing, referred to as multiple-dose activated charcoal (MDAC), results in the increased elimination of drugs/toxins that have already entered the systemic circulation, independent of their initial route of administration, whether intravenously, intramuscularly, or orally. An understanding of the rationale for the use of MDAC is crucial for the appropriate management of seriously poisoned patients.

An understanding of the rationale for the use of multiple-dose activated charcoal is crucial for the appropriate management of seriously poisoned patients.

BACKGROUND

The use of charcoal by the medical community dates back to 1550 BC. Hippocrates and Pliney both cite the use of charcoal for various ailments. The first recorded systemic

[†] Division of Toxicology, Department of Emergency Medicine, Mercy Catholic Medical Center, and The Medical College of Pennsylvania, Philadelphia, Pennsylvania

4   3

studies on the use of charcoal as a specific antidote were performed by Bertrand in the 1800s and demonstrated a beneficial effect of AC for arsenic poisoning. Touery further substantiated the significant antidotal capacity of the substance when he survived a lethal dose of strychnine by simultaneously ingesting AC. In the early 1900s multiple repeated doses of AC were suggested as a possible mechanism to reduce serum lipid concentrations in uremic patients. The modern age of AC began in the 1940s with the *in vitro* work of Anderson, who demonstrated the unique adsorbent capacity of AC and the antidote's efficacy with various ingested drugs. Clinical application of these principles, however, lagged behind the consequential laboratory evidence of the effectiveness of AC. Activated charcoal was rarely utilized on a consistent basis for the treatment of toxic ingestions until the 1960s. Cooney believed that the reasonable explanation for this phenomenon was that the medical community inadequately understood the pharmacokinetic principles associated with AC and therefore many clinicians were reluctant to use it. In the 1950s burnt toast, with a comparable appearance to the naked eye, was suggested as an alternative oral adsorbent in poisonings. This archaic concept adversely affected progress in the utilization of AC as an antidote, but as more knowledge was gained, AC eventually emerged as a mainstay in medical toxicology.[3]

ACTIVATED CHARCOAL PREPARATIONS

Charcoal is a fine, light black powder that is initially prepared by pyrolysis (also termed destructive distillation), a process by which organic material, usually wood pulp, is heated to temperatures between 600°C and 900°C in the absence of air. Metallic chlorides are often used to increase the porous quality of the material. The charcoal is then "activated" by exposing it to steam, carbon dioxide, or strong acids that remove any previously adsorbed contaminants and decrease particle size. The end result is the production of extremely small charcoal particles with a massive network of pores. The number and size of these pores determine the surface area of the charcoal and hence its adsorptive or binding qualities.[3,4] The standard AC compounds presently marketed contain a surface area of approximately 1,000 m^2/g. Newer forms of "super-activated" charcoal (eg, Super-Char) have been described to have a surface area from 2,500 to 3,500 m^2/g.[5] Unfortunately, due to formulation difficulties, none of these super-activated charcoals are currently available. Commercial preparations are available from numerous manufacturers and include plain AC powder, AC premixed with the cathartic sorbitol, and AC in an aqueous solution.

ADMINISTRATION OF ACTIVATED CHARCOAL

Oral AC is generally well accepted by children and most cooperative adults, but the gritty consistency makes it difficult for many patients to drink a full therapeutic dose. Palatability is enhanced by thoroughly mixing the powder to avoid lumps, drinking it through a straw from an opaque or covered container, or adding flavorings such as saccharin, a cola drink, or cherry or chocolate syrup. Sorbitol will also enhance patient acceptance, but this potent cathartic may produce excessive diarrhea.[6] Adding milk or ice cream to AC preparations may decrease adsorptive capacity.[7] Ultimately, if patients are either unwilling or unable to drink an AC slurry, it can be administered via a nasogastric tube. Ideally, for most ingestions a 10:1 ratio of AC to drug/toxin is recommended. Although the specific amount of drug ingested is rarely accurately known in an overdose, the standard recommended initial dose of AC is 1 g per kg of body weight because this dose is considered relatively safe and efficacious.

Although the specific amount of drug ingested is rarely accurately known in an overdose, the standard recommended initial dose of AC is 1 g per kg of body weight because this dose is considered relatively safe and efficacious.

CURRENT CLINICAL USE

Both clinical and experimental evidence have led physicians to routinely administer oral AC as the first-line treatment for most toxic ingestions, often replacing gastric emptying with AC therapy alone.[8,9] Recently, the status of AC has changed from adjunctive therapy to the primary or sole medical intervention for many deliberate or accidental drug ingestions. The use of AC appears to carry fewer risks of serious medical complications than either ipecac-induced emesis or gastric lavage.[10] Numerous authors have demonstrated equal clinical effectiveness and similar clinical outcomes, and even the superiority of AC, when this oral antidote is compared to a gastric emptying procedure in both experimental and clinical investigations.[11–13] For example, in a simulated overdose model, Curtis et al. demonstrated that AC plus a cathartic decreased salicylate absorption better than ipecac-induced emesis (70% vs 56%, respectively).[14] In a human volunteer overdose model, McNamara et al. demonstrated that AC plus a cathartic and ipecac-induced emesis were equally effective in re-

The use of AC appears to carry fewer risks of serious medical complications than either ipecac-induced emesis or gastric lavage.

Gastric emptying should not be abandoned in instances where the ingested drug/toxin is not adsorbed by AC, and emesis/lavage should always be considered in instances in which a life-threatening overdose is suspected and the time and clinical scenario allow for removal of a significant amount of unabsorbed drug/ toxin.

ducing acetaminophen absorption.[15] Relatively large clinical trials evaluating the outcome of drug overdose by Comstock et al. and Kulig et al. have also suggested that routine ipecac-induced emesis and gastric lavage are of questionable clinical benefit when compared to charcoal alone unless lavage is performed within 1 hour of ingestion.[11,12] Merigian et al. recently reported that a gastric emptying procedure had no additional benefit over AC alone, even in the treatment of symptomatic drug overdose, and further noted that the additional use of gastric lavage in patients given oral AC may actually increase pulmonary complications.[16] While AC alone may be recommended for the treatment-selected overdoses, this concept is still under evaluation and requires further study. Gastric emptying should not be abandoned in instances where the ingested drug/toxin is not adsorbed by AC, and emesis/lavage should always be considered in instances in which a life-threatening overdose is suspected and the time and clinical scenario allow for removal of a significant amount of unabsorbed drug/toxin.

COMPLICATIONS AND ADVERSE EFFECTS

While there are no absolute contraindications to oral AC, the routine administration of this antidote may not be totally benign.

While there are no absolute contraindications to oral AC, the routine administration of this antidote may not be totally benign and a number of caveats concerning its clinical use should be mentioned. Approximately 10–15% of patients given AC alone will vomit spontaneously, a clinically significant problematic effect in the patient at risk for pulmonary aspiration.[17,19] Spontaneous emesis is probably even higher in patients with an ileus, in those who have taken a drug known to produce vomiting (eg, theophylline, acetaminophen, hydrocarbons, salicylates), if nauseating antidotes are used (acetylcysteine), if sorbitol is added, or if a large bolus of poorly admixed AC is rapidly administered. Although AC itself is relatively nontoxic to the lungs, aspiration of swallowed charcoal introduces stomach acid and oral bacteria into the pulmonary system with the potential for a significant sequela. Large amounts of thickened AC can cause physical airway obstruction (especially in infants) and the black coloration may hamper attempts at tracheal intubation by obscuring important landmarks. Activated charcoal administration will also interfere with the endoscopic evaluation of the esophagus and stomach.

Krenzelok reviewed seven fatalities related to AC aspiration and concluded that in only one case was there a clear association between pulmonary aspiration and a fatal outcome. This was an unusual case of delayed bronchiolitis obliterans and death 14 weeks after aspiration in a patient with a tricyclic antidepressant overdose who had aspirated an AC/sorbitol combination.[17] Other rarely reported serious or life-threatening complications of AC administration include intestinal obstruction[18] and empyema after esophageal perforation.[19] These complications are exceedingly uncommon and have only been noted in isolated case reports.

Although diarrhea and constipation have both been attributed to AC, these effects are more likely due to the overly aggressive use of cathartics or the inherent antiperistaltic properties of ingested drug/toxins.[20] Some of the more serious complications ascribed to AC therapy have actually been due to the cathartics added to AC mixtures. Cathartics are commonly administered with AC to aid in the transit of toxin and to propel the adsorbent through the gut. The efficacy of cathartics remains to be precisely defined, but the complications of excessive cathartic use are well known. Multiple dosing of cathartic mixtures (sorbitol- or magnesium-containing products) are rarely indicated.[20,21] A single dose of sorbitol quickly produces significant diarrhea and can avoid the ensuing fluid and electrolyte imbalances that may result from multiple doses of this hyperosmolar sugar solution, which may be clinically significant. This is especially relevant in infants, the elderly, and those with cardiovascular instability. Magnesium toxicity may occur from repeated doses of magnesium-based cathartics, especially in patients with renal impairment.[22]

The pulmonary and gastrointestinal complications of AC use can be minimized by performing endotracheal intubation in patients at risk for aspiration, being certain that the tips of nasogastric tubes used for AC administration are in the stomach, administering well-mixed dilute solutions of AC, using smaller intermittent dosing regimens instead of large boluses and avoiding multiple doses of cathartics. Finally, AC should be avoided in the presence of a caustic ingestion since its use precludes immediate endoscopy and adsorption of caustics is minimal.

BINDING CHARACTERISTICS OF ACTIVATED CHARCOAL

Activated charcoal has been proven to significantly adsorb many drugs/toxins (Table 1) with notable exceptions being acids/alkalis, elemental metals (lead, lithium, boron, iron), petroleum distillates, cyanide, alcohols, and certain pesticides (parathion, DDT, N-methyl carbamate).[9,23] Although these substances have traditionally been labeled as "not well adsorbed" to AC, the specific binding properties

TABLE 1 Drugs that Are Effectively Bound by AC in the GI Tract of Humans and/or Animals

acetaminophen	ethchlorvynol	phenobarbital
aconitine	furosemide	phenylbutazone
d-amphetamine	glutethimide	phenylpropanolamine
amitriptyline	hexachlorophene	phenytoin
atropine	isoniazid	procainamide
barbital	kerosene	propantheline
benzene	malathion	propoxyphene
carbamazepine	mefenamic acid	quinine
chlordane	mercuric chloride	salicylates
chloroquine	methyl salicylate	secobarbital
chlorpromazine	nadolol	sodium valproate
chlorpropamide	nicotine	strychnine
digitoxin	nortriptyline	theophylline
digoxin	paraquat	tetracycline
disopyramide	pentobarbital	tolbutamide
doxepin	phencyclidine	yohimbine

Unless specific contraindications exist, it is reasonable to routinely administer AC when these poorly bound substances are ingested.

have not been rigorously studied *in vitro*, thus, unless specific contraindications exist, it is reasonable to routinely administer AC when these poorly bound substances are ingested.

The adsorptive capacity of AC appears to depend on several variables: gastric/intestinal pH, gastric contents, amount of drug/toxin ingested, and most importantly, time since ingestion. Activated charcoal adsorbs drugs most efficiently in their dissolved, undissociated state. Thus, salicylates and other similar weak acids are more completely adsorbed in the acidic milieu of the stomach, whereas the adsorption of tricyclic antidepressants and phenylpropanolamine is enhanced in the small intestine where the pH of gastrointestinal contents is more alkaline.[24]

Various substances in the stomach, such as gastric juices or food, may decrease the effectiveness of AC by as much as 50% when studied *in vitro*. These factors, as well as the ingestion of drugs/toxins with anticholinergic properties, also tend to slow gastric motility, thereby somewhat overcoming the lack of adsorption by increasing the time that AC is in contact with the substance to be bound. In short, the actual effectiveness of AC in the presence of a "full stomach" is highly variable.[25]

The amount of drug/toxin present versus the amount of AC administered will also affect binding properties. The adsorptive capacity is directly related to the amount of AC in contact with the drug/toxin, hence it is best to err on the side of generous AC administration. The maximum amount of drug/toxin adsorbed by AC is in the general order of 100 to 1,000 mg of drug per gram of AC. Thus, clinically, a 10 to 1 ratio of AC to drug/toxin has been traditionally recommended. Increasing this ratio will usually enhance the potential for completeness of the adsorption of the drug/toxin, although there is probably wide variation among specific substances.

The efficacy of AC in decreasing absorption is inversely related to the length of time prior to the administration of AC.[2,26] Absorption may begin as soon as a drug/toxin reaches the gut lumen, so that a delay of even a few minutes may result in a more toxic level. One reason why AC therapy is probably as clinically effective as a gastric emptying procedure is that many clinical situations involve a substantial time delay prior to the performance of lavage or emesis, thereby allowing for significant drug/toxin absorption. For this reason, some authors administer AC within 5–10 minutes of ipecac use if they choose this gastric emptying technique.[27] Other authors recommend an AC-lavage-AC routine, in which the initial dose of AC would theoretically bind to gastric contents. This hinders ongoing absorption of material and allows the AC and adsorbed drug/toxin to be evacuated by lavage. A repeat dose of AC would be given to adsorb any further material unaffected by the lavage procedure. This immediate use of AC takes advantage of the almost instantaneous adsorption that occurs when AC is in contact with an adsorbable substance. It seems to be a distinct clinical disadvantage to delay AC for 30 minutes while lavage is completed (and drug continues to be absorbed) or to wait 2–3 hours to give AC due to ipecac-induced emesis.

The efficacy of AC in decreasing absorption is inversely related to the length of time prior to the administration of AC.

MULTIPLE-DOSE THERAPY AND THE GASTROINTESTINAL DIALYSIS PRINCIPLE

MECHANISM OF ACTION

Activated charcoal administration may lower systemic levels of drugs/toxins by mechanisms other than the primary decrease in gastrointestinal absorption. Levy initially termed the process whereby orally administered AC enhanced the total body clearance of systemic drugs as "gastrointestinal dialysis." Multiple doses of AC administered at set time intervals have been experimentally shown to favorably enhance the nonrenal clearance of many orally administered drugs. The same mechanism may similarly increase the elimination in intentional drug overdose as well as in cases of iatrogenic intravenous drug overdose (Fig. 1).

Repetitive dosing of AC has been postulated to decrease the elimination half-life of already absorbed drugs through several mechanisms. For example, with theophylline, MDAC almost doubles nonrenal clearance.[1] The efficiency

Multiple doses of AC administered at set time intervals have been experimentally shown to favorably enhance the nonrenal clearance of many orally administered drugs.

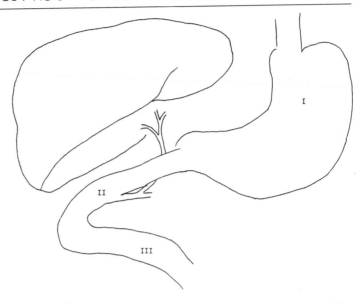

FIGURE 1   Sites of action of MDAC in the gastrointestinal tract. I. prevention of gastrointestinal absorption by initial adsorption of ingested drug; II. adsorption of drug secreted by the biliary system preventing reabsorption; III. adsorption of drug secreted and/or passively diffused through gastrointestinal cell membranes preventing reabsorption.

of this process is probably related to the physical properties of drugs/toxins, the ratio of drug/toxin to AC, and the physiology of the gastrointestinal tract among other factors. Many drugs/toxins passively diffuse or are actively secreted unchanged or as active metabolites into the gastrointestinal lumen. Any drug/toxin or metabolite in the serum that crosses the gastrointestinal cell membranes back into the gut can be bound to AC. Once adsorbed by the AC, the substance will then be unable to be reabsorbed into the systemic circulation unless desorption from AC occurs.[28]

Activated charcoal functions as an adsorbent "sink" at several sites in the gut.[4] First, AC can interrupt enterohepatic circulation of drugs/toxins/metabolites that are actively secreted in the bile. Substances demonstrated to exhibit this property include estrogens, dapsone, digitoxin, organic mercurials, arsenicals, indomethacin, and perhaps tricyclic antidepressants. This process contributes in a minor fashion to the overall gastrointestinal decontamination process. For example, Storstein noted that although multiple doses of AC doubled the rate of digitoxin elimination, only 7% of an intravenous dose of digitoxin was recovered from bile duct secretions.[29]

Secondly, AC can adsorb drugs/toxins/metabolites that enter the gut by active secretion. Aronow postulated that phencyclidine is secreted by the gastric mucosa into the gastric lumen. Theoretically, phencyclidine given intravenously will be secreted into gastric fluid, bind to AC, and then be excreted by the feces.[23]

The third mechanism relates to the fact that most unionized drugs/toxins/metabolites that are not protein-bound can pass from the blood across the gastrointestinal cell membrane by simple passive diffusion into the gastrointestinal lumen. If an excess of AC is present in the gut, a persistent concentration gradient will develop. This will enable a constant passive diffusion of drugs/toxins/metabolites from the systemic circulation into the gut lumen, thereby increasing systemic clearance. Furthermore, ion trapping as postulated by the pH partition hypothesis will concentrate unionized substances in the gut as these agents develop polarity.[2,30]

Finally, MDAC therapy may be indicated to prevent intestinal desorption. Activated charcoal and most drugs/toxins form a reversible bond that may be disrupted under specific conditions, such as pH changes. A substance that has been initially adsorbed by a single dose of AC may subsequently be released from the AC while still in the gut. Desorption would enable the unbound substance to be absorbed by the systemic circulation. For example, in the acidic environment of the stomach, weak acids such as salicylates bind two to three times more avidly to AC than in the more distal, alkalotic milieu of the intestines. Filippone et al. have shown that 30% of AC-bound salicylates are released into the intestinal lumen if only a single dose of AC is used, but little is desorbed when two or more doses are administered.[31]

Only a few specific drugs/toxins/metabolites have been rigorously evaluated as possible candidates for MDAC therapy in overdose situations (Table 2). It is hypothesized that substances that exhibit the following characteristics would be "eligible" for MDAC: a small volume of distribution (under 1 l/kg); a low plasma protein binding; a biliary or gastric secretion; or formation of active recirculating metabolites. In general, the criteria that dictate the effectiveness of hemodialysis and hemoperfusion can similarly be applied to determine the effectiveness by which MDAC

It is hypothesized that substances that exhibit the following characteristics would be "eligible" for MDAC: a small volume of distribution (under 1 l/kg); a low plasma protein binding; a biliary or gastric secretion; or formation of active recirculating metabolites.

TABLE 2   Drugs and Toxins That Demonstrate Significant Increased Clearance in Humans and/or Animals by Multiple-dose Activated Charcoal

carbamazepine	nadolol
dapsone	phenobarbital
digitoxin	phenylbutazone
disopyramide	phenytoin
N-acetylprocainamide	theophylline

may enhance systemic clearance of a drug/toxin. Exceptions to this are drugs/toxins that do not cross the gastrointestinal mucosa.[26] For example, aminoglycosides do not cross the gastrointestinal mucosa as evidenced by a lack of absorption when administered orally.[32,33] Although only a few drugs have been extensively studied, MDAC is highly recommended since the benefits of MDAC therapy far outweigh the potential morbidity and mortality of serious overdoses.

DOSING REGIMEN

In order to maintain a readily available source of AC in the intestinal lumen to facilitate gastrointestinal dialysis, several authors suggest an initial dose of 1–2 g per kg body weight, to be followed by 0.5–1.0 g per kg every 4 hours.

In order to maintain a readily available source of AC in the intestinal lumen to facilitate gastrointestinal dialysis, several authors suggest an initial dose of 1–2 g per kg body weight, to be followed by 0.5–1.0 g per kg every 4 hours.[34–36] Although the ideal regimen is unknown, Park et al. found a statistically insignificant difference in theophylline clearance when the same total dose of AC was given every 4 hours as compared to giving one–fourth of the total dose every hour.[37] Neuvonen noted that in clinical practice, dosage regimens for MDAC therapy have been based primarily on convenience.[2] In cases where patients are uncooperative or vomiting is problematic, it is possible to add charcoal to an aqueous solution and deliver the antidote by continuous slow infusion via a nasogastric tube. A suggested dose is 0.25–0.5 g/kg/h.[34–36] Clinical parameters, such as patient cooperation, degree of obtundation, the presence of an ileus, and the presence and amount of vomiting, will usually dictate the ideal dosing schedule.

SPECIFIC INDICATIONS FOR MULTIPLE DOSE THERAPY

It is important to note that although MDAC therapy has been shown to increase drug clearance, the specific beneficial effect of this therapy on the final clinical outcome is not well substantiated for most overdoses. Even if the clearance of a drug/toxin is doubled, it may not necessarily follow that mortality, overall complications, time to extubation, or length of stay are significantly decreased. Nevertheless, the principle is at least theoretically sound and, under the proper clinical circumstances, MDAC is a well-accepted therapeutic modality.[29,38]

Theophylline fits the criteria that would enable successful use of MDAC in cases of systemic poisoning: it is secreted and diffuses across the gastrointestinal mucosa, it has a low volume of distribution (0.5 l/kg), and it is efficiently adsorbed by AC.

Theophylline is a commonly prescribed drug with a narrow therapeutic range. Theophylline overdose and MDAC therapy have been extensively studied. Theophylline fits the criteria that would enable successful use of MDAC in cases of systemic poisoning: it is secreted and diffuses across the gastrointestinal mucosa, it has a low volume of distribution (0.5 l/kg), and it is efficiently adsorbed by

AC.[35] *In vitro* studies have shown that 1 g of AC will bind 300 mg of theophylline. *In vivo* studies have shown that 40% of an oral dose of theophylline (7.7 mg per kg body weight) was adsorbed by 30 g of AC given within 30 minutes of theophylline ingestion.[39] Several authors report that MDAC given in the acute setting of theophylline toxicity increases clearance by as much as 50–70%.[2,39,40] Kulig et al. have postulated that while this occurs partially from the inhibition of enterohepatic circulation, the majority of the effect is achieved through gastrointestinal dialysis.[39] Ingestion of the newer preparations is in a slow-release form. Multiple-dose activated charcoal therapy may also be of value in the treatment of iatrogenic theophylline poisoning when an excessive dose is inadvertently administered intravenously.

The severe gastrointestinal effects (nausea and vomiting) seen with serious theophylline toxicity may limit the effectiveness of MDAC therapy. Antiemetics have been recommended but they are not uniformly effective; when they are effective, their side effects, including excessive sedation, hypotension, lowering of the seizure threshold and dystonic reactions, may limit their use. The ideal antiemetic is unknown. Therapeutic doses of standard drugs should be given before labeling specific compounds as ineffective. Amitai et al. recommend ranitidine (50 mg every 8 hours intravenously) as a treatment to ameliorate the nausea and vomiting caused by the theophylline-induced hypersecretion of gastric juices.[41] Although not a well-studied practice, some authors administer metaclopramide intravenously in doses often as high as those suggested for the control of vomiting in chemotherapy (1–2 mg/kg) in order to control vomiting in theophylline overdose. To decrease the emetic effect of charcoal itself, Ohning recommends administration of charcoal by constant infusion through a nasogastric tube (0.25–0.5 g of AC per kg body weight per hour).[42]

The use of MDAC for phenobarbital poisoning has also been extensively studied, and the gastrointestinal dialysis principle has been reported as successful in treating overdose in infants as young as 28 days. Like theophylline, phenobarbital also has pharmacokinetic properties amenable to gastrointestinal dialysis: the drug easily diffuses across the gastrointestinal mucosa, has a low volume of distribution (0.5 l/kg), and is well adsorbed to AC.[35,36] Following the intravenous infusion of phenobarbital to healthy volunteers (2.85 mg/kg), Berg has demonstrated that MDAC reduced the serum half-life from 110 hours to 45 hours.[28] Pond et al. evaluated the effects of MDAC in a randomized, prospective study of 10 comatose patients with significant phenobarbital overdoses who were in a

The use of MDAC for phenobarbital poisoning has also been extensively studied, and the gastrointestinal dialysis principle has been reported as successful in treating overdose in infants as young as 28 days.

critical care unit. The author noted that although the average half-life of phenobarbital was shortened from 93 hours to 36 hours, clinical improvements as measured by duration of coma and extubation times did not correlate.[38] Most clinical studies involving MDAC therapy and phenobarbital have involved a limited number of patients, thus the clinical efficacy of this intervention necessitates further analysis.

Digitalis glycoside elimination has also been shown to be increased by the use of MDAC.

Digitalis glycoside elimination has also been shown to be increased by the use of MDAC. Pond reported a case whereby the serum half-life of digitoxin was reduced from 162 to 18 hours.[43] Lalonde et al. evaluated the effect of MDAC on digoxin administered intravenously, noting a 47% increase in digoxin clearance. The authors hypothesized that this phenomenon was probably due to the interruption of the enterohepatic circulation.[44] Storstein, however, retrieved only 7% of an intravenous dose of digitoxin in bile duct secretions, suggesting that another mechanism may be involved (perhaps related to the active or passive diffusion of digitalis compounds into the gut).[30]

Studies of the use of MDAC for salicylate poisoning have yielded controversial data. Mofenson et al. and Boldy et al. reported no advantage of repeated charcoal dosing in enhancing salicylate clearance over urinary alkalization.[45,46] However, Hillman et al. and Barone et al. recommended MDAC, citing its superiority over conventional decontamination methods alone.[47,48] Recently, Kirshenbaum et al. studied the effects of MDAC on 10 volunteers who ingested 2,880 mg of aspirin in a controlled, crossover, two-limb protocol. They noted only a 9% serum and 18% urine salicylate level change after treatment. They stated that their results did not support the routine use or effectiveness of MDAC in salicylate poisonings.[49] However, this study used less activated charcoal with a longer dosing interval than is presently recommended and did not mimic a true overdose. Although clearance may be only slightly enhanced, this benefit may have theoretical relevance in overcoming the salicylate desorption that follows a single dose of AC.

While tricyclic antidepressant overdose may also be theoretically amenable to MDAC, clinical experience has been disappointing. Tricyclic antidepressants are weak bases and are primarily metabolized in the liver with the metabolites being secreted into the biliary tract (enterohepatic circulation).[35] Although adsorbed by AC, tricyclic antidepressants are not cleared from the systemic circulation as effectively as theophylline or phenobarbital for a number of reasons. Tricyclic antidepressants have a large volume of distribution and undergo a slow transfer from intracellular compartments to extracellular compartments.

This not only reduces the effectiveness of MDAC but also limits the clinical use of hemodialysis and hemoperfusion. Scheinin et al. have shown that repeated doses of activated charcoal increase the clearance of desmethyldoxepin, the main excreted metabolite of doxepin. The overall doxepin elimination, however, was only slightly influenced. Tricyclic antidepressants are highly lipid-soluble, resulting in a depot of drug in the intracellular compartments. Although Neuvonen et al. have only shown slight increases in tricyclic antidepressant elimination with MDAC, they recommend MDAC therapy in the treatment of a tricyclic antidepressant overdose, to interrupt enterohepatic circulation, and to prevent delayed gastrointestinal absorption due to the direct effect of tricyclic compounds on decreasing gut motility.[2]

CHARCOAL–ORAL ANTIDOTE INTERACTIONS

N-ACETYLCYSTEINE

Toxic acetaminophen ingestions pose a unique therapeutic dilemma with regard to initial AC use and MDAC therapy. Clearly, AC adsorbs acetaminophen in the gastrointestinal tract, but AC also interferes with the absorption of the acetaminophen antidote, N-acetylcysteine (NAC). Although most authors believe that there is little clinical disadvantage to routine AC administration for serious acetaminophen overdose, the decision to use either AC or NAC, or to use both concurrently, remains somewhat controversial. Several authors have demonstrated that activated charcoal (in a 10:1 charcoal to drug ratio) binds between 60% and 80% of ingested acetaminophen when given within 1 hour of ingestion.[2] Therefore, expeditious AC administration may decrease acetaminophen absorption, thereby transforming a potentially toxic ingestion into a nontoxic ingestion and eliminating the need for the NAC therapy. In their respective large retrospective studies, Smilkstein et al. and Rumack et al. have demonstrated the benefits of NAC if given within 8–12 hours of ingestion.[50,51] However, isolated NAC use does not address concurrent co-ingestions.

Although the consensus is that both AC and NAC are indicated in a potentially life-threatening acetaminophen overdose, the specific clinical use of these antidotes remains somewhat controversial. The issues concerned with the combination of AC therapy and NAC have led several authors to evaluate the theoretical interactions between AC and NAC. Klein-Schwartz et al. have shown that AC adsorbs NAC at a 55–96% rate *in vitro*.[36] However, North et

Although Neuvonen et al. have only shown slight increases in tricyclic antidepressant elimination with MDAC, they recommend MDAC therapy in the treatment of a tricyclic antidepressant overdose, to interrupt enterohepatic circulation, and to prevent delayed gastrointestinal absorption due to the direct effect of tricyclic compounds on decreasing gut motility.

al. and Renzi et al. found minimal decreases in the NAC serum levels after AC administration *in vivo*.[52,53] To further confuse this topic, data by Ekins et al., although using very large doses of AC, contradicted previous studies by demonstrating a 40% reduction in total adsorption of NAC with concomitant AC administration.[54] In other studies, multiple-dose activated charcoal has had no effect on the systemic clearance of NAC by a gastrointestinal dialysis process.

The clinical significance of a potential decrease in serum NAC levels that may result from concomitant activated charcoal use has not been addressed. Neither the therapeutic serum levels of NAC required for the prevention of acetaminophen-induced hepatotoxicity[36] nor Smilkstein's review of over 11,000 acetaminophen overdoses suggests that the administration of AC adversely affects the efficacy of NAC as long as the acetaminophen antidote is given within 8 hours of an ingestion.[50] This data suggests that the amount of NAC that is currently recommended far exceeds the minimal dosage required to treat most acetaminophen overdoses. Thus, any adsorption of NAC to activated AC may become inconsequential. Because of the efficacy of AC in binding acetaminophen in mild to moderate ingestions, coupled with the high likelihood of co-ingestions, several sources recommend administration of a full dose of AC in all suspected acetaminophen overdoses.[35,36,53]

Because of the efficacy of AC in binding acetaminophen in mild to moderate ingestions, coupled with the high likelihood of co-ingestions, several sources recommend administration of a full dose of AC in all suspected acetaminophen overdoses.

IPECAC

The effect of AC on the emetic effect of ipecac has been studied. Although AC has been traditionally thought to inactivate ipecac if the two are given simultaneously, a number of studies have demonstrated that AC does little to interfere with the potency of ipecac if the adsorbent is given at least 10 minutes after a 60 ml dose of the emetic. Therefore, while it is not only reasonable to administer AC prior to lavage, the literature supports the nearly concurrent use of ipecac with a very limited delay prior to AC.[28]

OTHER ANTIDOTES

There is little evidence that AC interferes with the effectivenss of other oral antidotes, such as deferoxamine, dimercaptosuccinic acid (DMSA), sodium bicarbonate, Fuller's earth, ethanol, or starch. Clinical interactions between activated charcoal and these substances have not been well studied either *in vitro* or *in vivo*.

SUMMARY

Activated charcoal has an established role as a nonspecific adsorbent for many drugs, toxins, and their metabolites. Its routine use in drug overdose is undisputed. Activated charcoal alone may replace routine gastric emptying in selected cases. Multiple-dose AC therapy is also increasingly utilized as a noninvasive means of enhancing the removal of certain drugs/toxins already in the systemic circulation. Repetitive dosing is effective, inexpensive, safe, and relatively easy to administer, although the exact contribution to the clinical outcome is less clear. For most drugs/toxins, MDAC is considered adjunctive therapy. This modality should not replace the more efficient forms of toxin removal, such as hemodialysis and hemoperfusion, when they are indicated. However, MDAC should prevent continued absorption from the gut and further enhance elimination while stabilizing patients for these higher-risk methods of toxin removal, and should therefore be continued during such therapeutic interventions.

References

1. Levy G: Gastrointestinal clearance of drugs with activated charcoal. N Engl J Med 307(11):676, 1982

2. Neuvonen PJ, Olkkola KT: Oral activated charcoal in the treatment of intoxications: role of single and repeated doses. Med Toxicol Adverse Drug Exp 3(1):33, 1988

3. Cooney DO: Activated charcoal antidotal and other medical uses. Marcel Dekker, New York, 1980

4. Katona BG, Siegel EG, Claxton RJ: The new black magic, activated charcoal and new treatment uses. J Emerg Med 5:9, 1986

5. Krenzelok EP, Heller MB: Effectiveness of commercially available aqueous activated charcoal products. Ann Emerg Med 16:1340, 1987

6. Cooney D: Palatability of sucrose-sorbitol and saccharin sweetened activated charcoal formulations. Am J Hosp Pharm 37:237, 1980

7. Levy G, Soda GM, Lampan TA: Inhibition of ice cream on the antidotal efficacy of activated charcoal. Am J Hosp Pharm 32:289, 1975

8. Andelman RP: Changing priorities in gastrointestinal decontamination in toxic ingestions. Ann Emerg Med 17:385, 1988

9. Spyker DA: Activate charcoal reborn, progress in poison management. Arch Intern Med 145:43, 1985

10. Thompson AM, Robbins JB, Prescott LF: Changes in cardiorespiratory function during gastric lavage of drug overdoses. Hum Toxicol 6:215, 1987

11. Tenenbein M, Cohen S, Sitar DS: Efficacy of ipecac-induced emesis, orogastric lavage, and activated charcoal for acute drug overdoses. Ann Emerg Med 16:838, 1987

12. Comstock EG, Boisaubin EV, Comstock BS et al: Studies on the efficacy of activated charcoal following gastric lavage in acute drug emergencies. J Toxicol Clin Toxicol 19:219, 1982

13. Kulig K, Bar-Or D, Cantrill SV et al: Management of acutely poisoned patients without gastric emptying. Ann Emerg Med 14:562, 1985

14. Curtis RA, Barone J, Giacona N: Efficacy of ipecac and activated charcoal/cathartic: prevention of salicylate in a simulated overdose. Arch Intern Med 144:48, 1984

15. McNamara RM, Aaron CK, Gemborys M et al: Efficacy of charcoal cathartic versus ipecac in reducing serum acetaminophen in a simulated overdose. Ann Emerg Med 18:934, 1988

16. Merigian KS, Woodard M, Hedges JR et al: Prospective evaluation of gastric emptying in the self-poisoned patient. Am J Emerg Med 8:479, 1990

17. Krenzelok EP: Activated charcoal: a profile of repeated adverse effects. Clin Toxicol Forum 2:5, 1990

18. Watson, Cremer KF, Chapman JA: Gastrointestinal obstruction associated with multiple dose activated charcoal. J Emerg Med 4:401, 1986

19. Justiniani FR, Hippagaonkar R, Martinez LM: Charcoal containing empyema complicating treatment for overdoses. Chest 87:405, 1985

20. Neuvonen P, Olkkola K: Effects of purgatives on antidotal efficacy of oral activated charcoal. Hum Toxicol 5:255, 1986

21. Shannon M: Cathartics and laxatives: do they still have a place in management of the poisoned patient? Med Toxicol Adverse Drug Exp 1:247, 1986

2ʳ Smilkstein MJ, Smolinske S, Kulig KW et al: Severe hypermagnesemia due to multiple dose cathartic therapy. West J Med 148:208, 1986

    Jones J, McMullen MJ, Dougherty J et al: Repetitive doses of activated charcoal in the treatment of poisoning. Am J Emerg Med 5:306, 1987

ʹ. Nuevonen PJ: Clinical pharmacokinetics of oral activated charcoal in acute intoxications. Clin Pharmacokinet 7:465, 1983

25. Watson WA: Factors influencing the clinical efficacy of activated charcoal. Drug Intell Clin Pharm 21:160, 1987

26. Park GD, Spector R, Goldberg MJ et al: Expanded role of charcoal therapy in the poisoned and overdosed patient. Arch Intern Med 146:969, 1986

27. Freedman GE, Pasternak S, Krenzelok EP: A clinical trial using syrup of ipecac and activated charcoal concurrently. Ann Emerg Med 16:164, 1987

28. Berg MJ, Berlinger WG, Goldberg MJ et al: Acceleration of the body clearance of phenobarbital by oral activated charcoal. N Engl J Med 307:642, 1982

29. Storstein L: Studies on digitalis. III. biliary excretion and enterohepatic circulation of digitoxin and its cardioactive metabolites. Clin Pharmacol Ther 17:313, 1975

30. Pond SM: Role of repeated oral doses of activated charcoal in clinical toxicology. Med Toxicol Adverse Drug Exp 1:3, 1986

31. Filippone GA, Fish SS, Lacouture PG et al: Reversible adsorption (desorption) of aspirin from activated charcoal. Arch Intern Med 147:1390, 1987

32. Davis RL, Koup JR, Roon RA: Effect of oral activated charcoal on tobramycin clearance. Antimicrob Agents Chemother 32:274, 1988

33. Watson WA, Jenkins TC, Velasquez N: Repeated oral doses of activated charcoal and the clearance of tobramycin, a non-absorbable drug. J Toxicol Clin Toxicol 25:171, 1987

34. Haddad LM, Roberts JR: A general approach to the emergency management of poisoning. p. 2. In Haddad LM, Winchester JF (eds): Clinical management of poisoning and drug overdose. 2nd ed. WB Saunders, Philadelphia, 1990

35. Ellenhorn MJ, Barceloux DG: Gut decontamination. p. 53. In Ellenhorn MJ, Barceloux DG (eds): Medical toxicology diagnosis and treatment of human poisoning. 1st ed. Elsevier, New York, 1988

36. Smilkstein MJ, Price D, Flomenbaum NE: Gastrointestinal principles. p. 119. In Goldfrank LR, Flomenbaum NE, Lewin NA et al (eds): Goldfrank's toxicologic emergencies. 4th ed. Appleton and Lange, Norwalk, 1990

37. Park GD, Radomski I, Goldberg MJ et al: Efficacy of size and frequency of charcoal on theophylline clearance. Clin Pharmacol Ther 34:663, 1983

38. Pond S, Olson KR, Osterloh JD et al: Randomized study of the treatment of phenobarbital overdose with repeated doses of activated charcoal. JAMA 251:3104, 1984

39. Kulig K, Bar-Or D, Rumack B: Intravenous theophylline poisonings and multiple dose charcoal in an animal model. Ann Emerg Med 16:842, 1987

40. McKinnon RS, Desmond RV, Harmon PJ et al: Studies on the mechanisms of action of activated charcoal on theophylline pharmacokinetics. J Pharm Pharmacol 39:522, 1987

41. Amitai Y, Yeung AC, Moye J et al: Repetitive oral activated charcoal and control of emesis in severe theophylline toxicity. Ann Intern Med 105:386, 1986

42. Ohning BL, Reed MD, Blumer JL: Continuous nasogastric administration of activated charcoal for the treatment of theophylline intoxication. Ped Pharmacol 5:241, 1986

43. Pond S, Jacobs M, Marks J et al: Treatment of digitoxin overdose with oral activated charcoal. Lancet 27:823, 1980

44. Lalonde RL, Deshpande R, Hamilton PP et al: Acceleration of digoxin clearance by activated charcoal. J Clin Psychopharmacol 4:336, 1984

45. Mofenson HC, Caraccio TR, Greensher J et al: Gastrointestinal dialysis with activated charcoal and cathartic in the treatment of adolescent intoxications. Clin Pediatr 24:678, 1985

46. Boldy D, Vale JA: Treatment of salicylate poisoning with repeated oral charcoal. Br Med J 292:136, 1986

47. Hillman RJ, Prescott LF: Treatment of salicylate poisoning with repeated oral charcoal. Br Med J 291:1472, 1986

48. Barone JA, Raia JJ, Huang YC: Evaluation of the effects of multiple-dose activated charcoal on the absorption of orally administered salicylate in a simulated toxic ingestion model. Ann Emerg Med 17:34, 1988

49. Kirshenbaum LA, Mathew SC, Sitar DS et al: Does multiple dose charcoal therapy enhance salicylate excretion? Arch Intern Med 150:1281, 1990

50. Smilkstein MJ, Knapp GC, Kulig KW et al: Efficacy of oral *N*-acetylcysteine in the treatment of acetaminophen overdose. N Engl J Med 319(24):1557, 1988

51. Rumack BH, Peterson RG: Acetaminophen overdose: incidence, diagnosis, and management in 416 patients. Pediatrics 62:898, 1978

52. North D, Peterson R, Krenzelok E: Effect of activated charcoal administration on acetylcysteine serum levels in humans. Am J Hosp Pharm 38:1022, 1981

53. Renzi F, Donovan J, Morgan L et al: Concomitant use of activated charcoal and *N*-acetylcysteine. Ann Emerg Med 14:568, 1985

54. Ekins BR, Ford DC, Thompson MF: The effect of activated charcoal on *N*-acetylcysteine absorption in normal subjects. Am J Emerg Med 5:483, 1987

55. Arimori K, Kawano H, Nakano M: Gastrointestinal dialysis of disopyramide in healthy subjects. Int J Clin Pharmacol Ther Toxicol 27:280, 1989

56. Arimori K, Nakano M: Transport of procainamide and *N*-acetylprocainamide from blood into the intestinal lumen and intestinal dialysis by oral activated charcoal in rats with acute renal failure. J Pharmacobiodyn 11:504, 1988

57. Mauro LS, Mauro VF, Brown DL et al: Enhancement of phenytoin elimination by multiple-dose activated charcoal. Ann Emerg Med 16:1132, 1987

58. Arimori K, Nakano M: The intestinal dialysis of intravenously administered phenytoin by oral activated charcoal in rats. J Pharmacobiodyn 10:157, 1987

59. Siefkin AD, Albertson TE, Corbett MG: Isoniazid overdose: pharmacokinetics and effects of oral charcoal in treatment. Hum Toxicol 6:497, 1987

60. Hedges JR, Otten EJ, Schroeder TJ et al: Correlation of initial amitriptyline concentration reduction with activated charcoal therapy in overdose patients. Am J Emerg Med 5:48, 1987

61. Neuvonen PJ, Kivisto K, Hirvisalo EL: Effects of resins and activated charcoal on the absorption of digoxin, carbamazepine and fursemide. Br J Clin Pharmacol 25:229, 1988

ROLE OF HEMODIALYSIS AND HEMOPERFUSION IN THE TREATMENT OF INTOXICATIONS

LEAH BALSAM, MD[†]
GEORGE N. CORITSIDIS, MD[†]
DONALD A. FEINFELD, MD, FACP[††]

The treatment of poisoned patients involves several approaches, including the use of supportive care, removal of the noxious agent, and, when indicated, the administration of an antidote. Techniques such as accelerating the elimination of drugs/toxins by emptying the gastrointestinal tract and/or binding the drug/toxin with activated charcoal are routinely employed. (Throughout the rest of this chapter, the term "toxins" should be understood to include drugs.) In addition, the induction of a brisk diuresis coupled with urinary alkalization can result in more rapid elimination of specific toxins. More efficient, yet invasive, ways of extraction include various methods of extracorporeal removal of toxins. Hemodialysis and hemoperfusion have both been purported to remove numerous substances. However, these extracorporeal methods of substance removal are clinically indicated only in a limited number of poisonings.

This chapter discusses uses and limitations of extracorporeal removal of toxins. It must be emphasized, however, that these aggressive methods of toxin elimination do not

Aggressive methods of toxin elimination do not preclude standard techniques of detoxification.

[†] Attending Nephrologist, Nassau County Medical Center, East Meadow, New York, Instructor of Medicine, State University of New York at Stony Brook, Health Sciences Center, Stony Brook, New York

[††] Co-Director of Nephrology, Nassau County Medical Center, East Meadow, New York, Associate Professor of Medicine, State University of New York at Stony Brook, Health Sciences Center, Stony Brook, New York, Consultant in Nephrology, New York City Poison Control Center, New York, New York

preclude standard techniques of detoxification mentioned above: emptying the gut and administration of activated charcoal or antidotes. These methods should be continued throughout the extracorporeal treatment and afterwards until recovery is complete.

FACTORS LIMITING THE EFFECTIVENESS OF EXTRACORPOREAL TOXIN REMOVAL

In order to understand why hemodialysis and hemoperfusion are of limited usefulness in most poisonings, it is important to review certain variables that affect toxin removal from the body (see Table 1). The extraction ratio (E) of a substance by hemodialysis or hemoperfusion can be calculated as follows:

$$E = \frac{A - V}{A}$$

where A is the inflow plasma concentration and V is the outflow concentration of the substance in plasma entering and leaving the dialyzer, respectively.[1]

If plasma flow $= Q$ and clearance $= C$ (the theoretical volume of plasma completely cleared of a substance per unit time), then $C = QE$. A high clearance rate, however, is not in and of itself sufficient to guarantee effective toxin removal. There are numerous other factors involved in the effective elimination of toxins, the most important of which is volume of distribution.

The apparent volume of distribution (Vd) of a substance is that amount of water in which the administered sub-

A high clearance rate is not in and of itself sufficient to guarantee effective toxin removal. There are numerous other factors involved in the effective elimination of toxins, the most important of which is volume of distribution.

TABLE 1   Factors Affecting Efficiency of Extracorporeal Toxin Removal

Factor	Effect
Volume of distribution (Vd)	Substances with a high Vd (>1 l/kg) are not effectively removed from the body despite plasma clearance.
Molecular weight	High molecular weight substances (>150 d) are less effectively cleared.
Molecular charge	Ionized or polar molecules are more effectively cleared.
Protein or receptor binding	Tightly bound molecules are less effectively cleared.

stance must have been dissolved to give the observed steady-state plasma concentration.[2,3]

$$Vd = \frac{\text{total amount of substance in body}}{\text{concentration of drug in plasma}}$$

The Vd is a theoretical volume through which a substance is distributed; it does not necessarily correspond to a particular anatomic compartment or fluid space. In addition to being distributed in body water, a substance may disperse in fat or become bound by intracellular receptors. If a substance has a high Vd, the amount of a substance in the blood represents only a small fraction of the total body burden. For example, although both digoxin and cephapirin have very similar dialysis clearances (26 ml/min and 24 ml/min, respectively), removal of digoxin is much less efficient than that of cephapirin. Over a 6-hour dialysis session, approximately 20% of the total body burden of cephapirin is removed, while only 2% of digoxin is removed.[4] This is because digoxin has a much larger volume of distribution (11.7 l/kg) than does cephapirin (0.52 l/kg). (The digoxin in the plasma is substantially cleared; however, this clearance represents only a small percentage of the total amount of drug in the body.)

Other variables may limit the effectiveness of extracorporeal toxin removal. Factors affecting transport of toxins across dialysis membranes include molecular weight, lipid solubility, protein binding, and tight binding to the toxin's target tissues. Most substances move down a concentration gradient by passive diffusion. Higher molecular weight substances are less effectively dialyzed. Nonionized or nonpolar molecules are more lipid-soluble and are more likely to pass across cell membranes, while charged molecules tend to remain in the plasma and are more available to be removed by dialysis. The degree to which a substance is ionized depends on its pK and on the blood pH.[5] Similar to lipid solubility, protein binding of a molecule limits the amount of free molecules available for transport across dialysis membranes. The amount of a substance bound to protein can be affected by blood pH, renal failure, or competition with other molecules.[5]

Factors affecting transport of toxins across dialysis membranes include molecular weight, lipid solubility, protein binding, and tight binding to the toxin's target tissues.

MODALITIES OF EXTRACORPOREAL TOXIN REMOVAL

HEMODIALYSIS

Hemodialysis as a form of toxin elimination was first used in 1950 for salicylate poisoning.[6] This procedure involves the use of a semipermeable membrane to separate soluble

TABLE 2 Conditions
Necessary for
Hemodialysis or
Hemoperfusion

Adequate blood pressure
(>90 mmHg systolic)
Dialysis access to allow
blood flow of 150–250
ml/min
No unstable cardiac
arrhythmias

*Complications of
hemodialysis that
may occur include
bleeding or
thrombosis of the
vascular site,
peripheral bleeding
secondary to the use
of heparin, clotting in
the tubing or dialyzer,
hypotension due to
volume loss,
arrhythmias,
hypokalemia, air
embolus, infections,
and removal of
therapeutic
medications.*

substances from plasma. Once vascular access is obtained, the patient's blood is pumped through the dialyzer (the semipermeable membrane) in a direction that is counter to that of the dialysate. This promotes the diffusion of the toxic substance down its concentration gradient from the blood to the dialysate. Heparin is usually used to avoid clotting within the dialyzer.

It is the concentration gradient of the unbound toxin that provides the main driving force for the toxin's clearance. Hence, properties that predict enhanced elimination through hemodialysis include: low molecular weight, high water solubility, limited lipid solubility, and limited protein or tissue binding (ie, low volume of distribution) (Table 1).[5]

In order for hemodialysis to be performed, a number of conditions should be met (Table 2). The patient's blood pressure and cardiac reserve must be high enough to tolerate the fluid removal and generate adequate blood flow through the dialyzer. An adequate access must be placed, to allow a blood flow of 150–250 ml/min through the dialyzer. Unstable cardiac arrhythmias should be adequately suppressed. The platelet count should be monitored because platelets are lost in the dialyzer. Even if no heparin is used in the dialysis, platelet loss increases the risk for bleeding.

Complications of hemodialysis that may occur include bleeding or thrombosis of the vascular site, peripheral bleeding secondary to the use of heparin, clotting in the tubing or dialyzer, hypotension due to volume loss, arrhythmias, hypokalemia, air embolus, infections, and removal of therapeutic medications.[7] Hemolysis may occur if dialysis is continued for more than 6 hours. In addition, some patients may experience hypersensitivity to the dialyzer material or substances used to sterilize the dialyzer or tubing.[8]

HEMOPERFUSION

Hemoperfusion is a form of extracorporeal therapy whereby whole blood is passed through a sorbent-containing cartridge. Similar to hemodialysis, this procedure requires vascular access, a pump capable of blood flow rates of 200–300 ml/min, blood pressure monitoring, and heparin administration. The dialyzer membrane and the dialysate are simply replaced by the sorbent-containing cartridge.[9]

Sorbents such as activated charcoal, ion-exchange resins, and nonionic macroporous resins[9] have a large adsorptive capacity capable of binding toxic substances from the blood and provide better elimination of protein-bound substances than hemodialysis.[10] On the other hand, alcohols, due to their excellent clearance via hemodialysis and rapid saturation of charcoal, are a class of drugs for which hemoperfusion therapy is not indicated. (Since alcohols rapidly saturate the sorbent, effective hemoperfusion would require frequent cartridge changes.)

With such exposure to the blood compartment, a certain degree of biocompatibility is necessary. This biocompatibility has been accomplished by coating these sorbents with polymer membranes (eg, cellulose nitrate).[11] At present, the only hemoperfusion sorbent available in the United States is coated activated charcoal.

The risks of hemoperfusion are similar to those of hemodialysis, but there are a few additional ones largely related to the activated charcoal itself. When hemoperfusion devices were first utilized, particle embolization was a major risk.[9] Due to commercial washing and polymer coating techniques, embolization of activated charcoal particles is now insignificant.[12,13] These same improvements have also been effective in decreasing the pyrogen reactions and the marked degree of thrombocytopenia seen with hemoperfusion.[14] Currently, the expected fall in platelet count during treatment is less than 30%.[15]

Other side effects of hemoperfusion include hypoglycemia, hypocalcemia, and hypothermia, all of which need to be monitored and are easily corrected. Furthermore, in situations of long-term hemoperfusion, the possibility of trace metal and hormonal losses exist and should be evaluated during treatment.[11]

KINETICS OF ELIMINATION OF TOXINS BY HEMODIALYSIS AND HEMOPERFUSION

Most substances are handled in the body by first-order kinetics. A constant fraction of the substance is eliminated per unit time; therefore the amount removed is concentration-dependent. When the metabolic system is saturated during an intoxication, the toxin may be handled by zero-order kinetics. In this situation, a constant amount of toxin is removed per unit time, irrespective of concentration. Once hemodialysis or hemoperfusion is instituted, the kinetics will revert back to first order, due to the rapid removal of drug from the plasma.[3] For example, in a situation where hemodialysis is used in methanol intoxication, the drug is removed by first-order kinetics. If the level decreases initially from 200 mg/dl to 100 mg/dl over 3 hours, then, using first-order kinetics, one would expect to have

Sorbents such as activated charcoal, ion-exchange resins, and nonionic macroporous resins have a large adsorptive capacity capable of binding toxic substances from the blood and provide better elimination of protein-bound substances than hemodialysis.

a level of 50 mg/dl at the end of 6 hours. This is still a toxic level and further dialysis is required. If zero-order kinetics were erroneously used to estimate the methanol level at the end of 6 hours, one would expect that all of the methanol would have been removed and that dialysis could be terminated.

OTHER METHODS OF REMOVING TOXINS FROM THE BLOOD

PERITONEAL DIALYSIS

Peritoneal dialysis is a less effective technique of removing toxins than hemodialysis or hemoperfusion. In peritoneal dialysis, dialysate is placed in the peritoneal cavity. Toxins diffuse from the mesenteric capillaries across the peritoneal membrane; clearance is limited by the intrinsically slow rate of the mesenteric circulation.[5] The maximal clearance of urea is 30 ml/min, and most substances are removed much less rapidly than urea.[14] Therefore, peritoneal dialysis is almost never used in the management of drug overdoses or poisonings. It should never be considered an acceptable substitute for hemodialysis.

Peritoneal dialysis is almost never used in the management of drug overdoses or poisonings. It should never be considered an acceptable substitute for hemodialysis.

CONTINUOUS ARTERIOVENOUS HEMOFILTRATION

Continuous arteriovenous hemofiltration (CAVH), a modality used especially in critically ill patients to correct fluid and electrolyte abnormalities,[16] may have some theoretical advantages in intoxications. CAVH involves placement of two large bore catheters, usually one into a femoral artery and the other into a femoral vein. The blood from the femoral artery is routed to a hemofilter that is highly permeable and allows removal of large amounts of fluid. The remaining concentrated blood is returned to the patient via the femoral vein. Heparin must be infused continuously to prevent clotting in the filter and tubing. In order to perform CAVH, adequate blood pressure is necessary, as blood flow through the circuit is driven entirely by the patient's own blood pressure.[16,17] As water moves through the permeable membrane, solutes that can easily pass through the membrane are swept along with the water. This process is referred to as "solvent drag." Since at least 10–15 l/day can be removed though this process, large amounts of solutes can be cleared as well.[1] In addition, the continuous nature of this method can theoretically mitigate against the rebound effect commonly seen with drug extraction by hemodialysis or hemoperfusion.

There are several complications that may occur while performing CAVH. On placement or removal of the catheter, a hematoma may develop. In addition, distal ischemia may occur if the catheters are placed in stenotic vessels. Bleeding secondary to heparin, access site infarction, and fluid and electrolyte abnormalities are other potential problems that may arise during the performance of CAVH.[16]

It has been noted that CAVH can remove significant amounts of therapeutic drugs,[17,18] which has led to the suggestion that CAVH may be of benefit in drug toxicity.[19] However, literature addressing this issue is scarce. Domoto et al.[20] described four patients with renal failure who developed N-acetylprocainamide toxicity while receiving procainamide. Two patients who were treated with CAVH had a more rapid reduction in N-acetylprocainamide levels than the two who were treated with intermittent hemodialysis. A theoretical advantage for the use of CAVH would be the removal of large molecular weight compounds that are not removed well by hemodialysis or hemoperfusion. Mutzke et al.[21] examined the clearance of vancomycin via hemofiltration. By maintaining arterial blood flow at 300 ml/min, the clearance of the drug was increased to more than thirty times the endogenous clearance. However, at this time, since no controlled studies are available, CAVH cannot be recommended routinely as a substitute for hemodialysis or hemoperfusion.

CAVH may be of benefit in drug toxicity. However, literature addressing this issue is scarce.

FORCED DIURESIS AND URINE ALKALINIZATION

Forced diuresis and urinary alkalinization are only of limited benefit. The disadvantages of this method include the potential for causing fluid overload and acid–base disturbances.[22] In salicylate overdoses, however, this combination can greatly enhance net excretion of the drug since the ionized form of salicylate is trapped in the renal tubule. In contrast, in methanol overdose, a profound diuresis would be required in order to effectively remove the toxin. Methanol is generally metabolized by the liver; in methanol poisonings, ethanol or 4-methylpyrazole is given to inhibit its breakdown to toxic metabolites. The only means of elimination is by renal excretion. Methanol is not concentrated in the urine, as it is reabsorbed with water. Since the concentration of methanol in urine does not significantly exceed its concentration in blood, the volume of urine necessary to completely remove the toxin would approximate methanol's distribution space.[23] For example, in a 70 kg person with a Vd of 0.6 l/kg, 42 l of urine would be required to completely remove the methanol. Hemodialysis is, therefore, the only therapeutic choice.

SUBSTANCES FOR WHICH EXTRACORPOREAL REMOVAL IS OFTEN INDICATED

SALICYLATES

Renal excretion of salicylates can be substantially increased by inducing a large volume of alkaline urine as discussed above. There is a four-fold increase in clearance for each rise of one unit in urine pH.[24] Hemodialysis, however, is more efficient. Salicylates have a small Vd and a low molecular weight. In addition, in toxic states, protein binding in plasma decreases from 90% to 50%, which allows hemodialysis to remove the drug more effectively.[25] This is because the protein receptors become saturated, and only the free drug is dialyzable. Hemodialysis removes salicylates three to five times faster than diuresis,[26] five to seven times faster than normal renal excretion, and approximately twice as fast as hemoperfusion.[27] Another advantage of hemodialysis over hemoperfusion is its ability to correct fluid and acid–base abnormalities that occur with salicylism.[28] Hemodialysis is indicated in several situations: in cases where volume overload and/or renal failure are present and administration of fluid and sodium bicarbonate is precluded, in patients who clinically deteriorate

TABLE 3   Substances for Which Extracorporeal Removal is Often Indicated

Substance (preferred method)	Volume of Distribution (l/kg)	Indications for Extracorporeal Removal	
		Levels	Signs/Symptoms
Methyl alcohol (hemodialysis)	0.6	50 mg/dl	ocular disturbances, metabolic acidosis
Ethylene glycol (hemodialysis)	0.6	?	metabolic acidosis, neurological symptoms
Salicylate (hemodialysis)	0.2	80 mg/dl	clinical deterioration: coma, inability to tolerate administration of sodium salts
Lithium (hemodialysis)	0.8	4 mEq/l	cardiac arrhythmias, hypotension, confusion, delirium, coma
Theophylline (hemoperfusion)	0.5	80 mg/l (acute ingestion) 50–60 mg/l (chronic ingestion)	cardiac arrhythmias, seizures

(altered mental state, respiratory distress syndrome, or uncontrollable acid–base disturbance), and in overdoses in which plasma levels exceed 80 mg/dl.[5,28]

ALCOHOLS

The alcohols (methanol, ethylene glycol, isopropanol, ethanol) are also readily dialyzable because of their small Vd, high water solubility, and lack of protein binding. In addition, dialysis is often indicated when methanol and ethylene glycol are ingested in excessive amounts because their metabolites can cause significant toxicity.

Methanol is metabolized by alcohol dehydrogenase to formaldehyde, which in turn is rapidly metabolized by aldehyde dehydrogenase to formic acid. The slow metabolism of formic acid to CO_2 and water allows the toxin to accumulate. Formate and lactate are probably primarily responsible for the development of metabolic acidosis, optic nerve damage, and central nervous system and cardiac injury. In fact, the degree of acidemia is a better predictor of prognosis than the methanol level, probably because the acidemia reflects the amount of the toxic metabolite formate.[29] In order to retard the metabolism of methanol, ethanol should be administered as soon as the diagnosis is considered, since it has 10 times the affinity for alcohol dehydrogenase of methanol. It can be administered either orally or intravenously. One approach is to give a loading dose of 0.6 g/kg of 10% ethanol intravenously over 30–60 minutes. Concurrently, a maintenance dose of 100 mg/kg/h should be infused, increasing by approximately 7 g/h during hemodialysis in order to maintain a blood concentration of 100–200 mg/dl.[11,29] Since ethanol requirements may vary, its metabolism being especially dependent on the amount of alcohol usually ingested, ethanol levels should be monitored. The clearance of both methanol and formate is increased in hemodialysis ten-fold over renal clearance. Although some rebound in methanol levels does occur following dialysis, due to redistribution of methanol, hemodialysis can substantially reduce the total body burden of toxin.

Ethylene glycol is initially oxidized by alcohol dehydrogenase, which results in a series of toxic metabolites. The degrees of toxicity and metabolic acidosis correlate best with the accumulation of glycolic acid; however, due to the altered redox state and reversed ratio of NADH/NAD, lactic acid also significantly contributes to the acidosis.[28] Oxalic acid is another metabolite produced by the breakdown of ethylene glycol; the observation of oxalate crystals in the urine is often a clue to the presence of this overdose.[30]

Dialysis is often indicated when methanol and ethylene glycol are ingested in excessive amounts because their metabolites can cause significant toxicity.

Ethylene glycol poisoning should also be suspected if there is severe, high anion gap metabolic acidosis with a methanol level of zero and a high "osmolal gap" (measured osmolality − calculated osmolality > 20 mOsm/kg).[31] As in methanol toxicity, ethylene glycol poisoning is treated with the combination of administration of ethanol and hemodialysis. Ethanol has an affinity for alcohol dehydrogenase 100 times that of ethylene glycol. Early treatment with ethanol and hemodialysis can prevent the deposition of oxalate in the kidneys and prevent acute renal failure. It is also important to maintain good hydration during dialysis in order to prevent oxalate deposition. Preservation of renal function can increase the clearance of ethylene glycol by about 20%.[32]

LITHIUM

Lithium is a low molecular weight substance (molecular weight = 3 daltons) and is not protein-bound. Both these factors allow lithium overdoses to be treated effectively by hemodialysis. However, in lithium overdose, particularly with chronic poisoning, there is slow equilibration between intracellular and extracellular compartments. In fact, it may be the intracellular concentration of lithium that is the prime determinant of clinical toxicity.[34] Therefore, in order to lessen the rebound effect, dialysis should be extended to 6 hours and lithium levels should be followed. Repeated dialysis should be done until the lithium level remains in a safe range (0.6–1.2 mEq/l). Hemodialysis is indicated in patients with severe neurological or cardiovascular symptoms or blood levels greater than 4 mEq/l, especially in patients with renal failure in whom renal excretion is limited.[11]

THEOPHYLLINE

Theophylline has a small volume of distribution and is effectively removed by hemodialysis. However, since theophylline is approximately 60% protein-bound, it is even more efficiently removed by hemoperfusion.

Theophylline has a small volume of distribution and is effectively removed by hemodialysis. However, since theophylline is approximately 60% protein-bound, it is even more efficiently removed by hemoperfusion. A case report by Stegmayr[34] describes the treatment of a theophylline overdose with both hemodialysis and hemoperfusion on-line. It was felt that the combination of the two modalities reduces the risk of hypokalemia and hypocalcemia and increases the clearance of the drug. In most cases, however, charcoal hemoperfusion alone is sufficient. As both hemodialysis and hemoperfusion are invasive procedures, some authors recommend extracorporeal removal of the drug only if seizures, hypotension, or cardiac arrhythmias cannot be controlled by intensive supportive care.[35] Park et al., however, found a high morbidity and mortality associated with seizures.[36,37] Therefore, it is probably advisable to institute hemoperfusion if theophylline levels are high, even if the patient appears clinically stable. This is often the case when long-acting theophylline preparations are ingested. The following criteria can be used to institute hemoperfusion: (1) in acute ingestions, serum levels of greater than 80 mg/l; and (2) in chronic intoxication, serum levels of greater than 60 mg/l or concentrations of greater than 50 mg/l if the patient both (a) is greater than 60 years of age or has significant liver disease or heart failure and (b) cannot tolerate oral activated charcoal therapy.[37]

SUBSTANCES FOR WHICH EXTRACORPOREAL REMOVAL HAS BEEN SUGGESTED

CYCLOPEPTIDES

90% of deaths resulting from mushroom poisoning are either from *Amanita phalloides* (commonly found in Europe) or *A. verna* (found in the United States). The toxin involved, slow-acting α-amanitin, concentrates in the liver and causes massive liver necrosis through its inhibition of endonuclear RNA polymerase.[38] In general, as forms of treatment, hemoperfusion and/or hemodialysis have resulted

TABLE 4   Substances for Which Extracorporeal Removal Has Been Suggested

Toxin	Level of Ingestion Where ECT Indicated	Method	Condition
Amanatin	50 g (3 mushrooms)	Charcoal hemoperfusion	Up to 24 hours after ingestion
Ethanol	350 mg/dl	Hemodialysis	Especially, with evidence of liver failure
Isopropanol	400 mg/dl	Hemodialysis	Coma
Phenobarbital	10 mg/dl	Hemoperfusion or hemodialysis	Prolonged coma or cardiopulmonary complications not responsive to supportive intensive care
Short-acting barbiturates	5 mg/dl	Hemoperfusion	
Paraquat	–	Hemoperfusion	Up to 12 hours after ingestion
Procainamide/ N-acetylprocainamide	–	Hemoperfusion	In renal failure, with torsade de pointes

ECT = extracorporeal treatment.

in variable success. This is despite the fact that this water-soluble toxin is easily dialyzed and possesses a high affinity for charcoal.[39] The discrepancy likely reflects delays in treatment, often measured in days, that render treatment ineffective. Evidence for this is found in a report involving eight patients in whom hemoperfusion was undertaken within 24 hours of ingestion. Although seven of these patients had ingested lethal quantities, there were no deaths.[40] It is therefore recommended that activated charcoal hemoperfusion be considered if a lethal dose (more than 50 g) has been ingested and the patient presents early.

TRICYCLIC ANTIDEPRESSANTS

The tricyclic antidepressants' high lipid solubility and high protein and tissue binding result in a large volume of distribution that is reflected by their Vd of 20 l/kg. Therefore, although hemodialysis and hemoperfusion are efficient in their ability to clear these drugs from the plasma,[5] they are ineffective in significantly decreasing the body burden. This is the case even with early initiation of hemodialysis.[11] Reports of efficacy do exist, describing clinical improvement despite minimal total drug removal. Therefore, in situations of failing supportive treatment, hemodialysis may be considered as a last resort.[41,42] However, the seizures, hypotension, and cardiac arrhythmias that accompany tricyclic antidepressant toxicity generally preclude dialysis.

The seizures, hypotension, and cardiac arrhythmias that accompany tricyclic antidepressant toxicity generally preclude dialysis.

ETHANOL

Widely abused, ethanol is an associated intoxicant in over 30% of drug overdoses. Its effects on the central nervous system are closely related to blood levels; elimination is primarily via hepatic metabolism. At levels greater than 300 mg/dl, ethanol can cause hypoventilation or hypotension. In such cases, hemodialysis may be utilized, particularly if there is liver impairment. Although it is capable of increasing body clearance by 50%,[43] the need for dialysis in ethanol intoxication is extremely uncommon.

BARBITURATES

Phenobarbital is a long-acting, water-soluble barbiturate with a Vd of only 0.5 l/kg. In patient presentations involving high drug levels (more than 10 mg/dl), prolonged coma, or cardiopulmonary complications not responsive to intensive care, and especially if charcoal cannot be administered, hemodialysis or hemoperfusion may be warranted.[42] Otherwise, the preferred treatment is oral activated charcoal, emesis, gastric lavage, and supportive care. Alkaline diuresis greatly increases urinary excretion of the drug. In general, virtually all phenobarbital overdoses can be managed without dialysis.

Short-acting barbiturates are highly lipid soluble and more highly protein-bound. Hence, extracorporeal removal is more difficult and clears much less of the body drug burden. In short-acting barbiturate overdose, if extracorporeal removal must be done, the preferred treatment is charcoal hemoperfusion.[44] This is almost never needed, and conservative management is the rule. In all barbiturate poisonings, deterioration following discontinuation of treatment is possible, and hence repeated hemoperfusion may be necessary if it is done at all.

Virtually all phenobarbital overdoses can be managed without dialysis.

PARAQUAT

Paraquat ingestion results in extensive tissue distribution, which has rendered hemoperfusion and hemodialysis largely ineffective as modes of treatment. However, once extracorporeal treatment is initiated, levels are rapidly decreased, indicating good clearance from serum. Unfortunately, this toxin is very slow in equilibrating from other compartments, leaving tissue concentrations unaffected.[45]

Considering that there is a 70% mortality rate from paraquat poisoning and that most reports of unsuccessful hemoperfusion treatment have reflected treatment delay or ingestion of massive doses, some authors recommend hemoperfusion when the interval after ingestion is less than 12 hours.[46,47] Furthermore, as suggested by recent reports, success of hemoperfusion may also depend on repeated treatments to maintain enhanced clearance as paraquat equilibrates from tissue stores.[47,48]

ISOPROPANOL

Isopropanol or isopropyl alcohol ingestion is commonly reported in young children, derelicts, and suicidal adults. Eighty percent of the absorbed dose is metabolized to acetone, which is readily excreted via the lungs and kidneys. Its small volume of distribution and limited plasma protein binding make dialysis an effective form of elimination. However, hemodialysis is only warranted in patients presenting with hypotension and coma, when levels are greater than 400 mg/dl and the mortality rate may reach 45%.[49] Short of such a dramatic presentation, the mortality rate is negligible, and supportive treatment alone is generally recommended.

CHLORAL HYDRATE

Chloral hydrate is a non-barbiturate sedative-hypnotic which, via alcohol dehydrogenase, is converted to the pharmacologically active metabolite trichloroethanol. Complications of intoxication include central nervous system depression, respiratory arrest, hypothermia, gastric necrosis, and arrhythmias.[50] In massive overdoses, where saturation kinetics may increase the half-life from 8 hours to 35 hours, extracorporeal removal may be effective in removing up to 34% of body stores.[51] Therefore, hemoperfusion or hemodialysis should be considered in massive overdoses of chloral hydrate with central nervous system, cardiovascular, or respiratory dysfunction.[11]

Hemoperfusion or hemodialysis should be considered in massive overdoses of chloral hydrate with central nervous system, cardiovascular, or respiratory dysfunction.

PROCAINAMIDE/NAPA

Procainamide is an antiarrhythmic agent used for a wide variety of dysrhythmias. Its metabolite, the pharmacologically active N-acetyl procainamide (NAPA), is excreted by the kidney to a greater extent than procainamide (85% vs. 50%). Therefore, in renal insufficiency, decreased NAPA excretion can lead to intoxication. In fact, toxic NAPA levels have even been seen in patients on dialysis although NAPA clearance by dialysis is actually increased.[52] This is a result of the substantial tissue binding that further hampers the drug's elimination.

Hemoperfusion may be considered in the renal-insufficient patient where toxicity presents with such clinical manifestations as torsade de pointes.[52] With hemoperfusion, clearance of NAPA can be up to 36% greater than with hemodialysis.[53]

ETHICAL AND MEDICO-LEGAL CONSIDERATIONS IN EXTRACORPOREAL TOXIN REMOVAL

EXTRACORPOREAL TREATMENT IN THE UNSTABLE PATIENT

Some poisoned patients in whom the toxin might be appropriately removed extracorporeally may have a complication that makes the treatment problematic. As noted in Table 2, a patient should have adequate blood pressure, stable cardiac function, and vascular access. A temporary dialysis catheter should be inserted by the nephrologist or a surgeon; cardiac function should be maximized and arrhythmias controlled before treatment is begun.

Hypotension is the most common problem that might interfere with dialysis. Solute clearance is related to the flow of blood through the dialyzer, and at blood flows below 100 ml/min, the clearance becomes minimal.[54] Such blood flows cannot be maintained with systolic blood pressures less than 90 mmHg. In fact, a blood flow of 150–250 ml/min is preferable. If the poisoned patient's blood pressure is inadequate for hemodialysis or hemoperfusion, it is not safe to attempt the treatment and expose the patient to additional complications. In this situation, every effort should be made to raise the blood pressure to a level that will permit hemodialysis or hemoperfusion to be performed. Placement of a Swan-Ganz catheter will allow optimization of blood volume and cardiac function, as well as measurement of systemic vascular resistance. Administration of fluids or cardiotonic medications may improve the blood pressure. When necessary, pressors such as dopamine or norepinephrine may be used. As long as the blood pressure remains adequate (fluid removed during hemodialysis must be replaced), extracorporeal toxin removal can be performed. If the blood pressure cannot be maintained at the appropriate level, the patient will not benefit from the procedure.

As long as the blood pressure remains adequate (fluid removed during hemodialysis must be replaced), extracorporeal toxin removal can be performed. If the blood pressure cannot be maintained at the appropriate level, the patient will not benefit from the procedure.

AVAILABILITY OF EXTRACORPOREAL TOXIN REMOVAL

Just as it is important to avoid unnecessary invasive procedures in managing a poisoned patient, so it is equally vital that aggressive treatment be available when indicated. Patients with sustained toxic levels of the five substances that are removed well by extracorporeal methods—salicylate, methanol, ethylene glycol, lithium, and theophylline—require such treatment promptly, in order to prevent irreversible brain or cardiovascular injury. Delay in the institution of treatment may result in increased tissue toxicity. Therefore, a hospital that treats emergency patients should expect to encounter such intoxications and should be prepared to deal with them.

A receiving hospital for acutely ill patients should have the capacity to perform emergency hemodialysis and hemoperfusion within a short time after the need for the procedure is determined. This means having a nephrologist and any necessary ancillary dialysis personnel available on short notice 24 hours a day, 7 days a week. Necessary equipment, including hemoperfusion cartridges, should be

In situations where extracorporeal removal of toxins is not consistently available, the hospital should have a contingency plan for prompt transfer of patients to a facility where the procedure can be performed.

on-hand or readily obtainable. The directors of the Emergency Department and the Intensive Care Unit should plan for such emergencies with the hospital's nephrology staff.

In situations where extracorporeal removal of toxins is not consistently available, the hospital should have a contingency plan for prompt transfer of patients to a facility where the procedure can be performed. A working agreement should be made with the nephrologists at the receiving institution. This is particularly important for care of intoxicated pediatric patients, as the adult nephrologists at a hospital without a pediatric nephrologist may not be able to provide hemodialysis and hemoperfusion for infants and small children. Backup arrangements for such transfers should be made well in advance, so as not to delay a potentially life-saving treatment.

ACKNOWLEDGMENT

The authors thank Mrs. Vera Frankel and Mrs. Barbara C. Kern for assistance in completion of the manuscript.

References

1. Winchester JF: Active methods for detoxification. p. 154. In Haddad LM, Winchester JF (eds): Clinical management of poisoning and drug overdose. WB Saunders, Philadelphia, 1983

2. Winchester JF: Use of dialysis and hemoperfusion in treatment of poisoning. p. 437. In Daugirdas JT, Ing TS (eds): Handbook of dialysis. Little, Brown, Boston, 1988

3. Ambre J: Principles of pharmacology for the clinician. p. 18. In Haddad LM, Winchester JF (eds): Clinical management of poisoning and drug overdose. WB Saunders, Philadelphia, 1983

4. Gwilt PR, Perrier D: Plasma protein binding and characteristics of drugs as indices of their hemodialyzability. Clin Pharmacol Ther 2:154, 1978

5. Blye E, Lorch J, Cortell S: Extracorporeal therapy in the treatment of intoxication. Am J Kidney Dis 3:321, 1984

6. Doo PD, Walsh WP, Lyle LH et al: Acetylsalicylic acid intoxication: a proposed method of treatment. JAMA 146:105, 1951

7. Bregman H, Daugirdas JT, Ing TS: Complications during hemodialysis. p. 106. In Daugirdas JT, Ing TS (eds): Handbook of dialysis. Little, Brown, Boston, 1988

8. Wather RL, Klein E: Hypersensitivity in hemodialysis. Artif Organs 8:270, 1984

9. Winchester JF: Hemoperfusion. p. 305. In Drukker W, Parsons FM, Maher JF (eds): Replacement of renal function by dialysis. 2nd ed. Martinus Nijhoff, Boston, 1983

10. Rosenbaum JL, Winsten S, Kramer MS et al: Resin hemoperfusion in the treatment of drug intoxication. Trans Am Soc Artif Intern Organs 16:134, 1970

11. Cutler RE, Forland SC, Hammond PG et al: Extracorporeal removal of drugs and poisons by hemodialysis and hemoperfusion. Annu Rev Pharmacol Toxicol 27:169, 1987

12. Chang TMS: Semipermeable aqueous microcapsules (artificial cells): with emphasis on experiments in an extracorporeal shunt system. Trans Am Soc Artif Intern Organs 12:13, 1966

13. Andrade JD, Von Wagenen PA, Chen C et al: Coated adsorbants for direct blood perfusion. II. Trans Am Soc Artif Intern Organs 18:473, 1972

14. Winchester JF. Evolution of artificial organs: extracorporeal removal of drugs. Artif Organs 10:316, 1986

15. Winchester JF: Hemoperfusion in uremia. p. 387. In Giordano C (ed): Sorbents and their clinical applications. Academic Press, New York, 1980

16. Golper TA: Continuous arteriovenous hemofiltration in acute renal failure. Am J Kidney Dis 6:373, 1986

17. Golper TA, Pulliam J, Bennett W: Removal of therapeutic drugs by continuous arteriovenous hemofiltration. Arch Intern Med 145:1651, 1985

18. Golper TA, Wedel SK, Kaplan AA et al: Drug removal during continuous arteriovenous hemofiltration: theory and clinical observations. Artif Organs 8:307, 1985

19. Golper TA, Bennett W: Drug removal by continuous arteriovenous hemofiltration. Med Toxicol Adverse Drug Exp 3:341, 1988

20. Domato DT, Brown WW, Bruggersmith P: Removal of toxic levels of N-acetylprocainamide with continuous arteriovenous hemofiltration or continuous arteriovenous hemodiafiltration. Ann Intern Med 106:550, 1987

21. Matzke GR, O'Connel MB, Collins AJ et al: Disposition of vancomycin during hemofiltration. Clin Pharmacol Ther 40:425, 1986

22. Goldberg MJ, Spector R, Park GD et al: An approach to the management of the poisoned patient. Arch Intern Med 146:1381, 1986

23. Peterson RG, Peterson LN: Cleansing the blood. Pediatr Clin North Am 33:675, 1986

24. Morgan AG, Polak A: The excretion of salicylate in salicylate poisoning. Clin Sci 41:475, 1971

25. Wosilait WD: Theoretical analysis of the binding of salicylate by human serum albumin: the relationship between free and bound drug and therapeutic levels. Eur J Clin Pharmacol 9:285, 1976

26. Jorgensen HE, Wieth JO: Dialyzable poisons: hemodialysis in the treatment of acute poisoning. Lancet 1:81, 1963

27. James JA, Kimbell L, Read WT: Experimental salicylate intoxication: comparison of exchange transfusion intermittent peritoneal lavage and hemodialysis as means of removing salicylate. Pediatrics 29:442, 1962

28. Garella S: Extracorporeal techniques in the treatment of exogenous intoxications. Kidney Int 33:735, 1988

29. McCoy HG, Cipolle RJ, Ehlers SM et al: Severe methanol poisoning: application of a pharmacokinetic model for ethanol therapy and hemodialysis. Am J Med 67:804, 1979

30. Jacobsen D, Akesson I, Shefter E: Urinary calcium oxalate monohydrate crystals in ethylene glycol poisoning. Scand J Clin Lab Invest 42:231, 1982

31. Lund ME, Banner W, Finley PR et al: Effects of alcohols and selected solvents on serum osmolality measurements. J Toxicol Clin Toxicol 20:115, 1983

32. Cheng JT, Beysolow TD, Kaul B et al: Clearance of ethylene glycol by kidneys and hemodialysis. J Toxicol Clin Toxicol 25:95, 1987

33. Baldessarini RJ: Drugs used in the treatment of psychiatric disorders. p. 387. In Gilman A, Goodman LS, Rall TW, Murad F (eds): The pharmacological basis of therapeutics 7th ed. Macmillan, New York, 1985

34. Stegmayr BG: On-line hemodialysis and hemoperfusion in a girl intoxicated by theophylline. Acta Med Scand 223:565, 1988

35. Buckley BM, Braithwaite RA, Vale JA: Theophylline poisoning. Lancet 2:618, 1983

36. Park GD, Spector R, Roberts RJ et al: The use of hemoperfusion for theophylline intoxication. Am J Med 74:961, 1983

37. Goldberg MJ, Park GD, Berlinger WG: Treatment of theophylline intoxication. J Allergy Clin Immunol 78:811, 1986

38. Anonymous: Mushroom poisoning (editorial). Lancet 2:351, 1980

39. Winchester JF, Gelfand MC, Knepshield JM et al: Dialysis and hemoperfusion of poisons and drugs: update. Trans Am Soc Artif Organs 23:762, 1977

40. Wauters JP, Rossele C, Farquet JJ: Amanita phalloides poisoning treated by early charcoal hemoperfusion. Br Med J 2:1465, 1970

41. Pond SM: Principles of techniques used to enhance elimination of toxic compounds. p. 21. In Goldfrank LR, Flomenbaum NE, Lewin NA et al (eds): Goldfrank's toxicologic emergencies. Appleton & Lange, Norwalk, 1990

42. Goldfrank L, Flomenbaum N, Weisman R: Management of overdose with psychoactive medications. Emerg Med Clin North Am 2:63, 1984

43. Elliott RW, Hunter PR: Acute ethanol poisoning treated by hemodialysis. Postgrad Med J 50:515, 1974

44. Vale JA, Rees AJ, Woddop B et al: Use of charcoal hemoperfusion in the management of severely poisoned patients. Br Med J 1:5, 1978

45. Pond SM: Paraquat and diquat. p. 713. In Goldfrank LR, Flomenbaum NE, Lewin NA et al (eds): Goldfrank's toxicologic emergencies. Appleton & Lange, Norwalk, 1990

46. Douze JM, Van Heyst AN, Van Dijk A et al: Paraquat poisoning in man. Arch Toxicol 34:729, 1975

47. Pond SM, Johnston SC, Schoof DD et al: Repeated hemoperfusion and continuous arteriovenous hemofiltration in a paraquat poisoned patient. J Toxicol Clin Toxicol 25:305, 1987

48. Okonek S, Weilemann LS, Majdondzic J et al: Successful treatment of paraquat poisoning: activated charcoal per os and continuous hemoperfusion. J Toxicol Clin Toxicol 19:807, 1982–1983

49. Lacouture PG, Wason S, Abrams A et al: Acute isopropyl alcohol intoxication. Am J Med 75:680, 1983

50. Vaziri ND, Kumar KP, Mirahmodi K et al: Hemodialysis in treatment of acute chloral hydrate poisoning. South Med J 70:377, 1977

51. Stalken NE, Gambertoglio JG, Fukumitsu CJ et al: Acute massive chloral hydrate intoxication treated with hemodialysis: a clinical pharmacokinetic analysis. J Clin Pharmacol 18:136, 1978

52. Braden GL, Fitzgibbons JP, Germain MJ et al: Hemoperfusion for treatment of N-acetylprocainamide intoxication. Ann Intern Med 105:64, 1986

53. Rosansky SJ, Brady ME: Procainamide toxicity in a patient with acute renal failure. Am J Kidney Dis 6:502, 1986

54. Lazarus JM, Hakim RM: Medical aspects of hemodialysis. p. 2233. In Brenner BM, Rector FC Jr (eds): The kidney. WB Saunders, Philadelphia, 1991

SODIUM BICARBONATE

PAUL M. WAX, MD[†]
ROBERT S. HOFFMAN, MD, ABMT[††]

Sodium bicarbonate ($NaHCO_3$) is one of the most useful agents available for the treatment of the poisoned patient. Unlike more specific antidotes in which utility is usually limited to antagonizing a single drug or toxin, sodium bicarbonate is a nonspecific antidote effective in the treatment of a number of diverse poisonings. Its most valuable roles are in the treatment of patients with tricyclic antidepressant (TCA) and salicylate overdoses. These two poisonings are among the most frequently encountered and are associated with significant morbidity and mortality.[1] Sodium bicarbonate also serves as a useful adjuvant in the treatment of phenobarbital, chlorpropamide, and chlorophenoxy herbicide poisonings. Correcting the life-threatening acidosis generated by methanol and ethylene glycol intoxication and enhancing formate elimination are other important indications for sodium bicarbonate. More debatable indications include its use in the gastric lavage fluid for iron ingestions and in treating cocaine-induced wide-complex tachyarrhythmias.[2] Routine alkalinization of the urine for patients with drug- or toxin-associated myoglobinuria is also controversial. The use of sodium bicarbonate in the treatment of common nontoxicologic problems such as lactic acidosis, cardiac resuscitation, and diabetic ketoacidosis is even more questionable. Recent studies suggest much less utility for sodium bicarbonate in the treatment of these nontoxicologic disorders than previously thought.[3–5]

Multiple pharmacologic actions of sodium bicarbonate help explain its utility: altering drug ionization, changing sodium gradients, or buffering acidemia. Alkalinization of the blood and urine may alter the distribution and elimination of ionizable drugs. Ionization of weak acids, such as salicylate, phenobarbital, and chlorpropamide, occurs

Sodium bicarbonate (NaHCO₃) is one of the most useful agents available for the treatment of the poisoned patient.

[†] Senior Fellow, New York City Poison Control Center, Instructor Clinical Surgery/Emergency Medicine, New York University School of Medicine, New York, New York

[††] Associate Medical Director, New York City Poison Control Center, Instructor Clinical Surgery/Emergency Medicine, New York University School of Medicine, New York, New York

whenever the pH is greater than the pKa. Since cellular membranes are relatively impermeable to ionized compounds, alkalinization of the urine traps the ionized drug fraction in the urine while alkalinization of the blood prevents the movement of ionized drug into the tissues. Sodium bicarbonate may also prove beneficial via a direct sodium effect by increasing the sodium gradient and overcoming a sodium channel blockade. This action may be partly responsible for sodium bicarbonate's utility in treating TCA toxicity. Finally, sodium bicarbonate's ability to titrate acid makes it particularly helpful in reversing the life-threatening acidemia generated during methanol or ethylene glycol intoxication.

Sodium bicarbonate is usually administered as a hypertonic solution. The most commonly used preparations are an 8.4% solution (1 M) containing 1 mEq each of sodium and bicarbonate ions per milliliter (calculated osmolarity of 2,000 mOsm/l) and a 7.5% solution containing 0.892 mEq each of sodium and bicarbonate ions per milliliter (calculated osmolarity of 1,786 mOsm/l). Fifty-milliliter ampules of the 8.4% and 7.5% solutions contain 50 mEq and 44.6 mEq of $NaHCO_3$, respectively.[6] (For the remainder of this chapter, unless otherwise specified, one ampule of sodium bicarbonate will refer to 50 mEq amounts.)

TRICYCLIC ANTIDEPRESSANTS

Tricyclic antidepressant overdoses are among the most frequently reported ingestions, with the highest morbidity and mortality encountered in medical toxicology. Approximately 500,000 TCA overdoses occur annually.[7] Recent American Association of Poison Control Centers data shows that TCAs account for the largest number of reportable deaths.[11] Sodium bicarbonate's effect is perhaps most dramatic in the treatment of TCA toxicity. Along with gastrointestinal decontamination, the judicious use of sodium bicarbonate in the management of TCA poisoning may be life-saving. (For the remainder of the chapter, unless otherwise specified, TCA will refer to the first-generation cyclic antidepressants that contain a three-ring structure: amitriptyline, imipramine, doxepin, trimipramine, desipramine, nortriptyline, and protriptyline. These drugs all exhibit similar cardiac effects. Of the newer second-generation cyclic antidepressants, only maprotiline has shown similar cardiac effects. Other newer antidepressants such as amoxapine, trazadone, and fluoxetine have not been associated with significant cardiac toxicity.)[8,9]

The use of sodium bicarbonate for TCA overdose de-

Sodium bicarbonate's effect is perhaps most dramatic in the treatment of tricyclic antidepressant toxicity.

veloped as an extension of sodium bicarbonate use in the treatment of other cardiotoxic exposures. Sodium lactate (which is metabolized to sodium bicarbonate by cellular oxidative activity[10]) was used in the late 1950s for the treatment of quinidine toxicity.[11,12] Bellet noticed similarities in electrocardiographic findings between hyperkalemia and quinidine toxicity.[13] Both conditions adversely affect cardiac conduction and are manifested by a widening of the QRS complex. Since sodium lactate had previously been demonstrated to be useful in the treatment of hyperkalemia,[13] this agent was administered to a patient with quinidine toxicity who demonstrated hypotension and a marked widening of the QRS complex.[13] Normalization of the QRS complex and a rise in blood pressure resulted. Similar efficacy in the treatment of procainamide cardiotoxicity was also reported.[12] These clinical observations were demonstrated in dogs where quinidine-induced electrocardiographic changes and hypotension were consistently reversed by the infusion of sodium lactate.[14] Proposed mechanisms for the antagonistic actions of sodium lactate included a decrease in serum potassium concentration with a concomitant increase in pH,[14] a decrease in quinidine concentration,[14] and a direct sodium effect.[11]

With the introduction of the tricyclic antidepressants during the late 1950s and early 1960s, significant conduction disturbances, arrhythmias, and hypotension were reported.[15] The etiology of these cardiac disturbances appears to be multifactorial. The most commonly encountered cardiac manifestation is sinus tachycardia, which was seen in over 70% of TCA overdoses in one series.[16] Anticholinergic affects, alpha-adrenergic blockade, and biogenic amine (eg, norepinephrine) pump inhibition may all contribute to the development of the tachycardia. Conduction disturbances manifested by widening of the QRS, PR, and QT intervals, ventricular arrhythmias, and hypotension, are more ominous findings. The postulated mechanism for this finding involves a local anesthetic (or membrane-stabilizing) effect of the TCA on fast sodium channels located in the His-Purkinje system and ventricular muscle.[17,18] These observations are similar to those seen during other type IA antiarrhythmic intoxications and have been termed "quinidine-like" effects.[19] Direct binding of the TCA with the sodium channel receptor inhibits the rapid inward movement of sodium ions during depolarization. This results in a slowing of the upslope of the phase 0 action potential *in vitro* and is manifested, *in vivo*, by a widening of the QRS interval and decreased inotropy. Experimental animal models and clinical observations all demonstrate that a marked degree of QRS prolongation occurs prior to the development of serious ventricular arrhythmias.[20,21]

Work by Gaultier, Prudhommeaux, and Bismuth first demonstrated the potential for sodium lactate in the treatment of TCA toxicity.[22-24] Uncontrolled observations by Gaultier showed a decrease in mortality from 15% to less than 3% when sodium lactate was administered to patients with TCA poisoning.[25] In 1976 Brown was the first to report clinical success with the use of sodium bicarbonate in the treatment of a series of TCA-induced arrhythmias in children.[26] In this series, 9 out of 12 children who had developed multifocal PVCs, ventricular tachycardia, or heart block reverted to normal sinus rhythm with sodium bicarbonate therapy alone. Brown's experiments in amitriptyline (AMI)-poisoned dogs demonstrated resolution of arrhythmias upon alkalinization of the blood to a pH above 7.40.[26] Other methods of alkalinization including hyperventilation[27] and administration of a non-sodium buffer, trishydroxymethyl-amino-methane (THAM),[28] also appeared effective in reversing the arrhythmias. The exact mechanism for these beneficial effects was not clear; Gaultier[25] advocated a direct sodium effect (THAM did not work in his study) while Brown[29] advocated a pH-dependent effect. Brown further suggested in an *in vitro* study that alkalinization significantly decreased the proportion of pharmacologically active free drug by increasing protein binding of amitriptyline (82% protein-bound at pH 6.7 to 98% protein-bound at pH 7.5), theoretically making less free drug available to the tissue receptor sites.[28] Other proposed mechanisms for sodium bicarbonate's effect included lowering the serum potassium concentration and the intravascular volume expansion with resultant correction of hypotension.[30]

A better understanding of the mechanism and utility of sodium bicarbonate has come about through a series of additional animal experiments during the 1980s. In amitriptyline-poisoned dogs, Nattel et al. showed that sodium bicarbonate reversed conduction slowing and ventricular arrhythmias and suppressed ventricular ectopy.[31] When comparing sodium bicarbonate, hyperventilation, hypertonic sodium chloride, and lidocaine, sodium bicarbonate and hyperventilation proved most efficacious in reversing ventricular arrhythmias and narrowing QRS interval prolongation. Although lidocaine transiently antagonized AMI arrhythmias, this antagonism was only demonstrated at nearly toxic lidocaine dosages and was associated with hypotension. In these studies, hypertonic sodium chloride failed to reverse arrhythmias. Furthermore, prophylactic alkalinization protected against the development of ar-

In amitriptyline-poisoned dogs, Nattel et al. showed that sodium bicarbonate reversed conduction slowing and ventricular arrhythmias and suppressed ventricular ectopy.

rhythmias in a pH-dependent manner. The authors concluded that alkalinization was the most important mechanism of sodium bicarbonate therapy, offering both a prophylactic and therapeutic effect in treating TCA toxicity.

A similar study in desipramine(DMI)-poisoned rats also concluded that sodium bicarbonate was able to decrease the QRS interval.[30] In this study, the isolated use of sodium chloride was effective in decreasing QRS duration as well. Alkalinization (by discontinuing 10% CO_2 previously added to the inspired air), however, did not affect QRS duration. Thus, increased extracellular sodium concentration was thought to be a more consequential factor than pH change in reversing impaired cardiac conduction. The authors concluded that a direct effect of sodium in counteracting sodium channel inhibition may have occurred by increasing the sodium gradient across the cardiac membrane, thereby enhancing the driving force for sodium entry during phase 0.

In further experimental studies, *in vivo*, and on isolated cardiac tissue, Sasyniuk demonstrated that both alkalinization and sodium concentration modulate TCA effects on cardiac conduction.[32,33] While hypocapnia and sodium chloride each independently improved conduction velocity, this effect was greater when sodium bicarbonate was administered. Since TCAs are weak bases (high pKa), alkalinization increases the proportion of unionized drug. This increase in the proportion of unionized drug at the sodium channel may decrease drug-receptor binding[33] (possibly due to a redistribution of drug from the central compartment to the periphery because of less ion trapping in the blood), thus diminishing the TCA effect on cardiac conduction. Decreased ionization should not significantly decrease the rate of TCA elimination because of the small contribution of renal pathways to overall TCA elimination (less than 5%).[32]

Treatment modalities for TCA-induced hypotension have also been studied. Hypotension may result from both alpha-adrenergic blockade that causes vasodilation and sodium channel blockade that impairs myocardial contractility. Pentel showed that sodium bicarbonate or sodium chloride increased mean arterial pressure (MAP) in DMI-poisoned rats but hyperventilation or direct intravascular volume repletion with mannitol did not improve MAP.[30] Hence, it appears that sodium administration, by overcoming sodium channel blockade, is the most important factor in improving MAP.

Sodium bicarbonate seems to work independently of initial blood pH. Pentel showed that cardiac conduction improved after treatment with sodium bicarbonate or sodium chloride in both normal pH and acidemic animals.[30] Clinically, Molloy reported a patient with an imipramine overdose who responded to repeat doses of sodium bicarbonate despite the presence of alkalemia.[34] The ability of hyperventilation to improve cardiac conduction in patients with normal pH has also been demonstrated.[35]

The relationship of the serum potassium to the sodium bicarbonate effect is less clear. Sasyniuk proposed that a lowering of serum potassium, through the administration of sodium bicarbonate, may also be important in decreasing sodium blockade by causing membrane hypopolarization.[33] Nattel did not notice a change in serum potassium, however, after administration of sodium bicarbonate to correct TCA toxicity.[21] After comparing the effects of sodium bicarbonate solution with and without potassium, Pentel concluded that hypokalemia did not appear to be responsible for the sodium bicarbonate-induced reduction of TCA toxicity.[30]

While several authorities have suggested that sodium bicarbonate's efficacy is modulated via a pH-dependent change in protein binding that decreases the proportion of free drug,[28,36] recent evidence fails to support this hypothesis.[37] The administration of large doses of a binding protein alpha-1-acid glycoprotein (AAG) (to which TCAs show great affinity) to DMI-poisoned rats only minimally decreased cardiotoxicity.[37] Although the addition of AAG increased the concentration of total DMI and protein-bound DMI in the serum, the concentration of active free DMI did not decline significantly. A redistribution of TCA from peripheral sites may have prevented lowering of free DMI. The persistence of other TCA-associated toxicity such as the anticholinergic effects and seizures also argues against changes in protein binding modulating toxicity.[35] *In vitro* studies performed in a protein-free bath further support that sodium bicarbonate's efficacy is independent of protein binding.[32]

Hence, sodium bicarbonate appears to have a crucial antidotal role in TCA poisoning by partially reversing the fast sodium channel blockade caused by these drugs. The animal evidence supports two distinct and additive mechanisms for this effect: (1) a pH-dependent effect manifested by the production of an increased fraction of the more freely diffusible unionized drug that can be liberated from the sodium channel and (2) a sodium-dependent effect manifested by increasing the sodium gradient across the partially closed sodium channels. The actual contribution of each mechanism requires further clarification. Changes in serum potassium, drug concentration, or protein bind-

Sodium bicarbonate appears to have a crucial antidotal role in tricyclic antidepressant poisoning by partially reversing the fast sodium channel blockade caused by these drugs.

ing do not appear to have significant roles in modulating TCA toxicity.

INDICATIONS

While there are many anecdotal accounts supporting the efficacy of sodium bicarbonate in treating TCA cardiotoxicity in humans,[38] these reports are all uncontrolled observations; controlled studies are not available. The exact indications for the use of sodium bicarbonate after TCA overdose have not been studied. Sodium bicarbonate reverses the quinidine-like effects that produce the major life-threatening manifestations of TCA overdose. Other effects caused by the anticholinergic, alpha blockade, reuptake inhibition, and direct CNS properties of the TCAs are not affected by the administration of sodium bicarbonate.

In a prospective study, Boehnert and Lovejoy suggested that the maximal limb-lead QRS duration was the best predictor for seizures and ventricular arrhythmias in the TCA-poisoned patient.[20] They also noted that prolongation of the QRS interval (indicating TCA poisoning of the fast sodium channels) is a much more reliable indicator of toxicity than serum TCA levels. In this study, all patients with seizures had a QRS duration of at least 100 ms and all patients with ventricular arrhythmias had a QRS duration of at least 160 ms. Although criteria for treatment were not addressed, extrapolation of the study results is useful in guiding treatment strategy. Since the authors suggest that there is a critical QRS duration at which ventricular arrhythmias may occur (>160 ms), it seems reasonable that narrowing the QRS interval through the use of sodium bicarbonate or hyperventilation may prophylactically prevent the development of arrhythmias.[39] Patients with QRS intervals of 0.16 s or greater should be treated. Controversy exists, however, over the utilization of sodium bicarbonate in situations in which the QRS interval is less than 160 ms but greater than 100 ms. Although sodium bicarbonate has no proven efficacy in either the treatment or prophylaxis of TCA-induced seizures, seizures often cause acidemia, which rapidly increases the risks of conduction disturbances and ventricular arrhythmias.[30] Administrating sodium bicarbonate in situations in which the QRS duration is 100 ms or greater may establish a theoretical margin of safety in the event that the patient suddenly deteriorates by lessening the likelihood of subsequent arrhythmias without adding significant demonstrable risk. In situations in which the QRS duration is less than 100 ms (given the negligible risk of seizures or arrhythmias), prophylactic use

Although sodium bicarbonate has no proven efficacy in either the treatment or prophylaxis of TCA-induced seizures, seizures often cause acidemia, which rapidly increases the risks of conduction disturbances and ventricular arrhythmias. Administrating sodium bicarbonate in situations in which the QRS duration is 100 ms or greater may establish a theoretical margin of safety in the event that the patient suddenly deteriorates by lessening the likelihood of subsequent arrhythmias without adding significant demonstrable risk.

Sodium bicarbonate is indicated in situations in which impaired conduction (QRS prolongation to 100 ms or greater), ventricular arrhythmias, or hypotension exist. Since the potential benefits of alkalinization usually outweigh the risks, sodium bicarbonate should be administered regardless of whether the patient has an acidemic or normal pH.

of sodium bicarbonate is not indicated. Since cardiotoxicity may worsen during the first few hours after ingestion, sodium bicarbonate should be started immediately if QRS interval widening to 0.10 s or greater is noted. Because the risk of late deterioration in a patient who was previously normal rarely, if ever, occurs, the initiation of sodium bicarbonate in late presentations is less clear.[39]

Sodium bicarbonate is indicated in situations in which impaired conduction (QRS prolongation to 100 ms or greater), ventricular arrhythmias, or hypotension exist.[40] Since the potential benefits of alkalinization usually outweigh the risks, sodium bicarbonate should be administered regardless of whether the patient has an acidemic or normal pH. One to two mEq/kg body weight should be administered intravenously as a bolus over a period of 1–2 minutes.[40] Greater amounts may be required to treat unstable ventricular arrhythmias. Sodium bicarbonate should then be repeated as needed to achieve a blood pH of 7.50–7.55.[39,40] The end-point of treatment is a narrowing of the QRS interval. Excessive alkalemia (pH > 7.55) and hypernatremia, however, should be avoided. Since sodium bicarbonate has a brief duration of effect, a continuous infusion is usually required after the intravenous bolus. One to three 50 ml ampules may be placed in a liter of fluid and run at maintenance or more than maintenance, depending on the fluid requirements and blood pressure of the patient. If a multiple ampule infusion is contemplated, the sodium bicarbonate should be placed in a hypotonic solution such as 5% dextrose in water in order to limit the sodium load. Frequent evaluation of fluid status should also be performed to avoid precipitating pulmonary edema.

Hyperventilation may be a useful alternative to sodium bicarbonate in reversing the cardiotoxicity of TCAs. According to Bessen, hyperventilation provides a more rapid induction of alkalemia, can be more readily reversed through changes in the ventilatory settings, and avoids the sodium and osmolar load that may be particularly detrimental to the patients with compromised myocardial contractility.[35] This technique is certainly easy to perform in the intubated patient. As discussed above, however, animal models suggest that administration of sodium bicarbonate is more efficacious than alkalinization alone.[30,33] Furthermore, significant hypocapnia may lead to a reduction in coronary and cerebral bloodflow and further lower seizure threshold.[40] Hyperventilation may be advisable as a temporizing measure while preparing to administer sodium bicarbonate if an unstable patient is already intubated and requires immediate treatment; it is definitely preferred in the patient with coexisting pulmonary edema.

OTHER CARDIOTOXIC DRUGS

Sodium bicarbonate may also be useful in treating cardiotoxicity from other drugs that impair sodium channel functioning manifested by widened QRS complexes, arrhythmias, and hypotension. Demonstrable utility of sodium bicarbonate in treating type IA antiarrhythmics such as quinidine and procainamide has already been shown.[12,14] The use of sodium bicarbonate in treating conduction disturbances from an overdose of quinine (an optical isomer of quinidine) is also recommended.[41] Type IC antiarrhythmic agents (encainide, flecainide) have similar effects on depolarization, and sodium bicarbonate should also be used in their toxicity. Pentel has recently reported a case of an encainide overdose in which bradycardia, hypotension, and increased QRS duration all resolved after the administration of sodium bicarbonate.[42] In a dog model, Bajaj showed that conduction slowing from infusion of the encainide metabolite O-desmthyl encainide, could be partially reversed by administration of sodium bicarbonate and sodium chloride.[43] Sodium bicarbonate may also help in the management of amantadine,[44] phenothiazines,[45] and carbamazepine[46] overdoses, all of which have been associated with cardiac conduction abnormalities and arrhythmias. Its efficacy in these situations, however, is unknown. Recently, propoxyphene was shown to cause sodium channel blockade manifested by marked QRS widening.[47] Although untested, sodium bicarbonate may also have a therapeutic role in this situation.

Cocaine (a local anesthetic with membrane-stabilizing properties resembling other type I antiarrhythmics) may cause similar conduction disturbances.[2] In cocaine-intoxicated dogs, Parker recently demonstrated that sodium bicarbonate successfully reversed cocaine-induced QRS prolongation.[2] Unpublished observations suggest similar success in humans as well (Tucker W, personal communication, October 1990).

SALICYLATES

Although there is no known specific antidote for salicylate toxicity, the utilization of sodium bicarbonate in this situation may be life-saving. This therapy (as well as the use of multiple doses of activated charcoal) may ameliorate the need for more invasive treatment modalities such as hemodialysis. Sodium bicarbonate, through its ability to change the concentration gradient of the ionizable and unionizable fractions of salicylates, has proven utility in decreasing tissue (eg, brain) levels and enhancing urinary elimination of salicylates.

Sodium bicarbonate, through its ability to change the concentration gradient of the ionizable and unionizable fractions of salicylates, has proven utility in decreasing tissue (eg, brain) levels and enhancing urinary elimination of salicylates.

Salicylate is a weak acid with a pKA of 3.0[48]; according to the Henderson-Hasselbalch equation, at a pH of 3.0, equal concentrations of unionized and ionized salicylate exist. As pH increases, more of the drug is in the ionized form.[49] This change in ionization occurs in a logarithmic fashion such that 90% of the molecules are ionized at a pH of 4.0 and 99% are ionized at a pH of 50. Ionized molecules penetrate these lipid-soluble membranes less rapidly than unionized molecules due to the presence of polar groups on the ionized form.[50] Consequently, weak acids such as salicylates accumulate in alkaline milieu where the ionized forms predominate.[50]

Using sodium bicarbonate to "trap" salicylate in the blood (keeping it out of the brain) may be of assistance in preventing clinical deterioration of the salicylate-intoxicated patient.

Using sodium bicarbonate to "trap" salicylate in the blood (keeping it out of the brain) may be of assistance in preventing clinical deterioration of the salicylate-intoxicated patient. Hill has demonstrated that salicylate lethality is directly related to primary central nervous system dysfunction, which, in turn, corresponds to a "critical brain salicylate level."[48] Since intracellular pH is always lower than extracellular pH, the trapping of the ionized salicylates in the extracellular space is proportional to the intracellular-extracellular pH gradient.[51,52] At physiologic pH where a very small proportion of the salicylate is in the unionized form, a small change in pH will be associated with a significant change in amount of unionized molecules (eg, at a pH of 7.4, 0.004% of the salicylate molecules are in the unionized form, at a pH of 7.2, 0.008% of the salicylate is in the unionized form). Lowering the blood pH by inhaling a mixture of 20% carbon dioxide and 80% oxygen or infusing ammonium chloride[51] (thereby narrowing the intracellular-extracellular pH gradient) produces a shift of salicylate into the tissues. Hence, the metabolic acidemia that is observed in significant salicylate intoxications can be devastating.

Fortunately, in salicylate intoxication, the earliest and most common acid–base disturbance is a respiratory alkalosis, which results from a direct stimulation of the medullary respiratory center with a subsequent increase in tidal volume and respiratory rate. Alkalemia slows the entrance of salicylate into the brain by widening the arterial-cerebral spinal fluid pH difference. In salicylate poisoned rats, Hill showed that increasing the blood pH with sodium bicarbonate produced a shift in salicylate out of the tissues and into the blood.[53] This change in salicylate distribution did not result from enhanced urinary excretion since occlusion of the renal pedicles failed to alter these results. Acidemia with resultant aciduria, however, will tend to further inhibit elimination of salicylates, thus prolonging toxicity and possibly leading to worsening acidemia.[54]

"Ion trapping" in the urine is also helpful. Salicylate

elimination at low therapeutic concentrations consists predominately of first-order hepatic metabolism: conjugation with glycine to salicyluric acid, conjugation with glucuronide to salicylphenolic and acyl glucuronides, and hydroxylation to gentisic acid. At these low concentrations, without alkalinization, only about 10–20% of salicylate is eliminated unchanged in the urine.[55,56] With increasing concentrations under both therapeutic and toxicologic circumstances, two of these metabolic pathways become saturated and exhibit Michaelis-Menten kinetics (change elimination from first-order to zero-order kinetics).[57] With these metabolic changes, a larger percentage of elimination occurs as unchanged free salicylate. In an alkaline urine, urinary excretion of free salicylate becomes even more significant, accounting for 60–85% of total elimination.[55,56]

The exact mechanism of pH-dependent elimination has generated controversy. Morris first noted that alkali apparently enhanced the renal excretion of salicylate.[58] Smull reported a case in which the serum salicylate level fell markedly in a patient on high-dose salicylates for rheumatic fever who concomitantly took sodium bicarbonate for gastric discomfort.[59] Smith showed that falling serum salicylate levels after bicarbonate administration was associated with increased free salicylate in the urine and that urinary elimination appeared dependent on urinary pH.[60] A gradual increase in elimination was noted when the urinary pH was above 6.00, which increased rapidly above pH 7.00. The pH-dependent increase in urinary elimination was initially ascribed to "ion trapping": the filtering of both ionized and unionized salicylate while reabsorbing only the unionized salicylate.

Other authorities,[61,62] however, argue that limiting reabsorption of the ionizable fraction of filtered salicylate cannot be the primary mechanism responsible for enhanced elimination produced by sodium bicarbonate. Since the quantitative difference between the percentage of molecules trapped in the ionized form at a pH of 5.0 (99% ionized) and a pH of 8.0 (99.999% ionized) is small, decreases in tubular reabsorption cannot fully explain the rapid increase in urinary elimination seen above a pH of 7.0. "Diffusion theory" offers a reasonable alternative explanation. Fick's Law of Diffusion states that the rate of flow of a diffusing substance is proportional to its concentration gradient.[62] A large concentration gradient between the unionized salicylate in the peritubular fluid (and blood) and the tubular luminal fluid is found in alkaline urine. Since at a higher urinary pH a greater proportion of secreted unionized molecules quickly become ionized upon entering the alkaline environment, more salicylate (ie, unionized salicylate) must pass from the peritubular fluid into

The exact mechanism of pH-dependent elimination has generated controversy. Authorities argue that limiting reabsorption of the ionizable fraction of filtered salicylate cannot be the primary mechanism responsible for enhanced elimination produced by sodium bicarbonate.

Predominately increased tubular secretion, not decreased reabsorption, accounts for the increase in salicylate elimination observed in the alkaline urine.

Controversies regarding the indications for alkalinization, role of acetazolamide, and necessity of forced diuresis have persisted.

the urine in an attempt to reach equilibrium with the un-ionized fraction. In fact, as long as unionized molecules are rapidly converted to ionized molecules in the urine, equilibrium in the alkaline milieu will never be achieved. The concentration gradient of peritubular unionized salicylates to urinary unionized salicylates continues to increase with increasing urinary pH. Hence, predominately increased tubular secretion, not decreased reabsorption, accounts for the increase in salicylate elimination observed in the alkaline urine.[62] Furthermore, Macpherson showed that urinary alkalinization with sodium bicarbonate, acetazolamide or hyperventilation all achieved identical effects, which suggests that increased salicylate clearance was dependent on the urinary pH and independent of the systemic acid–base balance since acetazolamide produced significant systemic acidemia.[62]

Controversies regarding the indications for alkalinization, role of acetazolamide, and necessity of forced diuresis have persisted. While alkalinization undoubtedly works to lower serum salicylate levels and enhance urinary elimination, the risks associated with alkalinization in the management of salicylism have generated concern.[56,63–66] Problems such as excessive alkalemia,[67] hypernatremia,[63,66] hypokalemia,[67] hypocalcemia,[68] and fluid overload, as well as the potential delay in achieving alkalinization with sodium bicarbonate (as opposed to more rapid response achieved with hyperventilation) have all been raised.[56]

Some authorities have even suggested that the administration of sodium bicarbonate to adolescents and adults with prolonged hyperventilation and hypocapnia who have a pure respiratory alkalosis may result in tetany, encephalopathy, and death.[65,66] Patients with pure respiratory alkalosis often have alkaluria as well as alkalemia and do not require urinary alkalinization. In the more common scenario in which patients present with a mixed respiratory alkalosis and metabolic acidosis, sodium bicarbonate must be administrated cautiously. The young child, who rapidly develops a metabolic acidosis, often requires alkalinization, but should be at less risk for complications of this therapy.[64]

Administering acetazolamide, along with sodium bicarbonate, in order to alkalinize the urine has been advocated.[56,63,69] Acetazolamide works by inhibiting the enzyme carbonic anhydrase, thereby blocking the formation of carbonic acid in the kidney and decreasing the urinary excretion of hydrogen ions. As a result, increased secretion of bicarbonate, sodium, and potassium occurs. Acetazolamide was thought to be useful in treating salicylate intoxication because the urinary alkalinization was prompt[56,70] and could be performed in patients with contraindications to the use of sodium bicarbonate, such as patients with pulmonary edema. It was also thought to be particularly helpful in situations where the patient presented with a normal or alkalemic pH and was at risk for consequential alkalemia with the additional bicarbonate load. The decrease in hydrogen ion secretion into the urine, however, results in a metabolic acidosis and acidemia without aciduria, which enhances the movement of salicylates into the brain. Acetazolamide has been demonstrated to produce an increase in morbidity and mortality in animal studies,[53,54] as well as in human case reports.[71,72] Although some authorities still argue for selective use with sodium bicarbonate,[56,69,70,72] general use should be condemned.[73,74]

Sodium bicarbonate is indicated in the treatment of salicylate poisoning for most patients with evidence of significant systemic toxicity. Although some authors have suggested alkali therapy for asymptomatic patients with levels above 30 mg/dl,[75] these recommendations were made prior to the realization that multiple-dose activated charcoal may suffice as long as the patient remains asymptomatic. For patients suffering from a chronic intoxication, levels are not as helpful and may be misleading; clinical criteria remain the best indicators for therapy. A chest radiograph and arterial blood gas analysis to determine the alveolar-arterial oxygen gradient may be helpful in evaluating more subtle cases of acute or chronic intoxications. Patients with contraindications to sodium bicarbonate use, such as renal failure or pulmonary edema, may benefit from hyperventilation; extracorporeal removal may be required in some instances.

Dosing recommendations depend on the acid–base status of the patient. For the patient with acidemia, rapid correction is indicated with intravenous administration of 1–2 mEq/kg body weight of sodium bicarbonate.[74] Once the blood is alkalinized, or if the patient has already presented with a alkalemia, continued titration with sodium bicarbonate over 4 to 8 hours is recommended until the urine pH reaches 7.50.[76] Alkalinization can be maintained with a continuous sodium bicarbonate infusion of 100–150 mEq in 1 liter of 5% dextrose in water at 150–200 ml per hour (or about twice the maintenance requirements in a child). Obtaining a urinary pH of 8.0 is difficult but considered the goal.[74] Fastidious attention to the changing acid–base status is required. Systemic pH should be kept below 7.55 to prevent complications of alkalemia.

Hypokalemia can make urinary alkalinization particularly problematic.[67,75,77] In the hypokalemic patient, regardless of total body potassium stores, the kidney will preferentially reabsorb potassium in exchange for hydrogen ions. Alkalinization will be unsuccessful as long as hydrogen ions are excreted into the urine. Thus, appropriate potassium supplementation to achieve normokalemia may be required in order to alkalinize the urine.[73]

Until the past few years, proper urinary alkalinization was thought to require forced diuresis in order to maximize salicylate elimination.[67,78] Suggestions included administering enough fluid (2 l/h) in order to produce a urine output of 500 ml per hour.[78] This method of alkalinization, however, often leads to fluid retention. Excess fluid may be of particular concern in salicylate-poisoned patients who present with or are at high risk of pulmonary edema,[79–81] cerebral edema,[52,82] and renal failure.[76]

Recently, Prescott compared the following treatment strategies: sodium bicarbonate with forced diuresis, forced diuresis alone, and sodium bicarbonate alone.[83] The first two treatment groups received an average total fluid intake (orally and intravenously) of 8.43 and 8.66 liters in 16 hours, while the third treatment group received an average of 3.9 liters in the same time period. A significantly higher urinary pH was obtained with sodium bicarbonate (pH = 8.10) alone compared to forced alkaline diuresis (pH = 7.30) and forced diuresis (pH = 6.50),[83] perhaps due to a diluting effect of the high urine volume. Renal salicylate clearance was 23.5 ml/min in those patients receiving sodium bicarbonate alone, 17.5 ml/min for those receiving forced diuresis, and 4.4 ml/min for those receiving forced diuresis. Considering that salicylate clearance is logarithmically proportional to pH but only directly proportional to urinary flow rate, the pH effect is more valuable in increasing renal clearance.[83] Thus, forced alkaline diuresis appears unnecessary and is potentially harmful due to its unnecessarily large fluid load. Alkalinization, at a rate of approximately twice maintenance requirements, in order to achieve a urine output of 3–5 ml/kg/h is the goal.

Forced alkaline diuresis appears unnecessary and is potentially harmful due to its unnecessarily large fluid load.

PHENOBARBITAL

While cardiopulmonary support is the most critical intervention in the treatment of severe phenobarbital overdose,[84] sodium bicarbonate may be a useful adjunct to the general supportive care. The utility of sodium bicarbonate may be particularly important considering the long plasma half-life (about 100 hours)[85] of phenobarbital. Although analeptics such as amphetamine and picrotoxin had been used in the past to counteract the sedative effects of phenobarbital, complications such as arrhythmias, seizures, and aspiration pneumonitis were reported, and their use has since been discouraged.[86]

Phenobarbital is a weak acid (pKa of 7.24) that undergoes significant renal elimination. As in the case of salicylates, alkalinization of the blood and urine may reduce the severity and duration of toxicity. Waddell showed that a change in the blood pH affected phenobarbital distribution.[87] Acidemia increased the tissue to serum concentration of phenobarbital while alkalemia decreased the ratio. The median anesthetic dose for mice receiving phenobarbital increased by 20% with the addition of 1 g/kg of sodium bicarbonate (raising the blood pH from 7.23 to 7.41), suggesting decreased tissue levels associated with increased pH. Extrapolating the animal evidence to humans, Wadell suggested that phenobarbital-intoxicated patients in deep coma might develop a respiratory acidosis secondary to hypoventilation, with the acidemia enhancing the entrance of phenobarbital into the brain, thus worsening central nervous system and respiratory depression.[87] Alternatively, increasing the pH with bicarbonate and/or ventilatory support would enhance the passage of phenobarbital out of the brain, thus lessening toxicity.

Given the relatively high pKa of phenobarbital, significant phenobarbital accumulation in the urine is only evident when urinary pH is raised above 7.5.[88] As the pH approaches 8.0, a three-fold increase in urinary elimination occurs.[87] The urine to serum ratio of phenobarbital, while much higher in the alkaline urine than acidic urine, remains less than unity, thereby suggesting less of a role for tubular secretion than in salicylate toxicity. While increased urine flow rate also augments urinary elimination, the clearance is much higher in alkaline urine regardless of the flow rate.

Unfortunately, clinical studies examining the role of alkalinization in phenobarbital toxicity have been inadequately designed. Many are poorly controlled and fail to examine the effects of alkalinization independent of coadministered diuretic therapy. Mollaret showed a 59–67% decrease in duration of unconsciousness in patients with phenobarbital overdoses who were given alkali when compared to nonrandomized controls.[89] Myschetzky[90] showed that sodium lactate and urea therapy reduced mortality and frequency of tracheotomy to 50% of controls, while Lassen[84] demonstrated that similar therapy enhanced excretion and shortened coma.

Although undoubtedly useful in the treatment of phenobarbital intoxications, sodium bicarbonate is not indicated in the treatment of most other barbiturate intoxications. Significant renal elimination and a pKa well below 8.0 (the upper limit of urinary pH)[91] are required for sodium bicarbonate to be useful. Other commonly used barbiturates do not meet these criteria. Pentobarbital and secobarbital

Although undoubtedly useful in the treatment of phenobarbital intoxications, sodium bicarbonate is not indicated in the treatment of most other barbiturate intoxications.

have a pKa of 8.10, which does not permit production of an increased ionized fraction during routine alkalinization. Bloomer showed that a combination of sodium bicarbonate-mannitol therapy was effective in enhancing the elimination of phenobarbital but not pentobarbital or secobarbital.[88] The value of forced diuresis was also shown to be limited for pentobarbital due to its lack of significant urinary elimination.[91,92] Sodium bicarbonate dosing in the presence of phenobarbital intoxication is similar to that used in treating salicylate intoxication. Raising the urinary pH to 8.0 is imperative to obtain a significant effect. Sodium bicarbonate should not be used in the presence of significant renal or cardiopulmonary dysfunction.

CHLORPROPAMIDE

Alkalinization has also been shown to enhance the renal elimination of chlorpropamide.[93] Chlorpropamide is a weak acid (pKa of 4.80) and has a long half-life (30–50 hours). Since patients who ingest this agent in overdose are at risk for prolonged hypoglycemia, enhancing the elimination should shorten the duration of intoxication and lessen the risk of complications. In a recent human study using therapeutic doses of chlorpropamide, Neuvonen demonstrated that urinary alkalinization with sodium bicarbonate significantly increased renal clearance of the drug.[93] This study showed that nonrenal clearance was the more significant route of elimination at a urinary pH of 5.0–6.0 (only slightly above pKa), while at a pH of 8.00, renal clearance was 10 times that of nonrenal clearance[93]. Urinary acidification with ammonium chloride blocked almost all renal elimination. Alkalinization reduced the area under the curve almost four-fold and shortened elimination half-life from 50 hours to 13 hours; acidification increased the area under the curve by 41% and increased the half-life to 69 hours. Hence, with the addition of sodium bicarbonate, most of the drug was eliminated during the first 24 hours instead of the usual elimination time of 4–5 days. While not a study in overdose patients, this report suggests the utility of sodium bicarbonate as an adjunct in the management of chlorpropamide overdose.

The effect of alkalinization on elimination of other sulfonylureas is unknown. Although many of these agents are also weak acids with pKa levels of 4.8–5.8, they apparently exhibit predominantly hepatic metabolism at physiologic pH. Further study of the ability of alkalinization to increase renal clearance of these other agents is warranted.

CHLOROPHENOXY HERBICIDES

Alkalinization is also suggested in the treatment of poisonings from the weed killers that contain chlorophenoxy compounds such as 2,4-dichlorophenoxyacetic acid (2,4-D) or 2-4-chloro-2-methylphenoxy propionic acid (MCPP). Significant exposure to these herbicides may result in muscle weakness, peripheral neuropathy, coma, hyperthermia, and acidemia. These compounds are weak acids (pKa = 2.60 and 3.80 for 2,4-D and MCPP, respectively) that are excreted largely unchanged in the urine. Prescott reported that alkaline diuresis was associated with rapid clinical improvement in a patient poisoned with 2,4-D and MCPP[94]. Similarly, in an uncontrolled case series of 41 patients poisoned with a variety of chlorophenoxy herbicides, in the 19 patients who received sodium bicarbonate, alkaline diuresis significantly reduced the half-life of each compound by enhancing renal elimination.[95] In one patient, resolution of hyperpyrexia and metabolic acidosis and improvement in mental status was associated with a transient elevation of serum levels of these compounds, perhaps reflecting chlorophenoxy compound redistribution from the tissues into the more alkalemic blood, (although in Prescott's case report,[94] a fall in serum concentration was associated with clinical improvement). This limited data suggests that the increased ionized fractions of the weak-acid chlorophenoxy compounds produced by alkalinization appear to be trapped in both the blood and the urine (as demonstrated with salicylates and phenobarbital), thus ameliorating toxicity and shortening duration of effect.

TOXIC ALCOHOLS

Sodium bicarbonate may also be useful in the treatment of the acidemia associated with methanol and ethylene glycol ingestions. Metabolism of these alcohols to their toxic metabolites produces a high anion gap metabolic acidosis. The acidemia generated from methanol poisoning appears to be multifactorial, involving the production of formic acid as well as the accumulation of lactic acid. Lactic acid accumulation occurs as a result of formic acid inhibition of mitochondrial oxidative metabolism and changes in the NADH:NAD ratio, which favor the conversion of pyruvate to lactate.[96] Ethylene glycol causes an acidemia as a result of its conversion to glycolic and oxalic acid.[97] Lactate may accumulate in this setting as well. The degree of acidemia from either the ingestion of methanol or ethylene glycol

Sodium bicarbonate may have two important roles in treating toxic alcohol ingestions. First, administration of sodium bicarbonate will reverse the life-threatening acidemia. The second role for bicarbonate involves its ability to favorably alter the distribution and elimination of toxic metabolites.

can be profound. Not uncommonly, the pH will be less than 7.0 with a serum bicarbonate under 10 mEq/l and an anion gap over 35.0.[98] The severity of the acidemia appears to be related to the clinical course of these ingestions, and the development of visual disturbances after methanol ingestion may correlate with the degree of acidemia.[98] Furthermore, the extent of the acidemia, low serum bicarbonate, and anion gap all appear to directly correlate with the likelihood of survival.

Sodium bicarbonate may have two important roles in treating toxic alcohol ingestions. First, administration of sodium bicarbonate will reverse the life-threatening acidemia. The best treatment for any acidosis is to treat the underlying cause. In the case of methanol and ethylene glycol poisoning, definitive treatment requires administration of ethanol to halt the production of the toxic metabolites and emergent hemodialysis to remove parent compound and metabolites.[99] Without these definitive interventions, patients will continue to deteriorate due to the persistence and continued generation of organic acids. Nevertheless, as an immediate temporizing measure, sodium bicarbonate has an important role. In rats poisoned with ethylene glycol, the administration of sodium bicarbonate alone resulted in a four-fold increase in median lethal dose, perhaps due to decreased calcium excretion.[100] Clinically, titrating the exogenous acid with bicarbonate may be of great assistance in reversing the consequences of the severe acidemia, such as hemodynamic instability and multiorgan dysfunction.

The second role for bicarbonate involves its ability to favorably alter the distribution and elimination of toxic metabolites. This effect has only been investigated in methanol toxicity. Although still not extensively studied, it has been suggested that visual impairment associated with methanol toxicity improved with sodium bicarbonate therapy.[101] Martin-Amat[102] demonstrated that formic acid appeared to cause ocular toxicity independent of pH; hence, any improvement in toxicity after sodium bicarbonate was probably not directly a result of a decrease in acidemia. Others have suggested that decreased ocular toxicity may result instead from tissue redistribution of formic acid induced by rising pH.[96,102] The proportion of ionized formic acid can be increased by administering bicarbonate, which will trap formate in the blood compartment. Consequently, decreased visual toxicity may result not from a nonspecific correction of the acidosis but from the removal of the toxic metabolite from the optic nerve. In a case report, Jacobson suggests an association between the administration of sodium bicarbonate, correction of acidemia, and decrease in formic acid concentration, perhaps due to pH-dependent formate elimination[96]. A similarity exists between this hypothesis and the effects of sodium bicarbonate on salicylate and phenobarbital distribution and elimination. Further investigation is required to delineate the beneficial effects of sodium bicarbonate in the treatment of toxic alcohol ingestions.

Early treatment of acidemia with sodium bicarbonate is strongly recommended in cases of methanol and ethylene glycol intoxications.[99,103] This early use of sodium bicarbonate differs from the management of diabetic ketoacidosis and lactic acidosis where the threshold for bicarbonate use should be high. Sodium bicarbonate should be administered to toxic alcohol-poisoned patients with an arterial pH below 7.30.[104] More than 400–600 mEq of sodium bicarbonate may be required in the first few hours.[99] In cases of ethylene glycol toxicity, sodium bicarbonate administration may worsen hypocalcemia; therefore serum calcium should be monitored. Combating the acidemia, however, is not the mainstay of therapy, and concurrent administration of intravenous ethanol and preparation for hemodialysis is almost always indicated.

CHLORINE GAS

Nebulized sodium bicarbonate has recently been suggested as a useful adjunct in the treatment of pulmonary injuries resulting from chlorine gas inhalation.[105,106] Upon contact with water in the respiratory tree, chlorine gas is converted to hydrochloric acid and nascent oxygen, causing significant pulmonary mucosal irritation. Clinically, patients may present with cough, dyspnea, burning sensation, chest pain, bronchospasm, and pulmonary edema.[105] Inhaled sodium bicarbonate is purported to neutralize hydrochloric acid. While oral sodium bicarbonate is not recommended to neutralize acid ingestions because of the problems associated with the exothermic reaction and production of carbon dioxide in the relatively closed gastrointestinal tract, the rapid exchange of air with the environment should facilitate heat dissipation. Anecdotal experience suggests that nebulized bicarbonate therapy may lead to improvement of symptoms.[106] In a chlorine-inhalation sheep model, Chisolm demonstrated higher PO_2 and lower CO_2 in the animals treated with 4% nebulized sodium bicarbonate solution than in the normal, saline-treated animals. There was no difference, however, in 24-hour mortality or pulmonary histopathology. Further clinical studies are required to further assess the efficacy and safety of this treatment.

Nebulized sodium bicarbonate has recently been suggested as a useful adjunct in the treatment of pulmonary injuries resulting from chlorine gas inhalation.

IRON

Some authorities have recommended the use of sodium bicarbonate to limit iron absorption in the treatment of iron overdose.[107,108] An early study suggested that sodium bicarbonate converts soluble ferrous sulfate to insoluble ferrous carbonate at physiological doses.[109] Hence, adding bicarbonate to the lavage fluid was thought to promote formation of insoluble iron complexes, limiting gastrointestinal absorption and decreasing toxicity. Further advocacy for bicarbonate lavage arose as a result of reports of complications with phosphate lavage and resultant hypocalcemia.[110,111]

The efficacy of bicarbonate lavage in the treatment of iron ingestion has not been demonstrated.

The efficacy of bicarbonate lavage in the treatment of iron ingestion, however, has not been demonstrated. In an *in vivo* experiment, Czajka showed that 83% of iron remained in a soluble state after the addition of bicarbonate.[112] This study also revealed that decreasing absorbable iron appeared to be pH-dependent, regardless of solution. Hence, maintaining an alkaline-absorptive environment would be required to keep iron in the insoluble form; reverting to an acidic pH in the gastric milieu may promote increased solubility of the iron and promote additional absorption. Dean, in a rat study, failed to demonstrate a difference in serum iron levels between rats treated with intragastric instillation of sodium bicarbonate or distilled water.[114] Hypernatremia may result as a complication of repeated doses of oral sodium bicarbonate.[113] The use of sodium bicarbonate in the lavage solution appears unnecessary and perhaps dangerous, and is thus not recommended.[113,115]

RHABDOMYOLYSIS

Skeletal muscle injury (rhabdomyolysis) is a frequent complication of significant poisoning. This occurs as a direct toxic effect (eg, doxylamine, heroin) or indirect manifestation of muscle ischemia (eg, barbiturates, cocaine, carbon monoxide, ethanol withdrawal).[116,117] Subsequent myoglobinuria may lead to renal injury and accounts for approximately 10% of cases of acute renal failure.[117] Animal evidence suggests that renal injury from myoglobinuria is dependent on the pH of the urine.[118] At or below urine pH of 5.60, myoglobin dissociates into ferrihemate and globin[116]; ferrihemate is apparently toxic to the renal tubule.

Routine urinary alkalinization in patients with rhabdomyolysis as a means of preventing renal impairment and hyperkalemia has been suggested.[119–121] In an uncontrolled retrospective study, Eneas suggested that forced alkaline diuresis (with an intravenous infusion of 25 g of mannitol and 100 mEq of sodium bicarbonate in 1 l of 5% dextrose in water at a rate of 250 ml per hour for 4 hours as soon as possible after admission and after obvious volume deficits have been replaced) may prevent development of renal injury in some patients with rhabdomyolysis. Urinary pH, however, was not measured.[120] In a case series of traumatic rhabdomyolysis, Ron showed that a similar protocol appeared to prevent renal damage in patients who achieved a urine pH above 6.5 (taking, on average, 12 hours of therapy to achieve).[121]

Given the lack of strong clinical data, other authorities have questioned the necessity for sodium bicarbonate as long as the urine pH is kept above 6.0.[122,123] Fluid repletion and mannitol may increase the urine flow to 200–300 ml per hour, thus creating alkaline urine simply from a dilution effect.[122–124] Concerns about sodium bicarbonate precipitating tetany in patients already at risk for hypocalcemia have also been raised.[123] If it is not possible to keep the urine pH above 6.0 with fluid resuscitation and mannitol alone, however, alkalinization with sodium bicarbonate is indicated. Large amounts (eg, 300 mEq per day) may be required.

NONTOXICOLOGIC USES OF SODIUM BICARBONATE

Sodium bicarbonate has also been advocated for a variety of other critical care situations not directly pertaining to poisonings, such as hyperkalemia, lactic acidosis, cardiac resuscitation, and diabetic ketoacidosis. For most of these states, other than hyperkalemia, bicarbonate is given in an attempt to correct acidemia. Its use, however, in some of these conditions remains debatable and may actually prove detrimental.

SUMMARY

Despite the increasing tendency to avoid sodium bicarbonate administration in the critically ill acidemic patient, sodium bicarbonate remains an important agent in the treatment of a wide variety of drugs and toxins. In fact, its utility in the poisoned patient continues to expand. Not only is sodium bicarbonate effective in the treatment of poisonings by tricyclic antidepressants, salicylates, and phenobarbital, but it also shows promise in the treatment of toxicity from newer antiarrhythmics, cocaine, chlorophenoxy herbicides, and chlorine gas. In the severely poi-

Despite the increasing tendency to avoid sodium bicarbonate administration in the critically ill acidemic patient, sodium bicarbonate remains an important agent in the treatment of a wide variety of drugs and toxins.

soned patient such as those manifesting quinidine-like effects, sodium bicarbonate is specific therapy. In the more common causes of metabolic acidosis (eg, lactic acidosis), specific therapy such as antibiotics, volume resuscitation, and inotropic support is superior to bicarbonate administration.

References

1. Litovitz TL, Schmitz BF, Bailey KM: 1989 annual report of the American Association of Poison Control Centers national data collection system. Am J Emerg Med 8:394, 1990

2. Parker RB, Beckman KJ, Bauman JL, Hariman RJ: Sodium bicarbonate reverses cocaine-induced conduction defects. (Abstr) Circulation 80(4 Suppl 2):II-15, 1989

3. Cooper DJ, Walley KR, Wiggs BR, Russell JA: Bicarbonate does not improve hemodynamics in critically ill patients who have lactic acidosis. Ann Intern Med 112:492, 1990

4. Morris LR, Murphy MB, Kitabchi AE: Bicarbonate therapy in severe diabetic ketoacidosis. Ann Intern Med 105:836, 1986

5. Weil MH, Ruiz CE, Michaels S, Rackow EC: Acid–base determinants of survival after cardiopulmonary resuscitation. Crit Care Med 13:888, 1985

6. McEvoy GK (ed): AHFS drug information. American Society of Hospital Pharmacists, Bethesda, 1990

7. Frommer DA, Kulig KW, Marx JA, Rumack B: Tricyclic antidepressant overdose: a review. JAMA 257:521, 1987

8. Chiang WK, Ford M, Wav PM et al: Prospective evaluation of fluoxetine ingestions. (Abstr) Vet Hum Toxicol 32:348, 1990

9. Kulig K: Management of poisoning associated with "newer" antidepressant agents. Ann Emerg Med 15:1039, 1986

10. Mudge GH: Agents affecting volume and composition of bodily fluids. p. 848. In Gilman AG, Goodman LS, Gilman A (eds): Goodman and Gilman's the pharmacological basis of therapeutics. 6th ed. MacMillan, New York, 1980

11. Bailey DJ: Cardiotoxic effects of quinidine and their treatment. Arch Intern Med 105:13, 1960

12. Wasserman F, Brodsky L, Dick MM et al: Successful treatment of quinidine and procaine amide intoxication. N Engl J Med 259:797, 1958

13. Bellet S, Wasserman F: The effects of molar sodium lactate in reversing the cardiotoxic effect of hyperpotassemia. Arch Intern Med 100:565, 1957

14. Bellet S, Hamdan G, Somlyo A, Lara R: The reversal of cardiotoxic effects of quinidine by molar sodium lactate: an experimental study. Am J Med Sci 237:165, 1959

15. Callaham M: Tricyclic antidepressant overdose. JACEP 8:413, 1979

16. Noble J, Matthew H: Acute poisoning by tricyclic antidepressants: clinical features and management of 100 patients. Clin Toxicol 2:403, 1969

17. Groleau G, Jotte R, Barish R: The electrocardiographic manifestation of cyclic antidepressant therapy and overdose: a review. J Emerg Med 8:597, 1990

18. Henry JA, Cassidy SL: Membrane stabilizing activity: a major cause of fatal poisoning. Lancet 1:1414, 1986

19. Marshall JB, Forker AD: Cardiovascular effects of tricyclic antidepressant drugs: therapeutic usage, overdose, and management of complications. Am Heart J 103:401, 1982

20. Boehnert MT, Lovejoy FH: Value of the QRS duration versus the serum drug level in predicting seizures and ventricular arrhythmias after an acute overdose of tricyclic antidepressants. N Engl J Med 313:474, 1985

21. Nattel S, Keable H, Sasyniuk BI: Experimental amitriptyline intoxication: electrophysiologic manifestations and management. J Cardiovasc Pharmacol 6:83, 1984

22. Bismuth C, Pebay-Peyroula F, Frejaville JP et al: Nouveaux cas d'intoxication aigue par les derives tricycliques: traitmement par les sels de sodium. J Eur Toxicol 6:285, 1969

23. Gaultier M, Pebay-Peyroula F: Intoxication aigue par antidepresseurs tricyliques. La Revue du Praticien 21:2259, 1971

24. Prudhommeaux JL, Lechat P, Auclair MC: Etude experimentale de l'influences des ions sodium sur las toxicite cardiaque de l'imipramine. Therapie (Paris) 23:675, 1968

25. Gaultier M: Sodium bicarbonate and tricyclic-antidepressant poisoning. Lancet 2:1258, 1976

26. Brown TCK: Sodium bicarbonate treatment for tricyclic antidepressant arrhythmias in children. Med J Aust 2:380, 1976

27. Kingston ME: Hyperventilation in tricyclic antidepressant poisoning. Crit Care Med 7:550, 1979

28. Brown TCK, Barker GA, Dunlop ME, Loughnan PM: The use of sodium bicarbonate in the treatment of tricyclic antidepressant-induced arrhythmias. Anaesth Intensive Care 1:203, 1973

29. Brown TCK: Sodium bicarbonate and tricyclic-antidepressant poisoning. Lancet 1:375, 1977

30. Pentel P, Benowitz N: Efficacy and mechanism of action of sodium bicarbonate in the treatment of desipramine toxicity in rats. J Pharmacol Exp Ther 230:12, 1984

31. Nattel S, Mittleman M: Treatment of ventricular tachyarrhythmias resulting from amitriptyline toxicity in dogs. J Pharmacol Exp Ther 231:430, 1984

32. Sasyniuk BI, Jhamandas V: Mechanism of reversal of toxic effects of amitriptyline on cardiac purkinje fibers by sodium bicarbonate. J Pharmacol Exp Ther 231:387, 1984

33. Sasyniuk BI, Jhamandas V, Valois M: Experimental amitriptyline intoxication: treatment of cardiac toxicity with sodium bicarbonate. Ann Emerg Med 15:1052, 1986

34. Molloy DW, Penner SB, Rabson J, Hall KW: Use of sodium bicarbonate to treat tricyclic antidepressant-induced arrhythmias in a patient with alkalosis. Can Med Assoc J 130:1457, 1984

35. Bessen HA, Niemann JT: Improvement of cardiac conduction after hyperventilation in tricyclic antidepressant overdose. Clin Toxicol 23:537, 1985–86

36. Levitt MA, Sullivan JB, Owens SM et al: Amitriptyline plasma protein binding: effect of plasma pH and relevance to clinical overdose. Am J Emerg Med 4:121, 1986

37. Pentel PR, Keyler DE: Effects of high dose alpha-1-acid glycoprotein on desipramine toxicity in rats. J Pharmacol Exp Ther 246:1061, 1988

38. Hoffman JR, McElroy CR: Bicarbonate therapy for dysrhythmia and hypotension in tricyclic antidepressant overdose. West J Med 134:60, 1981

39. Smilkstein MJ: Reviewing cyclic antidepressant cardiotoxicity: wheat and chaff. J Emerg Med 8:645, 1990

40. Pentel PR, Benowitz NL: Tricyclic antidepressant poisoning: management of arrhythmias. Med Toxicol Adverse Drug Exp 1:101, 1986

41. Goldfrank LR, Osborn H: Quinine. p. 337. In Goldfrank LR, Flomenbaum NE, Lewin NA et al (eds): Goldfrank's Toxicologic Emergencies. 4th ed. Appleton and Lange, Norwalk, 1990

42. Pentel PR, Goldsmith SR, Salerno DM et al: Effect of hypertonic sodium bicarbonate on encainide overdose. Am J Cardiol 57:878, 1986

43. Bajaj AK, Woosley RL, Roden DM: Acute electrophysiologic effects of sodium administration in dogs treated with 0-desmethyl encainide. Circulation 80:994, 1989

44. Spoerke DG: Amantidine. In Poisindex. Vol. 66. Micromedex, Denver, 1990

45. Ellenhorn MJ, Barceloux DG: Neuroleptic drugs. p. 477. In Ellenhorn MJ, Barceloux DG (eds): Medical toxicology. Elsevier, New York, 1988

46. Seger D: Phenytoin and other anticonvulsants. p. 877. In Haddad LM, Winchester JF (eds): Clinical management of poisoning and drug overdose. 2nd ed. WB Saunders, Philadelphia, 1990

47. Whitcomb DC, Gilliam FR, Starmer CF, Grant AO: Marked QRS complex abnormalities and sodium channel blockade by propoxyphene reversed with lidocaine. J Clin Invest 84:1629, 1989

48. Hill JB: Salicylate intoxication. N Engl J Med 228:1110, 1973

49. Morgan AG, Polak A: The excretion of salicylate in salicylate poisoning. Clin Sci 41:475, 1971

50. Milne MD, Scribner BH, Crawford MA: Non-ionic diffusion and the excretion of weak acids and bases. Am J Med 24:709, 1958

51. Buchanan N, Kundig H, Eyberg C: Experimental salicylate intoxication in young baboons. J Pediatr 86:225, 1975

52. Done AK: Aspirin overdosage: incidence, diagnosis, and management. Pediatrics 62(Suppl):890, 1978

53. Hill JB: Experimental salicylate poisoning: observations on the effects of altering blood pH on tissue and plasma salicylate concentrations. Pediatrics 47:658, 1971

54. Kaplan SA, del Carmen FT: Experimental salicylate poisoning: observations on the effects of carbonic anhydrase inhibitor and bicarbonate. Pediatrics 21:762, 1958

55. Gutman AB, Sirota JH: A study by simultaneous clearance techniques of salicylate excretion in man: effect of alkalinization of the urine by bicarbonate administration; effect of probenecid. J Clin Invest 34:711, 1955

56. Reimold EW, Worthen HG, Reilly TP: Salicylate poisoning: comparison of acetazolamide

administration and alkaline diuresis in the treatment of experimental salicylate intoxication in puppies. Am J Dis Child 125:668, 1973

57. Levy G, Tsuchiya T: Salicylate accumulation kinetics in man. N Engl J Med 287:430, 1972

58. Morris N, Graham S: The value of alkali in salicylate therapy. Arch Dis Child 6:273, 1931

59. Smull K, Wegria R, Leland J: The effect of sodium bicarbonate on the serum salicylate level. JAMA 125:1173, 1944

60. Smith PK, Gleason HL, Stoll CG, Ogorzalek S: Studies on the pharmacology of salicylates. J Pharmacol Exp Ther 87:237, 1946

61. Berliner RW: The kidney. Annu Rev Physiol 16:269, 1954

62. MacPherson CR, Milne MD, Evans BM: The excretion of salicylate. Br J Pharmacol 10:484, 1955

63. Feurstein RC, Finberg L, Fleishman E: The use of acetazolamide in the therapy of salicylate poisoning. Pediatrics 25:215, 1960

64. Oliver TK, Dyer ME: The prompt treatment of salicylism with sodium bicarbonate. Am J Dis Child 99:553, 1960

65. Segar WE, Holliday MA: Physiologic abnormalities of salicylate intoxication. N Engl J Med 259:1191, 1958

66. Segar WE: The critically ill child: salicylate intoxication. Pediatrics 44:440, 1969

67. Lawson AAH, Proudfoot AT, Brown SS et al: Forced diuresis in the treatment of acute salicylate poisoning in adults. Q J Med 149:31, 1969

68. Fox GN: Hypocalcemia complicating bicarbonate therapy for salicylate poisoning. West J Med 141:108, 1984

69. Morgan AG, Polak A: Acetazolamide and sodium bicarbonate in treatment of salicylate poisoning in adults. Brit Med J 1:16, 1969

70. Liddell NE, Maren TH: CO_2 retention as a basis for increased toxicity of salicylate with acetazolamide: avoidance of increased toxicity with benzolamide. J Pharmacol Exp Ther 195:1, 1975

71. Cowan RA, Hartnell GG, Lowdell CP et al: Metabolic acidosis induced by carbonic anhydrase inhibitors and salicylates in patients with normal renal function. Br Med J 289:347, 1984

72. Schwartz R, Fellers FX, Knapp J, Yaffe S: The renal response to administration of acetazolamide (diamox) during salicylate intoxication. Pediatrics 23:1103, 1959

73. Gabow PA: How to avoid overlooking salicylate intoxication. J Crit Illness 1:77, 1986

74. Temple AR: Acute and chronic effects of aspirin toxicity and their treatment. Arch Intern Med 141:364, 1981

75. Whitten CF, Kesaree NM, Goodwin JF: Managing salicylate poisoning in children. Am J Dis Child 101:178, 1961

76. Snodgrass W, Rumack BH, Peterson RG, Holbrook ML: Salicylate toxicity following therapeutic doses in children. J Toxicol Clin Toxicol 18:247, 1981

77. Savege TM, Ward JD, Simpson BR, Cohen RD: Treatment of severe salicylate poisoning by forced alkaline diuresis. Br Med J 1:35, 1969

78. Dukes DC, Blainey JD, Cumming G, Widdowson G: The treatment of severe aspirin poisoning. Lancet 2:329, 1963

79. Hormaechea E, Carlson RW, Rogove H et al: Hypovolemia, pulmonary edema and protein changes in severe salicylate poisoning. Am J Med 66:1046, 1979

80. Proudfoot AT, Brown SS: Acidaemia and salicylate poisoning in adults. Br Med J 2:547, 1969

81. Zimmerman GA, Clemmer TP: Acute respiratory failure during therapy for salicylate intoxication. Ann Emerg Med 10:104, 1981

82. Temple AR, George DJ, Done AK, Thompson JA: Salicylate poisoning complicated by fluid retention. J Toxicol Clin Toxicol 9:61, 1976

83. Prescott LF, Balali-Mood M, Critchley JA et al: Diuresis or urinary alkalinisation for salicylate poisoning. Br Med J 285:1383, 1982

84. Lassen NA: Treatment of severe acute barbiturate poisoning by forced diuresis and alkalinisation of the urine. Lancet 2:338, 1960

85. Rall TW, Schleifer LS: Drugs effective in the therapy of the epilepsies. p. 436. In Gilman AG, Rall TW, Nies AS, Taylor TW (eds): Goodman and Gilman's the pharmacological basis of therapeutics. 8th ed. Pergamon Press, New York, 1990

86. Balagot RC, Tsuji H, Sadove MS: Use of an osmotic diuretic—THAM—in treatment of barbiturate poisoning. JAMA 178:1000, 1961

87. Waddell WJ, Butler TC: The distribution and excretion of phenobarbital. J Clin Invest 36:1217, 1957

88. Bloomer HA: A critical evaluation of diuresis in the treatment of barbiturate intoxication. J Lab Clin Med 67:898, 1966

89. Mollaret P, Rapin M, Pocidalo JJ, Monsallier JF: Treatment of acute barbiturate intoxication through plasmatic and urinary alcalinization. Presse Med 67:1435, 1959

90. Myschetzky A, Lassen NA: Urea-induced, osmotic diuresis and alkalization of urine in acute barbiturate intoxication. JAMA 185:116, 1963

91. Bloomer HA: Limited usefulness of alkaline diuresis and peritoneal dialysis in pentobarbital intoxication. N Engl J Med 272:1309, 1965

92. Mawer GE, Lee HA: Value of forced diuresis in acute barbiturate poisoning. Br Med J 2:790, 1968

94. Neuvonen PJ, Karkkainen S: Effects of charcoal, sodium bicarbonate, and ammonium chloride on chlorpropamide kinetics. Clin Pharmacol Ther 33:386, 1983

95. Prescott LF, Park J, Darrien I: Treatment of severe 2,4-D and mecoprop intoxication with alkaline diuresis. Br J Clin Pharmacol 7:111, 1979

95. Flanagan RJ, Meridith TJ, Ruprah M et al: Alkaline diuresis for acute poisoning with chlorophenoxy herbicides and ioxynil. Lancet 335:454, 1990

96. Jacobsen D, Webb R, Collins TD, McMartin KE: Methanol and formate kinetics in late diagnosed methanol intoxication. Med Toxicol Adverse Drug Exp 3:418, 1988

97. Gabow PA, Clay K, Sullivan JB, Lepoff R: Organic acids in ethylene glycol intoxication. Ann Intern Med 105:16, 1986

98. Pappas SC, Silverman M: Treatment of methanol with ethanol and hemodialysis. Can Med Assoc J 126:1391, 1982

99. Jacobsen D, McMartin KE: Methanol and ethylene glycol poisonings mechanism of toxicity, clinical course, diagnosis and treatment. Med Toxicol Adverse Drug Exp 1:309, 1986

100. Borden TA, Bidwell CD: Treatment of acute ethylene glycol poisoning in rats. Invest Urol 6:205, 1968

101. Roe O: Methanol poisoning: its clinical course, pathogenesis and treatment. Acta Med Scand 213:105, 1983

102. Martin-Amat G, McMartin KE, Hayreh MS, Tephly TR: Methanol poisoning: ocular toxicity produced by formate. Toxicol Appl Pharmacol 45:201, 1978

103. Herken W, Rietbrock N: The influence of blood-pH on ionization, distribution, and toxicity of formic acid. Naunyn Schmiedebergs Arch Pharmacol 260:142, 1968

104. Kulig K, Duffy JP, Linden CH, Rumack BH: Toxic effects of methanol, ethylene glycol, and isopropyl alcohol. Top Emerg Med 6:14, 1984

105. Chisholm CD, Singletary EM, Okerberg CV, Langlinais PC: Inhaled sodium bicarbonate therapy for chlorine inhalation injuries. (Abstr) Ann Emerg Med 18:466, 1989

106. Vinsel PJ: Treatment of acute chlorine gas inhalation with nebulized sodium bicarbonate. J Emerg Med 8:327, 1990

107. Henretig FM, Temple AR: Acute iron poisoning in children. Emerg Med Clin North Am 2:121, 1984

108. Robotham JL, Lietman PS: Acute iron poisoning: a review. Am J Dis Child 134:875, 1980

109. Murray MJ: Iron absorption. J Toxicol Clin Toxicol 4:545, 1971

110. Bachrach L, Correa A, Levin R, Grossman M: Iron poisoning: complications of hypertonic phosphate lavage therapy. J Pediatr 94:147, 1979

111. Geffner ME, Opas LM: Phosphate poisoning complicating treatment for iron ingestion. Am J Dis Child 134:509, 1980

112. Czajka PA, Konrad JD, Duffy JP: Iron poisoning: an *in vitro* comparison of bicarbonate and phosphate lavage solutions. J Pediatr 98:491, 1981

113. Banner W, Tong TG: Iron poisoning. Pediatr Clin North Am 33:393, 1986

114. Dean BS, Krenzelok EP: *In vivo* effectiveness of oral complexation agents in the management of iron poisoning. J Toxicol Clin Toxicol 25:221, 1987

115. Engle JP, Polin KS, Stile IL: Acute iron intoxication: treatment controversies. Drug Intell Clin Pharm 21:153, 1987

116. Curry SC, Chang D, Connor D: Drug- and toxin-induced rhabdomyolysis. Ann Emerg Med 18:1068, 1989

117. Koppel C: Clinical features, pathogenesis and management of drug-induced rhabdomyolysis. Med Toxicol Adverse Drug Exp 4:108, 1989

118. Perri GC, Gorini P: Uraemia in the rabbit after injection of crystalline myoglobin. Br J Exp Pathol 33:440, 1952

119. Better OS, Stein JH: Early management of shock and prophylaxis of acute renal failure in traumatic rhabdomyolysis. N Engl J Med 322:825, 1990

120. Eneas JF, Schoenfeld PY, Humphreys MH: The effect of infusion of mannitol-sodium bicarbonate on the clinical course of myoglobinuria. Arch Intern Med 139:801, 1979

121. Ron D, Taitelman U, Michaelson M et al: Prevention of acute renal failure in traumatic rhabdomyolysis. Arch Intern Med 144:277, 1984

122. Honda N: Acute renal failure and rhabdomyolysis. Kidney Int 23:888, 1983

123. Knochel JP: Rhabdomyolysis and myoglobinuria. Annu Rev Med 33:435, 1982

124. Frank LI, Admire RC: Rhabdomyolysis. Urol Clin North Am 9:267, 1982

PRIMER ON IMMUNOLOGY WITH APPLICATIONS TO TOXICOLOGY

MARY ANN HOWLAND, PharmD, ABAT[†]
MARTIN J. SMILKSTEIN, MD, ABMT[††]

Advances in immunology, particularly in the area of antibody formation and purification techniques, have paved the way for applications to toxicology. Model agents now in use include digoxin-specific immune Fab antibody fragments (Digibind), snake and spider antivenins, and botulinum antitoxin. Research is burgeoning and antibody development is being investigated for tricyclic antidepressants, colchicine, ricin, phencyclidine, and other potentially toxic agents. Many excellent reviews on antibody production and their clinical applications exist.[1–7] This paper will define the immunological principles and then emphasize them through the use of digoxin-specific antibodies and snake and spider antivenins.

A historical perspective on immunology must begin in the eleventh century with the event of the first written record describing the crude yet effective attempts at active immunization against smallpox.[8] In the eighteenth century, Jenner expanded the database with his treatise on Variolae Vaccinae. Subsequently, vaccines have been developed from natural and attenuated live organisms as well as killed organisms. These advances have been assisted by tissue culture techniques with improved production. Passive immunization began with von Behring's identification of antibodies for *Clostridium tetani* exotoxin in 1890. During World War I the production of equine tetanus antitoxin was developed, and by 1960 the transformation to a safer

Advances in immunology, particularly in the area of antibody formation and purification techniques, have paved the way for applications to toxicology.

[†] Clinical Professor of Pharmacy, St. John's University College of Pharmacy, Consultant, New York City Poison Control Center, New York, New York

[††] Assistant Professor Emergency Medicine and Trauma, University of Colorado Health Sciences Center, Denver, Colorado

human tetanus immunoglobulin had been made. Today, tissue culture and recombinant DNA techniques allow for the production of larger quantities of highly purified antibodies.[9]

PRODUCTION AND PURIFICATION OF ANTIBODIES

Passive immunization with antibodies has tremendous potential for treating toxin (drug) overdoses.

An antigen generates antibodies that are *anti* foreign *bodies*. Antibodies, when harnessed, can neutralize toxins. Therefore, passive immunization with antibodies has tremendous potential for treating toxin (drug) overdoses. Toxins most commonly taken in an overdose have molecular weights less than 1,000 daltons, and as such cannot incite direct antibody formation. Even digoxin, one of the larger drugs available, has a molecular weight of 780 daltons. Therefore, most agents with potential toxicity must be bound to larger carrier molecules that function as haptens in order to induce antibody formation.[2] Two types of antibodies are formed in this fashion: those against the drug and those against the carrier molecule. These antibodies are whole IgG immunoglobulins, and once the desired drug antibodies are separated, the next step is to obtain the smallest part of the IgG that can inactivate the drug yet be devoid of adverse effects. The IgG can be cleaved into two Fab components, which retain the ability to bind antigen, and one Fc component. The Fc fragment fixes complement, is immunogenic, and is thus unwanted. Current research is progressing in the evaluation of an even smaller, nonimmunogenic, antigen-binding fragment (Fv) of IgG, which at 25,000 daltons contains the smallest antigen-binding site.[10]

The current immunology literature contains many new and important paired terms used to describe antibodies. Among the most important are: heterologous (derived from a different species) vs homologous (derived from the same species); polyclonal (more than one cell line) vs monoclonal (single cell line); polyvalent (containing multiple antigen-binding sites) vs monovalent (containing a single antigen-binding site).

Once the initial phase of research for a specific drug antibody has been successful, the antibody's utility is determined by its ability to decrease drug toxicity with minimal adverse iatrogenic effects.

Once the initial phase of research for a specific drug antibody has been successful, the antibody's utility is determined by its ability to decrease drug toxicity with minimal adverse iatrogenic effects. The antibody must be able to attract the drug, capture it, render it inert, and hasten its elimination from the body, without resulting in an unac-

ceptable risk benefit ratio. These principles have been defined by Scherrman et al. and will be briefly described.[2]

In order for an antibody to be effective, it must reach the
drug before irreversible effects or irreversible binding takes
place. In addition, to achieve optimal affinity, the distribution and diffusion properties of the antibody should be
similar to the toxin, or such that mass action and the development of an equilibrium bring the drug to the antibody
in a timely fashion.[2] For example, the early and irreversible
effects of paraquat on the lung have limited all efforts at
antibody development for the treatment of paraquat toxicity.

Successful inactivation of the drug is dependent on binding affinity, dose requirements, and specificity issues. An-
tigen-antibody binding involves electrostatic forces, hydrogen bonds, and van der Waals forces. The affinity of
the antibody for the toxin should be higher than the affinity
of the toxin for the site of toxicity. The dose of antibody
required is influenced by the total body load of toxin, the
shape of the lethal dose curve (ie, a less than equimolar
dose of antibody might significantly decrease mortality),
and the amount of antibody that the body can tolerate without ill effects.[1] Figure 1 illustrates the effects of the shape
of the lethal dose curve.[2] A toxin with a steep lethal curve

In order for an antibody to be effective, it must reach the drug before irreversible effects or irreversible binding takes place.

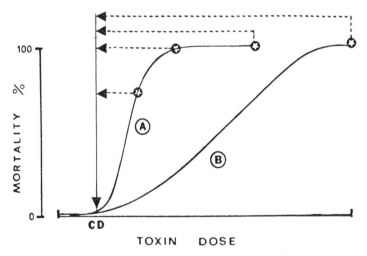

FIGURE 1 The effect of the shape of the lethal dose curve on
the dose of antibody required for neutralization. A toxin with
a steep lethal curve slope would require much less antibody
to neutralize that critical dose of toxin required to produce zero
mortality than a toxin with a shallow lethal curve slope. From
Scherrman JM, Terrien N, Urtizberea M et al: Immunotoxicotherapy: present status and future trends. J Toxicol Clin Toxicol 27:1, 1989. With permission.

slope would require much less antibody to neutralize the critical dose of toxin required to produce zero mortality than a toxin with a shallow lethal curve slope.

Once the toxin is bound to antibody, this toxin-antibody complex must be eliminated from the body before dissociation occurs. An additional concern relates to the mobilization from harmless and inaccessible deep compartments to active and toxic sites should toxin exceed antibody capacity.[2] For example, since the digoxin bound to digoxin-specific antibody is primarily eliminated by the kidneys, patients in renal failure are at risk for recurrent toxicity if dissociation occurs before elimination is completed.

Adverse effects of antibody administration center on acute and delayed immunologic reactions. The potential for immunogenicity is related to source, purity, size, and dose of the antibody, as well as the number of previous exposures to the antibodies.

Adverse effects of antibody administration center on acute and delayed immunologic reactions. The potential for immunogenicity is related to source, purity, size, and dose of the antibody, as well as the number of previous exposures to the antibodies.

Factors favoring the beneficial effects of passive immunization with antibodies for toxin toxicity would include high affinity, good access, good capacity, good elimination, good inactivation, and desirable reactivity or specificity on the part of the antibody.[2] Reversible binding, extracellular binding, slow onset of toxicity, and limited distribution by the toxin facilitates the application of antibodies as therapy.

DIGOXIN AND DIGOXIN-SPECIFIC Fab ANTIBODY FRAGMENTS

PHARMACOLOGY AND TOXICOLOGY OF DIGOXIN

William Withering is credited with recognizing the therapeutic benefits of foxglove and in detailing its toxic effects in a treatise published in 1785. In his account, he wrote that "the foxglove when given in very large and quickly repeated doses, occasions sickness, vomiting, purging, giddiness, confused vision, objects appearing green or yellow; increased secretion of urine, with frequent motions to part with it; slow pulse, even as low as 35 in a minute, cold sweats, convulsions, syncope death."[13]

In 1989, digoxin (as Lanoxin) was the second most commonly prescribed drug in America.[11] In the 1989 American Association of Poison Control Centers Report, cardiac glycosides accounted for 1,872 exposures, of which 175 cases resulted in moderate to severe toxicity and 17 resulted in death.[12]

DIRECT AND INDIRECT EFFECTS OF DIGOXIN

Digoxin has many indirect and direct effects on the heart. Clinicians take therapeutic advantage of the drug's positive inotropic and negative dromotropic actions on the AV node. The extensive research that has been undertaken to elucidate how digoxin causes its effects will be briefly discussed here.

Within the cardiac cell, the sodium/potassium enzyme system plays an important role in maintaining the electrical and ionic gradients in the heart. This enzyme actively extrudes three sodium (Na^+) ions in exchange for two potassium (K^+) ions.[14] An exchange site also exists where three extracellular Na^+ enter the cell and one calcium (Ca^{2+}) leaves the cell.[14] Inotropy is related to intracellular calcium concentration that is then coupled to actin and myosin to modulate the contraction process. The extracellular ratio of Ca^{2+}/Na^+ greatly influences inotropy,[15] and the extracellular concentration of potassium is also influential. Hypokalemia diminishes the potential for exchange; more sodium therefore remains in the cell and less calcium leaves the cell via the Na^+/Ca^{2+} exchange, and hence a greater inotropic effect due to the intracellular availability of calcium.[15] Digoxin binds to the external surface of the Na^+/K^+ ATPase enzyme, causing inhibition of this active process.[14] Therefore, like hypokalemia, less Na^+ is exchanged for K^+, more sodium remains in the cell and less calcium leaves the cell, making more calcium available intracellularly for coupling to actin and myosin in the contraction process.

The other direct actions of digoxin include effects on the sinoatrial (SA) node, atrioventricular (AV) node, Purkinje fibers, and atrial and ventricular muscle fibers.[13] Digoxin, in a dose-dependent fashion, can inhibit the generation of impulses from the SA node, slow conduction velocity through the AV node, and lengthen the effective refractory period.[13] The resting potential of the Purkinje fibers becomes less negative (closer to zero); phase 0 is slowed; the length of the action potential duration is shortened, thereby increasing membrane responsiveness; the rate of phase 4 depolarization is increased; and delayed after-depolarizations occur, thus causing automaticity to be augmented.[13] While the Purkinje fibers' action potential duration is diminished (giving rise to a shortened QT interval), conduction velocity is slowed and automaticity is enhanced secondary to delayed after-depolarizations.[13] The indirect effects of digoxin operate to increase vagal tone and the sensitivity of the SA node to acetylcholine

Digoxin, in a dose-dependent fashion, can inhibit the generation of impulses from the SA node, slow conduction velocity through the AV node, and lengthen the effective refractory period.

with a resultant reflex diminution in sympathetic tone.[13] However, when digoxin toxicity is present, efferent sympathetic activity is increased.[13]

DEVELOPMENT OF DIGOXIN-SPECIFIC Fab ANTIBODY FRAGMENTS

The development of digoxin antibody fragments to treat patients intoxicated with digoxin actually began with the development of digoxin antibodies for measuring serum digoxin concentrations by radioimmunoassay (RIA).[16] The RIA technique permitted the correlation between serum digoxin concentrations and clinical digoxin toxicity. One of the earliest prospective studies of patients receiving digoxin therapeutically demonstrated that toxic patients had statistically significant higher mean serum digoxin concentrations (2.3 ± 1.6 ng/ml) than nontoxic patients (1.0 ± 0.5 ng/ml), although considerable overlap was present (29% of the toxic group had levels less than 1.7 ng/ml while 15% of the nontoxic group had levels higher than 1.7 ng/ml).[17] Subsequent studies have reaffirmed the benefits of appropriate monitoring of serum digoxin concentrations.[18-20]

Butler and his colleagues suggested that purified digoxin antibodies with a higher affinity and specificity should be developed to treat digoxin toxicity in humans.[16] The digoxin molecule alone, with its molecular weight of 780 daltons, would be too small to be immunogenic. But digoxin, as in the case of most drugs, could function as a hapten when joined to an immunogenic protein carrier such as human serum albumin. Butler et al. then immunized sheep with this conjugate, thus generating antibodies. The antibodies were separated and highly purified in order to retain the digoxin antibodies while removing the antibodies to the protein carrier and all other extraneous proteins. The developed antibodies have a high affinity for digoxin and sufficient cross-reactivity with digitoxin to be useful for both agents. Moreover, the specificity is so significant that endogenous steroids, which resemble digoxin structurally, are not affected by antibody administration.

In order to demonstrate biological activity, *in vitro* studies were undertaken and followed with *in vivo* studies in animals.[21-24] Investigations proceeded and contributed significantly to the understanding of the pharmacodynamics and pharmacokinetics of the antibodies.[25-27] Intact IgG antidigoxin antibodies reversed digoxin toxicity in dogs, but the urinary excretion of digoxin was delayed, free digoxin was later released after antibody degradation, and the concern for hypersensitivity reactions was present. To be successfully and safely used on humans, the whole IgG antidigoxin antibodies were cleaved with papain, yielding two antigen-binding Fab fragments with a molecular weight of 50,000 daltons each and one Fc fragment.[25] The Fc fragment does not bind antigen, but increases the potential for hypersensitivity reactions and was therefore eliminated. The advantages of the Fab fragments compared to the whole IgG antibodies include a larger volume of distribution, a more rapid onset of action, a smaller risk of adverse immunologic effects, and a more rapid elimination.[25–27] Ultimately, the commercial product (Digibind) is a relatively pure Fab product that is very safe and extremely effective.

MECHANISM OF ACTION OF DIGOXIN-SPECIFIC ANTIBODIES

Fab digoxin-specific antibodies achieve the following effects: (1) immediately following IV administration, intravascular binding of free digoxin occurs; (2) diffusion into the interstitial space follows with binding of free digoxin; (3) a concentration gradient is then established that facilitates the movement of the free intracellular digoxin and the intracellular digoxin that is dissociated from its binding sites (the external surface of Na^+/K^+ ATPase enzyme) in the heart and throughout the body into the interstitial or intravascular spaces; (4) intravascular concentrations of inactive, antibody-bound digoxin rise substantially; and (5) the elimination kinetics of the Fab antibody-bound digoxin then depend on the patients' renal function and capacity for urinary elimination.

EFFICACY OF DIGOXIN-SPECIFIC ANTIBODIES

The largest body of evidence supporting the life-saving nature of the use of digoxin-specific Fab fragments for digitalis intoxication has recently been published.[28] One hundred twenty five patients with a median age of 65 (16 years or older) and 25 pediatric patients with a median age of 3 were treated. Forty-nine percent of the cases involved a single accidental or suicidal overdose, while the remaining cases involved patients on long-term digitalis therapy. Of the 150 patients, 148 were evaluated for cardiovascular manifestations of toxicity and 79 patients (55%) had high-grade AV block, 68 patients (46%) had refractory ventricular tachycardia, 56 patients (37%) had hyperkalemia, and 49 patients (33%) had ventricular fibrillation. Ninety percent of the patients responded. Complete resolution of all

The largest body of evidence supporting the life-saving nature of the use of digoxin-specific Fab fragments for digitalis intoxication has recently been published.

signs and symptoms of digoxin toxicity within minutes to several hours of Digibind administration occurred in 80% of the cases. Of the 15 patients who did not respond, 14 were either moribund or found not to be digoxin toxic in retrospective analysis. Bespeaking the spectacular effects of digoxin-specific Fab antibodies is the fact that of the 56 patients brought to cardiac arrest by digoxin, 54% survived hospitalization compared with a 100% mortality before the advent of these fragments.[28,29]

SAFETY OF DIGOXIN-SPECIFIC Fab FRAGMENTS

Digoxin-specific Fab antibody fragments are not only effective, they are also very safe.

Digoxin-specific Fab antibody fragments are not only effective, they are also very safe. In the multicenter study of 150 patients, the only acute clinical manifestations were: six patients (4%) developed hypokalemia, four patients (3%) experienced worsening of their congestive heart failure, and one several-hour-old neonate developed transient apnea.[28] Although the concern about allergic reactions and/ or serum sickness exists, no reactions were reported in any of the patients in this series. However, in the postmarketing surveillance study of Digibind that included 451 patients, two patients with a prior history of allergy to antibiotics developed rashes.[30] One of these patients developed a total body rash, facial swelling, and a flush during the infusion. The second patient experienced a pruritic rash. Two other adverse reactions (thrombocytopenia and shaking chills) were probably unrelated to the use of Digibind.[30]

INDICATIONS FOR DIGOXIN-SPECIFIC Fab ANTIBODIES

The manifestations of digoxin toxicity are generally exaggerations of the pharmacologic effects or altered by the following circumstances: (1) a single large dose (suicidal or accidental) or chronic dosing and accumulation; (2) the presence or absence of cardiac pathology; and (3) the age of the patient.

In order to define the indications for digoxin-specific Fab antibodies, the signs and symptoms of digoxin toxicity must be recognized.[31,32] The manifestations of digoxin toxicity are generally exaggerations of the pharmacologic effects or altered by the following circumstances: (1) a single large dose (suicidal or accidental) or chronic dosing and accumulation; (2) the presence or absence of cardiac pathology; and (3) the age of the patient (see Tables 1 through 4). Although the groups cannot definitely discriminate by these characteristics, in general, pediatric patients with normal hearts tolerate higher mg/kg dosages of digoxin than do adults. Potassium levels in these children tend to remain in the therapeutic range. Serum potassium concentrations result from a balance between the degree and extent of inhibition of the Na^+/K^+ ATPase pump and the

TABLE 1   Adult Acute Intoxication–Normal Cardiovascular System

Common cardiac abnormalities
  High degree of AV block
  Ventricular ectopic activity, bigeminy, salvoes
  Ventricular fibrillation
  Ventricular tachycardia
  Paroxysmal atrial tachycardia with block
  Sinus bradycardia
Non-cardiac abnormalities
  Nausea and vomiting
  High digoxin serum concentrations
  Rising potassium concentrations
Requires large total body load of digoxin
  Oral ingestion $\geq$ 6 mg

ability of the kidneys to excrete K^+.[31,32] Healthy children may maintain the renal excretion of potassium except in extreme circumstances. Adults and children with diseased hearts become digoxin toxic at lower total body loads than their respective healthy counterparts. Consequently, patients with diseased hearts receiving digoxin therapeutically are usually unable to tolerate high body burdens of digoxin before becoming intoxicated. In the chronically exposed, the extent of Na^+/K^+ ATPase enzyme inhibition in the heart and throughout the body is less extensive than in the patient with the acute overdose prior to the development of symptoms. Many patients who chronically receive digoxin also receive diuretics, which may also contribute to smaller rises in serum potassium levels in these patients. Adult patients who ingest a large single dose of digoxin or digitoxin have extensive Na^+/K^+ ATPase in-

TABLE 2   Adult Chronic Intoxication–Abnormal Cardiovascular System

Cardiac abnormalities
  Change in cardiac rhythm
  High grade AV block
  AV junctional rhythm
  Ventricular ectopic activity
  Ventricular tachycardia
  Ventricular fibrillation
  Sinus bradycardia, SA exit block or sinus arrest
Non-cardiac abnormalities
  Anorexia, nausea, vomiting
  Confusion
  Visual symptoms
  Moderate digoxin serum concentrations
  Lower total body load of digoxin than in acute overdose
  Low to normal potassium concentrations (normal renal function)
  High potassium concentrations (presence of renal compromise)

TABLE 3   Pediatric Acute Intoxication–Normal
Cardiovascular System

Cardiac abnormalities
  Often not life-threatening
    bradycardia
    first- or second-degree AV block
    ST-segment depression
    junctional rhythm with SA block or arrest
  Severest cases
    AV junctional tachycardia alternating with slow ventricular
      rate
    Ventricular fibrillation
Non-cardiac abnormalities
  Potassium serum concentrations often within therapeutic
    range
  Vomiting and lethargy common

hibition and consequently have significant elevations in potassium. Under these circumstances, before the advent of digoxin Fab fragments, rises in potassium above 5.5 mEq/l indicated a high probability of death.[29]

Prior to the development of digoxin-specific immune antibodies, the treatment for digoxin toxicity was gastric evacuation; activated charcoal; atropine; phenytoin and/or lidocaine; attention to electrolytes, especially potassium and magnesium; pacemaker insertion; and the avoidance of electrical cardioversion. Although the relative importance of these modalities has changed, these treatments continue to be of value. Gastric evacuation is especially important with the acute single overdose and should be accomplished as soon as possible after ingestion. Gastric lavage is preferred over ipecac-induced emesis because of time constraints. This procedure need not be employed if the patient has already vomited. Activated charcoal should be administered in all cases. Repeat-dose activated charcoal is especially useful in patients with renal failure and in those patients who have ingested digitoxin, because of an enhanced enterohepatic circulation.[41–44]

The effects of hypokalemia resemble digoxin and predispose the patient to conduction blocks and reentry or

Prior to the development of digoxin-specific immune antibodies, the treatment for digoxin toxicity was gastric evacuation; activated charcoal; atropine; phenytoin and/or lidocaine; attention to electrolytes, especially potassium and magnesium; pacemaker insertion; and the avoidance of electrical cardioversion. Although the relative importance of these modalities has changed, these treatments continue to be of value.

TABLE 4   Pediatric Chronic Intoxication–Abnormal
Cardiovascular System

Neonatal
  Sinus bradycardia, lethargy, feeding difficulty
Young children
  Slow rhythms, conduction defects, less often
Ventricular ectopy
Digoxin levels
  Mild to moderately elevated
Potassium
  Levels rise but absolute number depends on renal function

automatic rhythms.[15] In addition, hypokalemia increases
the myocardial uptake of digoxin. These similar effects explain the increased sensitivity to digoxin of patients with
hypokalemia. At therapeutic levels of digoxin, potassium
supplementation is beneficial for hypokalemia but should
be done carefully and with continuous monitoring. In the
presence of hypokalemia, atrial or ventricular tachyarrhythmias are more responsive than conduction blocks to
potassium. By contrast, if a patient is digitalis toxic, hyperkalemia causes depolarization of cells and can exacerbate conduction blocks and/or reentrant arrhythmias.[15]
Hyperkalemia is commonly found in the presence of acute
digoxin poisoning; as potassium levels exceed 5.5 mEq/l,
the risk of lethal refractory arrhythmias increases dramatically.[29] Thus, attention must be paid to the serum potassium level, as both hypokalemia and hyperkalemia cause
devastating consequences.

Phenytoin and lidocaine are both categorized as class IB
antiarrhythmics. *In vitro* and *in vivo* studies support the
use of these two agents in the presence of certain digitalis-
induced rhythm disturbances.[15] Phenytoin suppresses
ventricular arrhythmias at relatively low doses (200–400
mg), with higher doses ameliorating atrial tachycardia with
block.[15]

Atropine, by reversing the indirect parasympathetic effects of digoxin, may be useful in ameliorating sinus brad-
ycardias, AV block or SA exit block. However, atropine is
usually only effective in patients with mild digoxin intoxication. It may also be helpful in reversing the vagal effects
induced by lavage or vomiting. An external pacemaker can
be useful in patients with second- or third-degree AV
block. Endocardial pacemaker insertion can theoretically
increase the risks of arrhythmias in an already irritable
myocardium. If digoxin toxicity is consequential and hyperkalemia is substantial, pacemaker efficacy is limited.[15]

Digoxin-specific immune antibody fragments are indicated for potentially life-threatening digoxin or digitoxin
toxicity.[45] Patients with progressive bradyarrhythmias (including severe sinus bradycardia), or second- or third-degree heart block unresponsive to atropine and with severe
ventricular arrhythmias including ventricular tachycardia,
or ventricular fibrillation should be treated with digoxin-
specific immune antibody fragments. Any patient with a
potassium concentration exceeding 5 mEq/l should also be
treated. Acute ingestions of ≥4 mg in a child will probably
require antibody treatment. A rapid progression of clinical
signs and symptoms such as cardiac, gastrointestinal, and
a rising potassium in the presence of an acute overdose
suggests a potentially life-threatening ingestion and the
need for digoxin antibodies.

In a patient with an unknown ingestion who is clinically ill with characteristics suggestive of digoxin intoxication that may be caused by digoxin, calcium channel blockers, and beta-blockers, digoxin antibodies should be administered early in the management, certainly prior to calcium use. In this way, the effects of digoxin can be reversed, potentially obviating the need for calcium and certainly lessening the danger of administering calcium to a patient intoxicated with digoxin. Digoxin toxicity causes intracellular myocardial hypercalcemia, and the administration of exogenous calcium may further exacerbate conduction abnormalities.

Under clinical circumstances in which it is difficult to distinguish between digoxin intoxication and intrinsic cardiac disease, the administration of digoxin antibodies can clarify the dilemma. These indications are summarized in Table 5.

TIME OF ONSET OF RESPONSE TO DIGOXIN ANTIBODY FRAGMENTS

In the multicenter study of 150 patients, the mean time to initial response from the completion of the digoxin antibody infusion (accomplished over a period of 15 minutes to 2 hours) was 19 minutes (0–60 minutes) and the time to complete response was 88 minutes (30–360 minutes).[28] Time to response was not affected by age, concurrent cardiac disease, or the presence of a chronic or acute ingestion.[28]

DOSING OF DIGOXIN-SPECIFIC IMMUNE ANTIBODY FRAGMENTS

The dose of antibodies depends on the total body load of digoxin. Estimates of total body load (TBL) can be made in three ways: (1) estimate the quantity of digoxin ingested in the acute ingestion and assume 80% bioavailability (x mg ingested $\times$ 0.8 = TBL), (2) obtain a serum digoxin

---

TABLE 5 Indications for Administration of Digoxin-specific Fab Fragments

Severe ventricular arrhythmias
Progressive bradyarrhythmias unresponsive to atropine
Potassium level $\geq$ 5 mEq/l in setting of suspected digoxin toxicity
Rapidly progressive cardiac or gastrointestinal symptoms, or a rising potassium level
To solidify the diagnosis

concentration and incorporate the volume of distribution (Vd) of digoxin and the patient's body weight in kilograms using a pharmacokinetic formula, or (3) use an empiric dose based upon the average requirements for an acute or chronic overdose in an adult or child (Table 6) (sample calculations for each of these methods are demonstrated in Figures 2 and 3). Each vial of Digibind contains 40 mg of purified digoxin-specific Fab fragments that will bind approximately 0.6 mg of digoxin or digitoxin. If the quantity of ingestion cannot be estimated reliably, then it may be safest to use the largest calculated estimate or at least be prepared to increase dosing should resolution be inadequate. Inaccuracies in estimation can occur for a number of reasons, including faulty histories, serum digoxin concentrations determined during the acute phase of distribution thus overestimating requirements, and the fact that a Vd of 6 l/kg is merely a population estimate and varies considerably in individuals and in certain disease states.

ADMINISTRATION AND PHARMACOKINETICS

It is recommended that Digibind be administered intravenously over 30 minutes through a 0.22 μm membrane filter.[45] The 40 mg Digibind vial must be reconstituted with 4 ml of sterile water for intravenous injection, furnishing an isoosmotic solution. This preparation can be further di-

TABLE 6 Empiric Dosing Recommendations of Digibind

Acute ingestion
  Adult: 10–15 vials
  Child: 10–15 vials
Chronic toxicity
  Adult: 2–3 vials
  Child*: ¼–½ vial

* Package insert contains table for infants and children with corresponding serum concentrations.

Adult

weight: 70 kg

ingestion: 100 0.25 mg digoxin tablets

Calculation:

$$0.25 \text{ mg} \times 100 = 25.0 \text{ mg ingested dose}$$

$$25.0 \text{ mg} \times 0.80 \text{ (80\% bioavailability)} = 20.0 \text{ mg (absorbed dose)}$$

$$0.6 \text{ mg (reversed per vial)} = 33.3 \text{ vials}$$

Child

weight: 10 kg

ingestion: 100 0.25 mg digoxin tablets

Calculation:

same as for adult: child will require 33.3 vials

FIGURE 2   Sample calculation based on the history of digoxin ingestion.

Adult

weight: 70 kg

serum digoxin concentration = 10 ng/ml

Vd = 6 l/kg

Calculation:

$$\frac{\text{total body load (mg)}}{0.6 \text{ mg/vial}} = \text{no. vials} = \frac{\text{serum digoxin concentration} \times \text{Vd} \times \text{pt wt}}{1000^* \times 0.6 \text{ mg/vial}}$$

$$\text{no. vials} = \frac{10 \text{ ng/ml} \times 6 \text{ l/kg} \times 70 \text{ kg}}{1000 \times 0.6 \text{ mg/vial}}$$

$$\text{no. vials} = 7$$

Child

weight: 10 kg

serum digoxin concentration: 10 ng/ml

Vd: 6 l/kg

Calculation:

$$\text{no. vials} = \frac{10 \text{ ng/ml} \times 6 \text{ l/kg} \times 10 \text{ kg}}{1000 \times 0.6 \text{ mg/vial}}$$

$$\text{no. vials} = 1$$

* 1000 is a conversion factor to change ng/ml to mg/l.

FIGURE 3   Sample calculation based on the serum digoxin concentration.

luted with sterile isotonic saline (for small infants). Once reconstituted it should be used immediately or within 4 hours if refrigeration occurs .[45] In the presence of an unstable clinical situation, the Digibind is given by intravenous (IV) bolus.

In 1976, Smith et al. described the first clinical use of digoxin-specific antibody fragments in humans.[46] Within 1 hour after digoxin-specific Fab fragments were administered, free (unbound and active) digoxin dropped to an undetectable level and did not rise until 9 hours later, reaching a peak of only 2 ng/ml at 16 hours and remaining at approximately 1.5 ng/ml for the next 40 hours.[46] Total (free plus bound) digoxin, which was 17.6 ng/ml before digoxin Fab fragments, rose to 226 ng/ml 1 hour after the start of the infusion, remained there for 11 hours, and then fell over the next 44 hours with a half-life of 20 hours.[46] Fab concentrations peaked at the end of the infusion and then apparently exhibited a biphasic or triphasic decline (probably reflecting the distribution into different compartments) and excretion and catabolism. An analysis of renal elimination based on an incomplete collection suggested that digoxin was only excreted in the bound form during the first 6 hours, but by 30 hours after Fab all digoxin was free digoxin.

In 1986, Schaumann et al. studied the pharmacokinetics of Fab fragments in 17 patients with acute suicidal ingestions of digoxin.[47] Data from 11 of the patients were used to calculate a median total-body Fab fragment clearance of 24.5 ml/min, of which 13.6 ml/min was renal clearance.[47] The apparent distribution volume for the Fab fragments varied from 25.4 l to 54 l, depending on the time at which the calculation was made.[47] In the first 11 patients, the digoxin Fab dose ranged from 400 to 480 mg (10–12 vials) and was infused over a period of ½ to 5 hours.[47] In the last 6 patients, 160 mg (4 vials) was given as a loading dose over 15 minutes followed by an additional 160 mg given over 7 hours.[47] If the digoxin Fab fragments are given so rapidly that elimination occurs before redistribution of digoxin occurs from the binding sites, then the total amount of Fab fragments actually bound to digoxin will be less than predicted or optimal and digoxin levels may once again increase. In the first 11 patients, the percentage of bound to unbound Fab was about 50% and free digoxin concentrations appeared earlier and the maximum levels were higher than in the last 6 patients. In those six patients who received a loading dose followed by a maintenance infusion, the percentage of bound Fab was 70%, indicating a more optimal match between Fab fragments and digoxin. Free digoxin levels reappeared between 12 and 24 hours, and maximum levels only averaged 2.2 ng/ml (0–4.4 ng/ml).[47]

Schaumann's findings suggest some important points.[47] The first point is that it makes more sense to give a loading dose of Fab followed by a maintenance infusion. This technique optimizes the binding of digoxin to Fab. The loading dose immediately captures digoxin already in the vascular space and digoxin that can be rapidly redistributed to the vascular space. The maintenance dose provides enough Fab fragments to continue to draw digoxin from the tissues into the serum to be bound. It appears that in the acute intentional overdose setting, four to six vials given as a loading dose, followed by 0.5 mg/min for 8 hours and then 0.1 mg/min for about 6 hours, should be safe and effective and efficient.[47] However, more patients should be studied in this fashion and the protocol validated before this approach can be adopted. Another point suggested by the study is that the distribution volumes for Fab fragments indicate that they may enter the cells in spite of a molecular weight of 50,000 daltons.[47]

MEASUREMENT OF DIGOXIN SERUM CONCENTRATIONS

Most hospital laboratories are not equipped to determine free serum digoxin concentrations. Therefore, once digoxin-specific Fab antibody fragments are administered, serum digoxin concentrations can no longer be clinically useful since they represent free plus bound digoxin.

Most hospital laboratories are not equipped to determine free serum digoxin concentrations. Therefore, once digoxin-specific Fab antibody fragments are administered, serum digoxin concentrations can no longer be clinically useful since they represent free plus bound digoxin.[48-52] If the correct dose of Fab fragments is administered, the free serum digoxin concentrations should be near zero. Free digoxin concentrations begin to reappear from 5 to 24 hours or longer after Fab administration, depending on the antibody dose, the infusion technique and the patient's renal function. In view of the inability to measure free digoxin, the patient's cardiac status must be carefully monitored for signs of recurrent toxicity.

Other pitfalls in the measurement and utility of digoxin serum concentrations include endogenous and exogenous factors. Endogenous digoxin-like immunoreactive substances (DLIS) have been described in infants, in the third trimester of pregnancy, and in patients with renal and hepatic failure.[39,53-58] Endogenous DLIS, when free or weakly bound, as in these circumstances, are measurable by the typical RIA assay and can account for factiously high digoxin serum concentrations being reported when the patient is not being treated with digoxin. The role of DLIS in the body has not been fully elucidated, but DLIS do have an effect on both the sodium potassium pump and the digoxin-glycoside receptor site,[39] and have been implicated as a causative factor in hypertension and renal disease. Exogenous factors relate primarily to the measurement techniques and their interpretation.[59] Digoxin is metabolized to compounds with varying levels of cardioactivity.[60] Some metabolites cross-react and are measured by RIA while others are not. The *in vivo* production of these metabolites varies in patients and may depend on intestinal metabolism by gut flora, as well as renal and liver clearance.

Patients with renal insufficiency will have altered digoxin and Fab fragment pharmacokinetics.[61-68] Initially, Fab will bind digoxin and free digoxin levels will be zero. However, compared to patients with normal renal function, these patients will have much longer Fab and digoxin elimination half-lives. Free digoxin levels will gradually rise and may not peak for a week. Distribution kinetics may also be altered. Therefore, in these patients, and perhaps in patients with hepatitis, vigilance for a secondary phase of digoxin toxicity is in order.

Hemodialysis and charcoal hemoperfusion have no role

in the management of digoxin intoxication. Without the use of Fab fragments, these procedures are not indicated because digoxin has too large a molecular weight for hemodialysis to be successful. In addition, digoxin has too large a volume of distribution to make either approach feasible except as a temporizing measure as most of the drug is extravascular. With Fab fragments, hemodialysis is ineffective and hemoperfusion is superfluous. Even in anephric patients, the Fab fragments are effective although return of symptoms may occur 7–14 days later, possibly indicating the need for another dose of Fab fragments. Hemoperfusion through columns with antidigoxin antibodies bound to agarose polyacrolein microsphere beads has been accomplished, but the availability of Fab fragments in the United States makes this modality outmoded.[69,70] The principles that make charcoal hemoperfusion less than ideal (Vd of digoxin, extracorporeal access, anticoagulation) also apply to this technique. Continuous arteriovenous hemofiltration in an experimental model has failed to remove the digoxin-Fab complex.[71]

The future for digoxin-specific Fab antibody fragments lies in developing an even smaller antigen-binding fragment and then manufacturing a consistent product through the use of monoclonal antibody techniques. Experimental studies in animals using monoclonal antibodies have already begun with much success.[72]

ANTIBODIES TO ANTIDEPRESSANTS

When the cyclic antidepressants are used inappropriately, a significant amount of morbidity and mortality result. These drugs represent an ideal group with which to assess the merits and disadvantages of antidotal antibodies and to determine the evolution of current research. Desipramine is a representative agent of this group. Its properties include: a molecular weight of 266 daltons, 82% protein binding, 20 l/kg Vd, toxic serum concentrations at 1,000 ng/ml, reversible binding to the myocardium, and a rapid onset of toxicity. In order for antibodies to be safe and effective, we must ensure toxin inactivation, toxin extraction from sites of toxicity, enhanced toxin elimination, and minimal adverse effects. As the tricyclic antidepressants possess a significant structural resemblance, an antibody with cross-reactivity among the comparable agents would be desirable. One potential limiting factor would be the dose requirement of Fab. Assuming that an equimolar dose of Fab would be needed, we could estimate the amount of

The future for digoxin-specific Fab antibody fragments lies in developing an even smaller antigen-binding fragment and then manufacturing a consistent product through the use of monoclonal antibody techniques.

Fab needed with the following formula:

$$\text{Total body load in mg} = \frac{\text{SDC} \times \text{Vd} \times \text{kg wt}}{1000}$$

$$= \frac{1000 \text{ ng/ml} \times 20 \text{ l/kg} \times 70 \text{ kg}}{1000}$$

$$= 1400 \text{ mg}$$

$$\frac{\text{MW of Fab}}{\text{MW of drug}} = \text{ratio needed}$$

$$\frac{50000}{266} = 188:1$$

where SDC equals serum drug concentration. Therefore, $1400 \times 188 = 26.32$ g of Fab are needed.

Thus, using an equimolar amount of Fab would require approximately 26 grams of Fab. This is an amount that is excessive, is probably exceedingly expensive, and places the patients at too great a risk. Even under the worst circumstances in suicidal ingestions of digoxin, the maximal amount of digoxin Fab fragments required is 400–800 mg!

Research is exploring whether much smaller doses (much less than equimolar) could be used to improve the outcome or whether Fab administration could be coupled with other extracorporeal techniques such as ultrafiltration.[73–76]

IMMUNOTHERAPY AND IMMUNODIAGNOSIS OF ENVENOMATION

Immunotherapy of biotoxin-mediated poisoning has been important for over a century, beginning with the use of crude antisera to neutralize the causative toxins of tetanus, botulism, and diptheria. In addition to improvements in these antitoxins, the last 60 years have led to the development of antivenins to treat envenomation by snakes, spiders, scorpions, fish, jellyfish, and others.

The following discussion is intended to summarize the current status of immunodiagnosis and immunotherapy in envenomation, and to briefly describe some future advances.

IMMUNOTHERAPY OF ENVENOMATION

For the overwhelming majority of antivenins produced thus far, there is no debate that they effectively neutralize the target toxin. However, tremendous concern exists about the risk-to-benefit ratio of such treatment.

For the overwhelming majority of antivenins produced thus far, there is no debate that they effectively neutralize the target toxin. However, tremendous concern exists about the risk-to-benefit ratio of such treatment. Although current technology is capable of producing pure, safe, and effective antivenins, these are not yet available for most toxins.[77]

In order to obtain sufficient amounts of antibody to venoms, equine-derived antisera have traditionally been used. Although there are several methods of antibody isolation and purification, the end product is still horse protein. As a result, immediate anaphylaxis (IgE mediated), anaphylactoid reactions (non-IgE mediated), and delayed serum sickness (antigen excess) are well-described consequences of therapy.[78]

While human-derived antibodies have obvious therapeutic advantages, they have only been seriously pursued in the case of tetanus and botulinus antitoxins due to cost and other complications. All current commercial antivenins are derived from animals[79]; all snake antivenins are equine-derived.[77] Horses are gradually immunized with venom, bled periodically, and the antibody-containing serum is taken for processing. The Wyeth polyvalent crotalid antivenin, for example, then undergoes a series of steps including pepsin digestion, ammonium sulfate precipitation, and filtration.[77] The end product has relatively more IgG antibody and less albumin and extraneous proteins than crude serum, but it still contains considerable amounts of the unwanted fractions (Fig. 4). Purification by immunosorbent affinity chromatography, production of mouse monoclonal antibodies, animal-human hybrid antibodies, human antibodies, Fab fragments, and other techniques is possible,[6,77] but very expensive to initiate. Although an estimated 50,000 fatalities due to snake bite occur each year internationally,[80,81] these are caused by a staggering number of different species, necessitating myriad individual antivenins.[79] Until newer methods can be made less time-consuming and expensive, large-scale commercial production of purified antivenins is unlikely. This is particularly true in the United States, where less than 20 people a year die from venomous snakebites.[82,83]

General Principles of Antivenin Use

Adverse Effects
The adverse effects of antivenin can be best classified into general etiologic categories: IgE-mediated anaphylaxis, non-IgE-mediated anaphylactoid, and antigen-excess-induced serum sickness. These three causes result in two clinical presentations: immediate and delayed. Anaphylaxis occurs when antigen combines with IgE antibodies bound to mast cells and basophils. These cells then degranulate, releasing histamine, leukotrienes, kinins, kallikrein, prostaglandins, platelet activity factor,

The adverse effects of antivenin can be best classified into general etiologic categories: IgE-mediated anaphylaxis, non-IgE-mediated anaphylactoid, and antigen-excess-induced serum sickness.

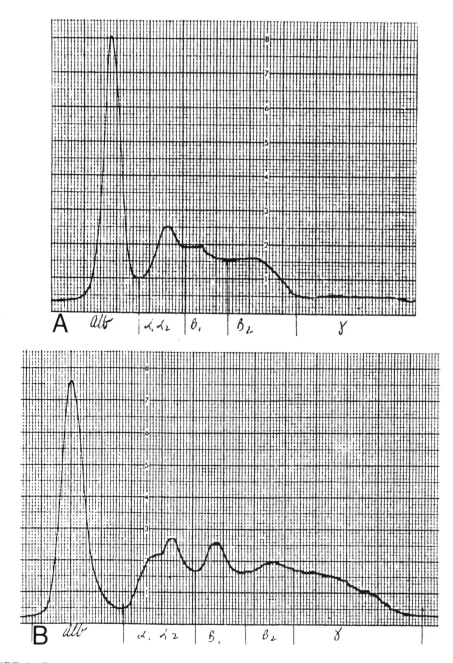

FIGURE 4 Protein electrophoresis profiles of equine-derived (A) skin test material (normal serum, Merck Sharpe & Dohme), (B) Latrodectus antivenin (crude hyperimmune serum, Merck Sharpe & Dohme). Note relative increase in immunoglobulins and decrease in other fractions with more advanced purification. (*Figure continues.*)

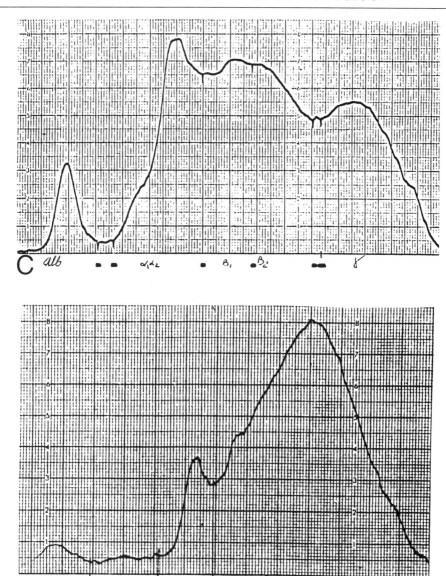

FIGURE 4 (*continued*) (C) Crotalid antivenin (ammonium sulfate precipitation, filtration, Wyeth), and (D) Latrodectus antivenin (pepsin digestion, ammonium sulfate precipitation, filtration, Commonwealth Serum Laboratories).

and hydrolytic enzymes, among others. Release of these substances occurs in anaphylactoid reactions as well, but the degranulation is triggered by other mechanisms involving complement activation, the fibrinolytic or coagulation systems, the kinin-generating system, or a combination thereof.[84]

While the basis for anaphylaxis (IgE-mediated) and anaphylactoid (non-IgE-mediated) reactions are different, the clinical manifestations are the same. Reactions may involve some or all of the following: skin flushing, urticaria, edema, sneezing, tachypnea, stridor, bronchospasm, nausea, vomiting, vasodilation, decreased cardiac inotropy, cardiovascular collapse, and death. These may appear immediately upon starting the antivenin infusion or with a delay of 2–15 minutes. Anaphylaxis from antigens other than antivenin has been reported as long as 2.5 hours after antigen exposure.[84] Although many patients demonstrate easily recognized signs such as urticaria or wheezing, others initially complain only of anxiety or mild nausea, symptoms that are difficult to distinguish from those caused by envenomation. It is clear that life-threatening anaphylaxis can occur without skin rash or wheezing.[85]

Delayed serum sickness can result from relatively large doses of any foreign protein. Animal-derived antivenin, including the immunoglobulins directed at the venom, acts as a source of antigens to trigger this reaction. The dose causes an "antigen excess" and stimulates the production of antibodies in the recipient after 4–10 days. These antibodies then form soluble complexes with the antigen (antivenin), and these complexes may then diffuse into vascular membranes throughout the body and fix and activate complement, thus initiating widespread vasculitis. The sites and amounts of immune-complex deposition determine the severity and manifestations of illness.[86,87]

Symptoms usually are most often noted 7–14 days after antigen exposure, although previously sensitized individuals may become ill after only 2–4 days, and onset of illness is commonly as late as 21 days. Classic symptoms include fever, skin rash, lymphadenopathy, and arthralgias. Renal involvement, including proteinuria and hematuria, is common, yet actual renal failure or permanent renal impairment is very rare. Other potentially serious signs have been reported but are quite unusual: myocarditis, generalized vasculitis, peripheral neuritis, glomerulonephritis, and Guillain-Barre syndrome.[86,87]

Unlike immediate reactions, the severity of which are determined by the pattern of release of endogenous mediators, the severity of serum sickness is largely dependent on the dose of antigen. Prior to the use of human-derived tetanus antitoxin, it was noted that 80 ml of equine antitoxin would virtually always cause serum sickness, while the incidence dropped to 5–10% if only 5–10 ml were given. The dose relationship probably explains why the incidence of serum sickness may exceed 70% in patients who receive multiple vials of crotalid antivenin, while few patients treated with single-vial black widow antivenin treatment develop delayed reactions.[86,87]

Administration of Antivenin Prior to the administration of antivenin, three goals should be met. First, a careful, well-documented analysis of the evidence of envenomation and the rate of progression must be meticulously, but quickly, performed. Second, evidence must be sought to establish whether or not the person to be treated may be more likely to suffer an adverse response to antivenin. A careful history is most useful and should consider atopic illness (eczema, urticaria, asthma, hay fever), exposure to horses (hobbies, occupational, pets), allergies to horses or horse products, and previous treatment with equine serum products.

Skin or conjunctival testing is controversial but clearly is not an accurate predictor of response to antivenin. Some studies suggest that 10–40% of patients still develop immediate reactions after negative skin tests and that patients with positive skin tests may have no reaction to antivenin.[78,88] Some have speculated that this is because the skin test is not performed with antivenin but usually uses crude horse serum, which is not antigenically equal to the actual antivenin (Fig. 4). Even if the antivenin itself is used for skin testing, one vial may differ antigenically from another. Furthermore, the skin test dose can potentially sensitize, leading to future reactions, or cause anaphylaxis itself. As a result of these observations, skin testing should be considered unreliable and absolutely should not be done unless the decision to treat with antivenin has been made.

Unfortunately, skin testing remains the only test available and is widely recommended despite its shortcomings.[80,89,90] If one feels compelled to do skin testing, the actual antivenin may be used in addition to or instead of the crude horse serum intended for this purpose. The package insert for the Wyeth crotalid antivenin kit suggests intradermal injection of 0.02–0.03 ml of the skin test material (supplied as a 1:10 dilution) or of the antivenin (requires reconstitution followed by a 1:10 dilution before injection). It must be understood that these dosages are not well studied. Many authors suggest lower doses (0.01 ml) or greater dilution (1:100) if the antivenin is used for skin testing.[89] If horse allergy is suspected, then neither material should be used unless diluted to at least 1:100. After injection, the site is observed for 15–30 minutes for development of erythema, edema, wheal formation, or itching.

The final goal before giving antivenin is preparation of the patient. Antivenin should only be given in a setting where immediate cardiopulmonary resuscitation can be performed and with personnel who are experienced in the emergency management of the critically ill present. Equipment, drugs, and skilled personnel needed for endotra-

Studies suggest that 10–40% of patients still develop immediate reactions after negative skin tests and that patients with positive skin tests may have no reaction to antivenin.

Antivenin should only be given in a setting where immediate cardiopulmonary resuscitation can be performed and with personnel who are experienced in the emergency management of the critically ill present.

cheal intubation, cricothyroidotomy, large-bore intravenous catheterization, fluid resuscitation, cardiac monitoring, administration of vasopressors, epinephrine, diphenhydramine, and corticosteroids should be present. At least two large-bore intravenous lines should be established. The tubing to be used for the antivenin should enter one of the patient's lines as close as possible to the patient, preferably directly into the catheter. This precaution is important if a reaction does occur in order to avoid a large amount of antivenin remaining in the tubing that might then be flushed into the patient even if the tubing carrying antivenin is disconnected. Pretreatment with diphenhydramine, methylprednisolone, and/or epinephrine is also controversial. There is no evidence that these modalities prevent immediate reactions, and thus their routine use is not logical. In patients who are at greatest risk (strong atopic history, previous horse allergy, or positive skin test), many would pretreat despite the lack of supporting data.

Based on patient history, skin testing, or the response to the initiation of antivenin infusion, some patients will be identified as being at high risk for an immediate reaction. The decision to forego or discontinue antivenin in an individual represents a difficult risk-benefit decision that requires the informed understanding and consent of the patient. It is our belief that regardless of the risk of anaphylaxis, antivenin should still be recommended when a real limb or life threat is evident, but that lesser indications may warrant withholding antivenin. For example, on a practical level, this means that moderate or severe envenomation by a diamondback rattlesnake should be treated with antivenin despite the risk of immediate reaction, whereas black widow spider envenomation should not.

Each vial of antivenin should be reconstituted according to the package insert and then diluted prior to administration. If possible, each vial should be diluted in 50–200 ml of saline, for example, five vials of crotalid antivenin should be administered in 250–1,000 ml of saline. It is speculated that at least some anaphylactoid reactions can be prevented by dilution, since a lower concentration should decrease the likelihood of widespread complement activation.[91] Therefore, dilution into the largest volume that can be safely given in a timely manner seems advisable. With low doses of antivenin, 200 ml per vial is usually not a problem, however, if 20–30 vials of antivenin are required, fluid overload considerations may necessitate less dilute solutions.

Regardless of the suspected risk of an immediate reaction, the infusion should always be started very slowly and then increased if no adverse clinical manifestations are present.

Regardless of the suspected risk of an immediate reaction, the infusion should always be started very slowly and then increased if no adverse clinical manifestations are present, until the patient is receiving the equivalent of one vial over approximately 20 minutes. Using this basic formula, a five-vial infusion should take between 1½ and 2 hours. An obvious problem with this regimented approach is treating immediately life-threatening severe envenomation. If such a patient needed 30 vials of antivenin, 10 hours would be required for the infusion.

In these cases, the infusion should be gradually increased, given as rapidly as the patient will tolerate, until clinical improvement and stabilization are achieved. At that point, the remainder of the infusion should be given at the standard rate.

Treatment of Adverse Effects If evidence of an immediate reaction appears, the infusion should be stopped and the patient should receive intravenous diphenhydramine (1 mg/kg) and subcutaneous epinephrine (1:1,000; 0.1 ml/kg up to 0.5 ml). Intravenous steroids are controversial since some authors believe that they are of limited value in treating these reactions and may worsen the effects of envenomation.[80] We believe that they should be used to treat severe antivenin reactions and would administer either methylprednisolone (1–2 mg/kg; up to 125 mg) or hydrocortisone (4 mg/kg; up to 250 mg). If severe symptoms of anaphylaxis are evident, airway management may be required and intravenous epinephrine considered (1:10,000 if cardiac arrest; 1:100,000 or more dilute, otherwise). If antivenin is to be continued because of a significant life or limb threat, it should be restarted very slowly, if possible after a 30-minute delay to allow some effect of medication, and with an epinephrine continuous infusion mixed and ready in the second intravenous line. If further adverse reaction is evident, but antivenin is still required, the antivenin is given as rapidly as tolerated while supportive care including oxygen, airway support, volume expansion, and epinephrine infusion are optimized.

Serum sickness is nearly always a self-limited illness that, although very distressing to the patient, resolves spontaneously in 2–3 weeks, and poses no significant long-term threat.[86,87] The mildest cases may require only oral diphenhydramine hydrochloride (1 mg/kg per dose up to 50 mg, every 6 hours) to control symptomatic skin rash. Patients with more widespread symptoms will benefit from oral prednisone. Hospitalization is rarely needed but is a consideration if significant renal impairment is evident or if joint symptoms are disabling.

Prophylactic steroids have been suggested in other settings to diminish symptoms after a known exposure likely to cause serum sickness. This is a particularly serious consideration for patients who receive many vials of antivenin, since nearly all will develop serum sickness. Because corticosteroids may exacerbate the initial effects of envenomation, there is little experience or analysis regarding prophylactic use to prevent delayed serum sickness. Once the acute effects of envenomation are clearly resolving, that is, after a few days, we see no reason not to begin a short course of oral prednisone, however, this is controversial.

Treatment of Specific Envenomations

Snakebite Envenomation   Treatment of snake bite envenomation has generated tremendous controversy, yet it is clear that antivenin therapy is the most effective means of limiting the adverse effects of snake venoms. For those venoms against which antivenin is available, there is no debate regarding efficacy; the controversy focuses upon their safety. Since many snake bites produce either no envenomation or trivial envenomation, the decision to use a therapy with a potential for morbidity or mortality can be difficult. Underutilization of antivenin after serious envenomation and unnecessary use of antivenin have both led to patient morbidity and mortality.[80]

Crotalid Snakebite Envenomation. The family Crotalidae accounts for 95% of poisonous snake bites in the United States. These snakes include true rattlesnakes (genus *Crotalus*), pigmy rattlesnakes and massasaugas (genus *Sistrurus*), and cottonmouths and copperheads (genus *Agkistrodon*). Although all are capable of causing serious envenomation, the eastern and western diamondback rattlesnakes (*C. adamanteus* and *C. atrox*, respectively) are more likely to cause severe toxicity, while life-threatening problems from copperheads (*A. contortix*) or cottonmouths (*A. piscivorus*) are quite unusual. A discussion of the venom characteristics and clinical presentation of these envenomations is beyond the scope of this discussion, but excellent reviews are available.[80,89,90]

Although there are significant differences between the venoms of various crotalids, they share antigenic properties. Antivenin (Crotalidae) Polyvalent (Wyeth) is an equine-derived product from horses immunized with venoms of eastern and western diamondback rattlesnakes, South American rattlesnake (*C. durissus terrificus*), and the fer-de-lance (*Bothrops atrox*). Because of the antigenic similarities, this antivenin is not only effective for the venoms of the four species used for immunization, but also for all other crotalids found in the United States, Central and

South American bushmaster species, and certain Asian species of *Agkistrodon*.

Precise indications for Crotalid antivenin are controversial, however, rough classification of the severity of envenomation provides a useful framework for treatment decisions. We favor the use of five classifications (Table 7). No antivenin is indicated for crotalid bite victims if findings suggest no or minimal envenomation. For mild envenomation, five vials is an appropriate starting dose. For moderate toxicity, 10 vials is a typical dose, and at least 15 vials should be used in cases of severe envenomation. These are obviously only general guidelines and are only useful when adjusted based on the expertise of the treating physician or consultant.[92] It is probably never indicated to use less than five vials, since lower doses are either inadequate or unnecessary yet still carry significant risk of immediate, life-threatening adverse reactions. At the opposite end of the spectrum, 20 vials is probably the minimum starting dose for patients in extremis with immediately life-threatening toxicity that does not quickly respond to other supportive measures. Because the only endpoint of therapy is clinical response, there is no maximum dose. Although the use of as many as 75 vials has been reported,[93] this is extraordinary, even for severe envenomations.

In view of the potential adverse effects of the antivenin, it is important to realize that even some cases of significant envenomation can be managed with supportive care alone.[94] This applies most to patients with soft tissue edema without significant vital sign or hematologic abnormalities. If there are no indications of compartment syndrome and no large areas of tissue necrosis, even massive edema may resolve without antivenin with meticulous observation. The progression of cardiovascular and hematologic complications are less predictable and potentially

In view of the potential adverse effects of the antivenin, it is important to realize that even some cases of significant envenomation can be managed with supportive care alone.

TABLE 7   Framework for Grading the Severity of Crotalid Envenomation

Grade	Description	Antivenin Dose
0 (none)	Fang marks only; no local or systemic signs of envenomation.	none
1 (minimal or trivial)	Nonprogressive edema or ecchymosis at the bite site only; no systemic signs of envenomation.	none
2 (mild)	Slowly progressive edema and/or limited ecchymosis at the bite site and/or metallic taste as only systemic manifestation.	>5 vials
3 (moderate)	Rapidly progressive edema and/or more extensive ecchymosis and/or non-life-threatening abnormalities of vital signs, coagulopathy, hemolysis, or neurologic dysfunction.	>10 vials
4 (severe)	Limb-threatening progressive edema or ecchymosis and/or life-threatening abnormalities of vital signs, coagulopathy, hemolysis, or neurologic function.	>15 vials

more devastating, and most authors agree that early, aggressive use of antivenin is the only advisable course of action if systemic envenomation is apparent. Expectant management, observation, and supportive care without antivenin should be considered, particularly when a strong atopic history is obtained, or when a past history of allergy to horses or equine-derived products is obtained. When clearly life- or limb-threatening envenomation is evident, antivenin should be used, regardless of allergic history or skin testing results (see above).

The timing of antivenin use has also been a topic of controversy. Although antivenin use within 4 hours is more effective in neutralizing venom and preventing the cascade of events triggered by envenomation,[82] there is still a role for late antivenin use. Although antivenin use more than 24 hours after envenomation is far less effective, it is still logical, regardless of the delay since the event of the bite, in any case in which life- or limb-threatening signs continue to progress. For example, slow progression of edema alone 36 hours after envenomation probably does not justify use of antivenin, but a falling hematocrit and an increasing coagulopathy might.

As stated above, there are marked differences between species in terms of the likelihood of serious envenomation and in the type of envenomation produced. Nonetheless, the same system of evaluation and treatment guidelines apply to nearly all crotalids. The most significant exception is perhaps the Mojave rattlesnake (*C. scutulatus*), which some authors suggest should be treated presumptively with at least 10 vials of antivenin because of the likelihood of serious delayed neurologic manifestations without significant local evidence of envenomation.[89]

Elapid Snakebite Envenomation. There are two elapids found in the United States: the western coral snake (*Micrurus euryxanthus*), found in Arizona and New Mexico, and the eastern coral snake (*M. fulvius*), found in the southeastern states from North Carolina, throughout the Gulf states, to Texas. Symptoms of western coral snake bite are generally mild and require only supportive care, whereas the eastern coral snake is clearly capable of causing death. Unlike crotalid envenomation, coral snake bite causes little or no tissue injury at the bite site. The venom is a potent neurotoxin, however, capable of causing paresthesias, fasciculations, nausea and vomiting, diplopia, bulbar paralysis, weakness, respiratory failure, and death. Onset of limb weakness and paresthesias is usually within 1–2 hours, but central signs may be delayed 10 or more hours.[80,83,89]

Wyeth Laboratories produces a horse-derived antivenin for *M. fulvius* that appears to be quite effective, particularly if used soon after envenomation. Because early use is more effective, serious toxicity is delayed, and local bite signs are not reliable predictors of severity, most authors recommend the use of antivenin whenever there is evidence of envenomation by *M. fulvius* and before serious signs are evident. An initial dose of three to six vials is usually adequate, additional antivenin may be indicated for multiple bites or sustained bites when larger venom doses are suspected.[80,89]

Black Widow Spider Envenomation (Latrodectism)

Determining the appropriate role for antivenin to treat *Latrodectus* envenomation may be the most difficult problem faced when treating common envenomations. Despite common misconceptions, there is essentially no risk of permanent tissue or limb dysfunction, and there have been no recent reports of death from widow spider envenomation. Unfortunately, this information does little to comfort the victim of a bite.

The venom causes the uncontrolled release of synaptic transmitter vesicles, which results in variety of signs and symptoms. Acetylcholine release is probably responsible for diaphoresis, as well as muscular fasciculations, cramps, and sustained, painful contractions. Marked hypertension, which is common, is thought to be secondary to norepinephrine release. Older reports of altered mental status, seizures, and respiratory arrest may be due to similar effects in the central nervous system. It is commonly accepted, although not studied, that only infants, the elderly, and those with cardiovascular or cerebrovascular disease are actually at risk for life-threatening complications.[95,96]

Pharmacotherapy, including intravenous calcium chloride or calcium gluconate, benzodiazepines, methocarbamol, and opioid analgesics, is often effective, however relief is generally transient in cases of severe envenomation.[96] These patients may experience agonizing pain, hypertension, and profuse diaphoresis for several days. A single vial of Antivenin (*Latrodectus mactans*) (Merck Sharpe & Dohme), will provide rapid, nearly complete resolution of symptoms in virtually all cases, however, the antivenin does carry the same risks as other equine antisera products and fatal reactions have occurred.

Given that the treatment is potentially more dangerous than the envenomation, the role of antivenin remains controversial. The most conservative recommendation is that antivenin use only be considered in cases that are obviously life-threatening (hypertensive crisis, respiratory compro-

*Determining the appropriate role for antivenin to treat **Latrodectus** envenomation may be the most difficult problem faced when treating common envenomations.*

mise, or seizures), but such cases are extraordinarily rare, if they occur at all. A more moderate position is to also consider antivenin in cases of obvious envenomation in infants, the elderly, or those with known cardiovascular or cerebrovascular disease.

It is our belief that antivenin is often appropriate even when there is no actual threat to life. We consider antivenin therapy when severe envenomation is evident (eg, onset of severe symptoms within 1 hour of a bite, failure of aggressive pharmacotherapy, sustained severe symptoms) and there is no evidence by history or skin testing of probable horse allergy. In such patients, careful informed consent is critical and administration of antivenin should only be done in the appropriate setting (see above). In our anecdotal experience, many patients opt for antivenin, despite the risk of anaphylaxis, rather than suffer intense pain for several days. Unlike other forms of life-threatening envenomation (eg, crotalid), there is generally no harm in trying to control symptoms of latrodectism with calcium, benzodiazepines, and opioids before resorting to the use of antivenin. Administration of antivenin should follow the guidelines described above.

Unlike other forms of life-threatening envenomation (eg, crotalid), there is generally no harm in trying to control symptoms of latrodectism with calcium, benzodiazepines, and opioids before resorting to the use of antivenin.

Other Envenomations (Native to the United States)

There are at least three other antivenins available to treat envenomation by animals native to the United States. Brown recluse spider (*Loxosceles reclusa*) antivenin is only available on an experimental basis from Vanderbilt University.[97] This is a rabbit-derived product that is isolated using affinity chromatography. Although no large-scale safety studies have been conducted, this method yields a highly purified product that would be expected to cause less adverse reaction than cruder products. Studies suggest that it is effective, however, the analysis of these results is limited by the typically late presentation of cases and by difficulties in proving brown recluse envenomation. Nonetheless, it is likely in the near future that recent, proven brown recluse bites (see *Immunodiagnosis of Envenomation*) will be treated with antivenin.

Many scorpions of the genus *Centuroides* can cause painful stings, but only *C. exilicauda* (includes former variants *C. gertschi*, *C. sculpturatus*, and *C. gracilis*) is known to cause serious toxicity. Found in the deserts of Arizona, New Mexico, and California, the sting of these scorpions can cause local pain, signs of sympathomimetic and/or parasympathomimetic excess, and neurologic manifestations including hyperactivity, bizarre posturing, roving eye movements, visual disturbance, hyperesthesia, muscle twitching, and seizures.[98]

A goat-derived antivenin is available only from Iatric Laboratories for patients within the state of Arizona. It appears to be effective, but since supportive care and pharmacotherapy are likely to prevent any permanent morbidity or mortality, the role of antivenin is controversial, as in the case of black widow spider envenomation.

Other Envenomations (International and Exotic)

In the United States, sources of envenomation requiring antivenin are limited to very few culprits, however, this is not the case internationally. There are hundreds of poisonous snakes, spiders, scorpions, marine animals, and fish causing significant health problems in other parts of the world. Table 8 lists many of the venoms thus far used to produce antivenins to these sources.

Envenomation by many of these may be encountered within the United States because of legal or illegal exotic pet ownership, research or zoo animal collections, or at international ports of entry. Most zoos and research facilities will stock a supply of antivenin and are excellent sources of help. For unknown agents, or to access supplies of antivenin from sources around the country, it is wise to immediately contact the nearest regional poison information center for access to the AAPCC/AAZPA antivenom index.

IMMUNODIAGNOSIS OF ENVENOMATION

There are several reasons why precise diagnosis of envenomation has not received much attention in the United States. Relatively few species are capable of causing dangerous envenomation in the United States, most are easily recognizable, and antivenin treatment rarely requires accurate identification. In contrast, there are areas of the world where many lethal, nondescript snakes coexist and proper antivenin treatment requires species identification. For this reason, attempts at immunodiagnosis of envenomation including the precipitin test, gel diffusion, countercurrent electrophoresis, radioimmunoassay (RIA), and enzyme-linked immunosorbent assay (ELISA) have been evolving.[99] Earlier tests have proved either slow or insensitive; RIA and ELISA remain active areas of study. The most sensitive is RIA, however it requires expensive equipment and about 24 hours to run.

The lower cost, easy use, stability of reagents, and rapidity (½–3 hours) of ELISA have made it the most important immunodiagnostic method for assessing envenomation. Plates or tubes coated with rabbit-derived anti-

For unknown agents, or to access supplies of antivenin from sources around the country, it is wise to immediately contact the nearest regional poison information center for access to the AAPCC/AAZPA antivenom index.

TABLE 8   Important Venoms Used in the Production of Antivenins*

Snakes
   Acanthophis antarctica: death adder
   Agkistrodon species (long-nosed pit viper, cantils, mumushis, Malayan pit viper, hundred-pace snake)
   Bitis species (gaboon viper, puff adder, river jack, rhinocros viper)
   Bothrops species (Urutu, fer-de-lance, amazon tree viper, jararaca, jararacussa, Maximillan's viper, jumping pit viper, Brazil's pit viper, cotiara)
   Bungarus species (Indian, Taiwan, and banded kraits)
   Cerastes species (Saharan sand viper, horned viper)
   Crotalus species (eastern diamondback[†], western diamondback[†], Central American, South American, Mexican black-tailed, tiger rattlesnakes)
   Dendroaspis species (eastern green, Jameson's, black, and western green mambas)
   Echis species (saw-scaled, carpet, Arabian vipers)
   Enhydrina schistosa: beaked sea snake
   Hemachatus hemachatus: South African spitting cobra
   Lachesis muta: bushmaster
   Micrurus species (eastern[†] coral Brazilian giant coral snakes)
   Naja species (Egyptian, forest, Indian, Taiwan or Chinese, Central Asian, Philippine, Malayan, Cape, and spitting cobras)
   Notechis scutatus: tiger snake
   Ophiophagus hannah: king cobra
   Oxyuranus scutellatus: taipan
   Pseudechis australis: mulga snake
   Pseudocerastes persicus: Palestine or Persian horned viper
   Pseudonaja texilis: common brown snake
   Trimeresurus species (habu, Chinese habu, green tree viper)
   Vipera species (asp, Russell's, sand, common, latifi, meadow, mountain, long-nosed, snub-nosed, European, Levantine, Orsini's, and Turkish vipers)
Spiders
   Atrax robustus: funnel-web spider
   Latrodectus species (black widow[†], red-back, shoe-button spiders)
   Loxosceles species (brown recluse spider[†])
Scorpions
   Androctonus species
   Buthotus species
   Buthus species
   Centruroides species[†]
   Leirus quiquestriatus
   Mesobuthus eupeus
   Odontobuthus doriae
   Parabuthus species
   Scorpio maurus
   Tityus species
Fish and marine invertebrates
   Chironex fleckeri: box jellyfish
   Scorpaena: scorpionfish
   Synanceia trachanis: stonefish
   Trachinus: weeverfish
   Uranoscopus: stargazers

* Not all-inclusive. Many antivenins are effective against other species.
† Native to the United States.

bodies against a variety of venoms are incubated with serum, urine, bleb aspirate, tissue extract, or other samples. After a wash, enzyme-linked antibodies are added, incubated, and washed. A reagent that reacts with the enzyme to yield a color change is then added and the presence or absence of venom is determined. This method has been widely used, and kits are available in Australia to distinguish between five of the most medically important snakes in that area.

Similar methodology is being developed in the United States for identification of venom and proof of envenomation from native snakes and spiders.[6,99] This is likely to have the most immediate impact on the management of envenomation by brown recluse spiders, mojave rattlesnakes, and eastern coral snakes. Antivenin therapy for these bites is currently problematic because of the difficulty in proving the type of envenomation (brown recluse) or the need to give potentially dangerous therapy before serious symptomatology is evident. Clearly, timely laboratory proof of envenomation would be useful.

For the remaining crotalids, scorpions, and the black widow spider, immunodiagnosis will increase in importance only when more refined antivenins become available. In the case of crotalid envenomation, a single antivenin is currently used to treat all United States species and the indications for dosing are based on clinical findings. Unless the available antivenins change, identification of the species or proof that venom is present would have no bearing on therapy. Other than proving that symptoms were, in fact, due to envenomation and not another disorder, immunodiagnosis would similarly not change current therapy of *Centuroides* stings or *Latrodectus* bites.

References

1. Butler V, Berser S: Antibodies to small molecules: biological and clinical applications. Adv Immunol 17:255, 1973

2. Scherrman JM, Terrien N, Urtizberea M et al: Immunotoxicotherapy: present status and future trends. J Toxicol Clin Toxicol 27:1, 1989

3. Colburn W: Specific antibodies and Fab fragments to alter the pharmacokinetics and reverse the pharmacologic/toxicologic effects of drugs. Drug Metab Rev 11:223, 1980

4. Haber E: Antibodies *in vivo*. Pharmacol Rev 34:77, 1982

5. Butler V: Antibodies as specific antagonists to toxins, drugs and hormones. Pharmacol Rev 34:109, 1982

6. Sullivan JB: Immunotherapy in the poisoned patient. Med Toxicol Adverse Drug Exp 1:47, 1986

7. Rolins DE, Blizgys M: Immunological approach to poisoning. Ann Emerg Med 15:1046, 1986

8. Plotkin SA, Mortimer EA (eds): Vaccines. WB Saunders, Philadelphia, 1988

9. Roitt I (ed): Essential Immunology. 5th ed. Blackwell Scientific Publications, Boston, 1984

10. Jones PT, Dear PH, Foote J et al: Replacing the complimentarity determining regions in a human antibody with those from a mouse. Nature 321:522, 1986

11. Simonsen L: What are the pharmacists dispensing most often? Pharmacy Times 56:56, 1990

12. Litovitz TL, Schmitz B, Baley K: 1989 Annual report of the American Association of Poison Control Centers National Data Collection Systems. Am J Emerg Med 8:394, 1990

13. Goodman Gilman A, Rall T, Nies A, Taylor P (eds): The pharmacologic basis of therapeutics. 8th ed. Pergamon Press, Elmsford, 1990

14. Smith TW: Mechanisms of action and clinical use. N Engl J Med 318:358, 1988

15. Smith TW, Antman EM, Friedman PL et al: Digitalis glycosides: mechanisms and manifestations of toxicity. Prog Cardiovasc Dis 27:21, 1984

16. Butler V, Chen J: Digoxin specific antibodies. Proc Natl Acad Sci U S A 57:71, 1967

17. Beller GA, Smith TW, Abelmann WH et al: Digitalis intoxication: a prospective clinical study with serum level correlations. N Engl J Med 284:989, 1971

18. Duhme DW, Greenblatt DJ, Kock-Weser J: Reduction of digoxin toxicity associated with measurement of serum levels: a report from the Boston collaborative Drug Surveillance Program. Ann Intern Med 80:516, 1974

19. Ordog GJ, Benaron S, Bhasin V: Serum digoxin levels and mortality in 5100 patients. Ann Emerg Med 16:32, 1987

20. D'Angio RG, Stevenson JG, Lively BT et al: Therapeutic drug monitoring: improved performance through educational intervention. Ther Drug Monit 12:173, 1990

21. Schmidt DH, Butler VP: Immunological protection against digoxin toxicity. J Clin Invest 50:866, 1971

22. Schmidt DH, Butler VP: Reversal of digoxin toxicity with specific antibodies. J Clin Invest 50:1738, 1971

23. Curd J, Smith TW, Jaton J et al: The isolation of digoxin specific antibody and its use in reversing the effects of digoxin. Proc Natl Acad Sci U S A 68:2401, 1971

24. Butler VP, Smith TW, Schmidt DH et al: Immunological reversal of the effects of digoxin. Fed Proc 326:2235, 1977

25. Butler VP, Schmidt DH, Smith TW et al: Effects of sheep digoxin: specific antibodies and their Fab fragments on digoxin pharmacokinetics in dogs. J Clin Invest 59:345, 1977

26. Lloyd BL, Smith TW: Contrasting rates of reversal of digoxin toxicity by digoxin: specific IgG and Fab fragments. Circulation 58:280, 1978

27. Smith TW, Lloyd BL, Spicer N et al: Immunogenicity and kinetics of distribution and elimination of sheep digoxin specific IgG and Fab fragments in the rabbit and baboon. Clin Exp Immunol 36:384, 1979

28. Antman EM, Wenger TL, Butler VP et al: Treatment of 150 cases of life-threatening digitalis intoxication with digoxin specific Fab antibody fragments: final report of multicenter study. Circulation 81:1744, 1990

29. Bismuth C, Gaultier M, Conso F et al: Hyperkalemia in acute digitalis poisoning: prognostic significance and therapeutic implications. J Toxicol Clin Toxicol 6:153, 1973

30. Postmarketing Surveillance Study of Digibind Interim Report to Contributors (July 1986–July 1987) Burroughs Wellcome

31. Eagle KA, Haber E, DeSanctis RW et al (eds): The practice of cardiology. 2nd edition. Little, Brown, Boston, 1989

32. Smith TW: New advances in the assessment and treatment of digitalis toxicity. J Clin Pharmacol 25:522, 1985

33. Smolarz A, Roesch E, Lenz E et al: Digoxin specific antibody (Fab) fragments in 34 cases of severe digitalis intoxication. J Toxicol Clin Toxicol 23:327, 1985

34. Ekins BR, Watanabe AS: Acute digoxin poisonings: review of therapy. Am J Hosp Pharm 35:268, 1978

35. Smith TW, Willerson JT: Suicidal and accidental digoxin ingestion: report of five cases with serum digoxin level correlations. Circulation 44:29, 1971

36. Lewander WJ, Gaudreault P, Einhorn A et al: Acute pediatric digoxin ingestion. Am J Dis Child 140:770, 1986

37. Springer M, Olson KR, Feaster W: Acute massive digoxin overdose: survival without use of digitalis specific antibodies. Am J Emerg Med 4:364, 1986

38. Zucker AR, Lacinda SJ, Das Gupta DS et al: Fab fragments of digoxin specific antibodies used to reverse ventricular fibrillation induced by digoxin ingestion in a child. Pediatrics 70:468, 1982

39. Hastreiter AR, John EG, Nander Hoist RL: Digitalis, digitalis antibodies, digitalis like immunoreactive substances, and sodium homeostasis: a review. Clin Perinatol 15:491, 1988

40. Presti S, Freidman D, Saslow J et al: Digoxin toxicity in a premature infant: treatment with Fab fragments of digoxin specific antibodies. Pediatr Cardiol 6:91, 1985

41. Lalonde RL, Deshpande R, Hamilton PP et al: Acceleration of digoxin clearance by activated charcoal. Clin Pharmacol Ther 37:367, 1985

42. Park GD, Goldberg MJ, Spector R et al: The effects of activated charcoal on digoxin and digitoxin clearance. Drug Intell Clin Pharm 19:937, 1985

43. Boldy DA, Smart V, Vale JA: Multiple doses of activated charcoal in digoxin poisoning. Lancet 2:1076, 1985

44. Pond S, Jacobs M, Marks J et al: Treatment of digitoxin overdose with oral activated charcoal. Lancet 2:1177, 1981

45. Digibind. p. 755. In: Physicians desk reference 1991. 45th ed. Edward R Barnhart Medical Economics Data, Oradell, 1991

46. Smith TW, Haber E, Yeatman L et al: Reversal of advanced digoxin intoxication with Fab fragments of digoxin specific antibodies. N Engl J Med 294:797, 1976

47. Schaumann W, Kaufmann B, Neubert P et al: Kinetics of the Fab fragments of digoxin antibodies and of bound digoxin in patients with severe digoxin intoxication. Eur J Clin Pharmacol 30:527, 1986

48. Gibb I, Adams PC, Parnham AJ et al: Plasma digoxin: assay anomalies in Fab treated patients. Br J Clin Pharmacol 16:445, 1983

49. Argyle JC: Effect of digoxin antibodies on TDX digoxin assay. Clin Chem 32:1616, 1986

50. Soldin S: Digoxin: issues and controversies. Clin Chem 32:5, 1986

51. Lemon M, Andrews DJ, Binks AM et al: Concentrations of free serum digoxin after treatment with antibody fraagments. Br Med J 295:1520, 1987

52. Hursting MJ, Raisys VA, Opheim KE et al: Determination of free digoxin concentrations in serum for monitoring Fab treatment of digoxin overdose. Clin Chem 33:1652, 1987

53. Graves SW, Brown B, Valdes R: An endogenous digoxin-like substance in patients with renal impairment. Ann Intern Med 99:604, 1983

54. Vasdez S, Johnson E, Longerich L et al: Plasma endogenous digitalis-like factors in healthy individuals and in dialysis-dependent and kidney transplant patients. Clin Nephrol 27:169, 1987

55. Kelly RA, O'Hara DS, Canessa MG et al: Characterization of digitalis-like factors in human plasma. J Biol Chem 260:11396, 1985

56. Frisolone J, Sylvia LM, Gelwan J et al: False positive serum digoxin concentrations determined by three digoxin assays on patients with liver disease. Clin Pharm 7:444, 1988

57. Karboski JA, Godley PJ, Frohna PA et al: Marked digoxin-like immunoreactive factor interference with an enzyme immunoassay. Drug Intell Clin Pharm 2:703, 1988

58. Vinge E, Ekman R: Partial characterization of endogenous digoxin-like substance in human urine. Ther Drug Monit 10:8, 1988

59. Koren G, Parker R: Interpretation of excessive serum concentrations of digoxin in children. Am J Cardiol 55:1210, 1985

60. Lindenbaum J, Rund D, Butler VP et al: Inactivation of digoxin by the gut flora: reversal by antibiotic therapy. N Engl J Med 305:789, 1981

61. Koren G, Deatie D, Soldin S: Agonal elevation in serum digoxin concentrations in infants and children long after cessation of therapy. Crit Care Med 16:793, 1988

62. Durham G, Califf RM: Digoxin toxicity in renal insufficiency treated with digoxin immune Fab. Prim Cardiol 1:31, 1988

63. Sinclair AJ, Hewick DS, Johnston PC et al: Kinetics of digoxin and anti-digoxin antibody fragments during treatment of digoxin toxicity. Br J Clin Pharmacol 28:352, 1989

64. Nollet H, Verhaaren H, Stroobandt R et al: Delayed elimination of digoxin antidolum determined by RIA. J Clin Pharmacol 29:41, 1989

65. Erdmann E, Mair W, Knedel M et al: Digitalis intoxication and treatment with digoxin antibody fragments in renal failure. Klin Wochenschr 67:16, 1989

66. Colucci R, Choses M, Kluger J et al: The pharmacokinetics of digoxin immune Fab, total digoxin and free digoxin in patients with renal impairment. Pharmacotherapy 9:175, 1989

67. Nuwayhid N, Johnson G: Digoxin elimination in a functionally anephric patient after digoxin specific Fab fragment therapy. Ther Drug Monit 11:680, 1989

68. Sherron PA, Gelband H: Reversal of digoxin toxicity with Fab fragments in a pediatric patient with acute renal failure. Symposium 1985–San Francisco, Burroughs Wellcome Sponsor.

69. Savin H, Marcus L, Margel S et al: Treatment of adverse digitalis effect by hemoperfusion through columns with antidigoxin antibodies bound to agarose polyacrolein microsphere beads. Am Heart J 113:1078, 1987

70. Marcus L, Margel S, Savin H et al: Therapy of digoxin intoxication in dogs by specific hemoperfusion through agarose polyacrolein microsphere beads: antidigoxin antibodies. Am Heart J 110:30, 1985

71. Quaife EJ, Banner W, Vernon D et al: Failure of CAVH to remove digoxin Fab complex in piglets. Clin Toxicol 28:61, 1990

72. Lechat P, Mudgett-Hunter M, Margolies M et al: Reversal of lethal digoxin toxicity in guinea pigs using monoclonal antibodies and Fab fragments. J Pharmacol Exp Ther 229:210, 1984

73. Pentel P, Pond SM, Schoof D: Redistribution into plasma of tracer doses of desipramine by anti-desipramine antiserum in rats. Biochem Pharmacol 2:293, 1987

74. Liu D, Purssell R, Levy JG: Production and characterization of high affinity monoclonal antibodies to cyclic antidepressant molecules. J Toxicol Clin Toxicol 25:527, 1987

75. Hursting M, Opheim K, Raisys VA: Tricyclic antidepressant specific Fab fragments alter the distribution and elimination of desipramine in the rabbit: a model for overdose treatment. J Toxicol Clin Toxicol 27:53, 1989

76. Pentel PR, Brunn GJ, Pond SM et al: Pretreatment with drug-specific antibody reduces desipramine cardiotoxicity in rats. (Abstr) Vet Hum Toxicol 1990

77. Sullivan JB: past, present, and future immunotherapy of snake venom poisoning. Ann Emerg Med 16:938, 1987

78. Jurkovich GJ, Lutherman A, McCullar K et al: Complications of *Crotalidae* antivenom therapy. J Trauma 28:1032, 1988

79. Chippaux JP, Goyffon M: Producers of antivenomous antisera. Toxicon 21:739, 1983

80. Russell FE: Snake venom poisoning. JB Lippincott, Philadelphia, 1980

81. Podgorny G: Venomous reptiles and arthropods of the United States and Canada. In Haddad LM, Winchester JF (eds): Clinical management of poisoning and drug overdose. WB Saunders, Philadelphia, 1983

82. Russell FE, Carlson RW, Wainschel J, Osborn AH: Snake venom poisoning in the United States: experience with 550 cases. JAMA 233:341, 1975

83. Russell FE: Snake venom poisoning in the United States. Ann Rev Med 31:247, 1980

84. Levy HH, Rozen MF, Morris JM: Anaphylactic and anaphylactoid reactions: a review. Spine 11:282, 1986

85. Smith PL, Kagey-Sobotka A, Bleeker ER et al: Physiologic manifestations of human anaphylaxis. J Clin Invest 66:1072, 1980

86. Naguwe SM, Nelson BL: Human serum sickness. Clin Rev Allergy 3:117, 1985

87. Erffmeyer JE: Serum sickness. Ann Allergy 56:105, 1986

88. Malasit P, Warrell DA, Chantharanich P et al: Prediction, prevention, and mechanism of early (anaphylactic) reactions in victims of snake bites. Br Med J 292:17, 1986

89. Sullivan JB, Wingert WA: Reptile bites. In Auerbach PS, Geehr EC (eds): Management of wilderness and environmental emergencies. 2nd ed. CV Mosby, St. Louis, 1989

90. Kunkel DB, Curry SC, Vance MV, Ryan PJ: Reptile envenomations. J Toxicol Clin Toxicol 21:503, 1983–84

91. Sutherland SK: Serum reactions: an analysis of commercial antivenoms and the possible role of anticomplementary activity in de novo reactions to antivenoms and antitoxins. Med J Austr 1:613, 1977

92. Russell FE: Treatment of rattlesnake bites. West J Med 141:245, 1984

93. Buntain WL: Successful venomous snakebite neutralization with massive antivenin infusion in a child. J Trauma 23:1012, 1983

94. Dart RC, Sullivan JB, Troutman W: Management of severe rattlesnake envenomation without antivenin. Vet Hum Toxicol 28:485, 1985

95. Maretic Z: Latrodectism: variations in clinical manifestations provoked by Latrodectus species of spiders. Toxicon 21:457, 1983

96. Rauber A: Black widow spider bites. J Toxicol Clin Toxicol 21:473, 1983–84

97. Rees R, Campbell D, Rieger E, King LE: The diagnosis and treatment of brown recluse spider bites. Ann Emerg Med 16:945, 1987

98. Banner W Jr: Scorpion envenomation. In Auerbach PS, Geehr EC (eds): Management of wilderness and environmental emergencies. 2nd ed. CV Mosby, St. Louis, 1989

99. Minton SA: Present tests for detection of snake venom: clinical applications. Ann Emerg Med 16:932, 1987

EVALUATION AND MANAGEMENT OF THE AGITATED PATIENT IN THE INTENSIVE CARE UNIT

KATHLEEN A. DELANEY, MD, ABMT[†]

Psychiatric syndromes are common in patients admitted to the intensive care unit, and their etiologies are multifold. Delays in the recognition of medical and surgical conditions in patients with chronic psychiatric diagnoses are common.[1] Failure to appreciate signs of physical illness at an early stage in the patient with chronic psychiatric illness may result in intensive care admission when the disease entity progresses to an obviously recognizable state.[1] In addition, acute disease processes often precipitate or exacerbate a preexisting functional psychiatric disorder. Persons with normal neuropsychiatric functioning, particularly the elderly, frequently demonstrate organic behavioral and cognitive disturbances in association with serious physical illnesses that do not involve the central nervous system.[2-5] Finally, behavioral and cognitive disturbances may reflect the direct effects of medical or structural disease on the brain. Such patients are appropriately admitted to the intensive care unit for diagnosis and treatment. This chapter will focus on the identification, diagnosis, and management of medically ill patients with acute organic brain syndromes.

RECOGNITION OF DELIRIUM

The term "organic brain syndrome" implies a toxic, metabolic, or structural abnormality that impairs normal brain function. The brain may be primarily affected (as in the patient with meningitis, brain tumor, or cerebrovascular

The term "organic brain syndrome" implies a toxic, metabolic, or structural abnormality that impairs normal brain function.

[†] Assistant Professor, Division of Emergency Medicine, University of Texas Southwestern Medical School, Dallas, Texas

accident) or secondarily affected (as in the patient with drug toxicity, vitamin deficiency, uremia, or sepsis).[2,3] The term "functional psychiatric disorder" implies an abnormal mental state due to an (usually preexisting) affective or thought disorder. The most important initial task in the evaluation of the patient with an altered mental status is the search for clues that may help to differentiate between a functional disturbance and one with an organic etiology. Such clues can often be found in a careful history, physical examination, and mental status examination. The differentiation of organic from functional disorders is somewhat artificial, as all neurologic and psychologic functions are dependent on neurochemical processes and hence are "organic" in their basis. In addition, it is now well recognized that some patients with organic brain disease may present with symptoms clinically indistinguishable from those of a functional psychiatric disorder.[6-11] Despite these uncertainties in patients with apparent functional presentations, clinical features elicited by the mental status examination allow ready identification of the patient with an acute organic brain syndrome or delirium. Patients whose examinations suggest delirium require urgent investigation for a treatable cause. Controlled studies report mortality rates in a general medical population as high as 13% for patients with delirium, compared to 6% in matched controls.[12] Raw mortality figures for delirious patients as high as 22% have been reported.[13] The increased mortality in delirious patients is correlated with the severity of the underlying illness.[4,5] Deaths in patients with unrecognized delirium are frequently attributed to preventable causes.[3,14,15]

Elderly patients are at significant risk of developing delirium as a consequence of illness. Delirium has been demonstrated in 40–50% of hospitalized patients over the age of 70.[16,17] A recent investigation of 229 hospitalized patients over 70 years of age detected delirium in 22% (this study excluded patients with metastatic disease and patients from nursing homes). Variables independently associated with the presence of delirium in this population were abnormal serum sodium, illness severity, chronic cognitive impairment, hyperthermia or hypothermia, and the use of psychoactive drugs.[4] These patients are at risk of falls and potential morbidity from medical interventions related to management of the behavioral disturbance. Restraints, psychotropic medications, nasogastric tubes, and urinary catheters predispose to thrombophlebitis and pulmonary embolism, aspiration pneumonia, urinary tract infection, and sepsis.[4,16]

The essential feature of delirium that distinguishes it from a functional psychiatric disorder is the global nature of cognitive impairment. The delirious patient has distur-

Clinical features elicited by the mental status examination allow ready identification of the patient with an acute organic brain syndrome.

bances in alertness, perception, thinking, attention, and memory.[2,11,14,15] The patient with a functional psychiatric disturbance has a specific selective impairment of thought processes with preservation of many other aspects of cognitive functioning. A normal level of alertness and orientation are always present in uncomplicated functional psychiatric illness, however difficult it may be to demonstrate the extent of orientation in the agitated psychotic patient. The delirious patient may be alternatively somnolent and difficult to arouse or hyperalert and combative. Agitation and confusion fluctuate and are particularly exacerbated at night. The patient with chronic dementia is distinguished from the delirious patient by the demonstration of a normal level of consciousness and relatively normal attention. A history of preexisting cognitive disturbance should also be present in the patient with chronic dementia.[2,12] In delirium, it is not uncommon to see progression from a hyperalert, agitated state to stupor and coma as a manifestation of increasing global neurologic impairment.[18] Sleep-wake disturbances such as insomnia or inappropriate drowsiness are always present in delirium.[2,7] Exaggerated or inappropriate responses to the environment are precipitated by diminished perceptive capacities. The patient may leap up to answer the doorbell (a telephone), mistake the folded bedclothes for his or her spouse, or engage in incoherent conversation with people who are not present. Although most commonly visual, misperceptions can occur in all sensory modalities. They may be illusions that the patient recognizes as false, or hallucinations, which the patient believes to be real.[2,7] Psychomotor disturbances are manifest as restlessness or repetitive picking at the bedclothes, restraints, or intravenous apparatus. A decrease in normal psychomotor activity may also herald the onset of delirium.[2,7] Agitated or disruptive behavior is present in fewer than half of delirious hospitalized elderly patients. Incontinence and an increased incidence of falls characterize the onset of delirium in many elderly patients.[4,16]

In the delirious patient, attention, memory, and orientation are impaired in proportion to the degree of the global insult. Disorientation to time appears first. The patient is as likely to be unable to recall the year as the month. This is followed by more severe disorientation to place, then to person. The patient who knows the date yet cannot recall his own name is unlikely to have an organic disturbance. As in the more chronic, global cognitive disturbance of dementia, distant memory is more preserved than is the memory of recent events.[18]

A normal level of alertness and orientation are always present in uncomplicated functional psychiatric illness.

Incontinence and an increased incidence of falls characterize the onset of delirium in many elderly patients.

*The delusions
associated with
delirium fluctuate and
suggest confusion of
thought rather than
the highly organized,
bizarre, and persistent
delusions that
characterize
schizophrenic illness.*

*Personality
disturbances
characterized by
paranoid or abusive
behavior may occur as
an initial
manifestation of an
evolving delirium and
distract the
evaluating physician
from the investigation
of serious underlying
disease.*

Impairment of intellectual processes is manifest as the inability to do calculations, the inability to perform abstractions and a loss of general knowledge.[3] The delusions associated with delirium fluctuate and suggest confusion of thought rather than the highly organized, bizarre, and persistent delusions that characterize schizophrenic illness.[2,7] The patient who states "I was dragged off my planet and brought to Bellevue by para-astronauts" (or astro-medics) demonstrates orientation and evidence of a complex delusional system typical of a psychotic patient. A delirious patient found on the street and brought by ambulance who states "My son drove me here from home" evidences disorientation and confusion inconsistent with a functional psychiatric diagnosis. The affect of the delirious patient, like the psychotic patient, is often angry, irritable, or fearful.[2] The organic patient's mood fluctuates, however, while the affect of the psychotic patient is generally consistent. The intoxicated or demented patient who moves rapidly from agitated anger to tears provides a familiar example of lability of affect in the patient with an organic brain syndrome.

Personality disturbances characterized by paranoid or abusive behavior may occur as an initial manifestation of an evolving delirium and distract the evaluating physician from the investigation of serious underlying disease. These patients are occasionally brought to the attention of a physician in a critically deteriorated state hours following arrest for disorderly conduct.

A simple and ordered screen for mental status abnormalities should be developed by each clinician. The Mini-Mental State examination as described by Folstein et al. is a simple test that generates a point score that can be used to follow subtle deterioration or improvement in the mental state. The method was tested and used to predict the absence of cognitive dysfunction in psychiatric patients.[19] Jacobs et al. developed a brief mental status examination that was used to identify the presence of cognitive dysfunction in patients on a medical ward.[20] A much more complex mental status examination appropriate to detailed neurological assessment of the organic patient is described by Strub and Black.[21]

The mental status examination should first assess the level of consciousness. The Glasgow Coma Scale was initially developed as a tool to predict outcome in patients with head trauma and has no predictive value in nontraumatized patients. However, its familiar components (eye opening, motor, and verbal responses) provide a useful means of describing the sensorium of any depressed patient and of following changes in the level of consciousness. It is a gross test and is not useful in patients with subtle impairment where the presence of organic disturbance is in question. Simple descriptors (lethargic, drowsy, stuporous, comatose) may also suffice for the individual examiner but do not allow accurate documentation or identification of changes over time when multiple examiners are involved.

The quality and coherence of spontaneous speech should be noted, as should any paucity of movement or the presence of purposeless or repetitive movements. The patient's affect should also be noted.

Orientation should not be assumed even in an apparently bright and verbal patient. Orientation to person is intact except in severely impaired patients. Questions assessing orientation to time start with the specific (day of the month) and proceed to the general (month, season, and year). Orientation to the patient's location (town, state) and situation (doctors, hospital) should also be determined.

Orientation should not be assumed even in an apparently bright and verbal patient.

Attention is tested by the immediate ability to repeat a series of numbers. Attention may be so impaired that no further meaningful assessment of mental status can be accomplished. More complex attention tasks, which should be intact in the completely normal patient, include the patient's ability to spell his or her name backwards and to subtract "serial sevens" from 100. "Serial sevens" also tests the ability to do calculations.

Short-term memory is tested by a capacity to recall three objects 5 minutes after the patient has been able to repeat them back to the examiner. Long-term memory and general knowledge are examined by asking about historical events compatible with the patient's age, national origin, and educational level. Abstraction can be tested by eliciting the meaning of proverbs ("A rolling stone gathers no moss" or "People who live in glass houses shouldn't throw stones"). Lesions of the non-dominant hemisphere are detected by constructional tasks (draw a clock, copy a star, Greek cross, triangle). The dominant hemisphere is tested by word-finding abilities (identify a pen or watch, "Name as many animals as you can" or "Name as many words as you can that start with 'H'"); verbal comprehension ("Touch your nose" or "Put the pen on the table between yourself and the glass"); complex repetition ("Repeat 'If he were to come I would go' or 'God save the commonwealth of Massachussets'"); reading comprehension (CLOSE YOUR EYES); and the ability to write a coherent sentence.

ORGANIC ETIOLOGIES OF APPARENT FUNCTIONAL PSYCHIATRIC ILLNESS

The differentiation between organic and functional illness is blurred by the recognition that very limited and selective cognitive impairment may also accompany localized organic disturbances. Specific organic disorders appear to predispose to specific organic brain syndromes.[7,8,11] The *Diagnostic and Statistical Manual of Mental Disorders* describes five organic brain syndromes where cognitive impairment is much more circumscribed than that seen in patients with delirium.[7] These are the amnestic, delusional, hallucinosis, affective, and personality syndromes.

Localized injury to the mammillary bodies, temporal lobes, or fornices results in an inability to learn new material accompanied by preservation of alertness, attention, some intellectual abilities, personality function, and a variable amount of old learned material. This is seen in patients with thiamine deficiency, vascular insufficiency, infarction, dysrhythmias or infection (especially herpes encephalitis) affecting the temporal lobes, and as a consequence of significant head trauma.[7,11,22] Although we associate thiamine deficiency with ethanol abuse, any patient who is nutritionally deprived due to anorexia, vomiting, malabsorption, or even dieting is at a risk of thiamine deficiency.[11,23] It has also been reported in hemodialysis patients due to dialysis of water-soluble thiamine.[24] Acute niacin deficiency precipitated by increased metabolism following administration of thiamine and pyridoxine in the nutritionally deprived patient may also result in delayed encephalopathy.[25]

Apparent psychotic episodes characterized by delusions of reference, persecution, or infestation can be seen in patients with vitamin B_{12} deficiency, temporal lobe epilepsy, post-ictal states, or dementia.[7,11,26,27] These patients may also experience auditory hallucinations and exhibit bizarre appearance and psychomotor disturbance such as hypervigilance and stereotyped repetitive behaviours. Attention, orientation, alertness, and other aspects of normal cognitive functioning are preserved.[7,11] It is important to recognize that the neuropsychiatric effects of vitamin B_{12} deficiency frequently appear prior to the development of suggestive hematologic manifestations such as macrocytosis and anemia.[28]

A number of drugs may provoke psychotic reactions that, in the absence of history, are difficult to distinguish clinically from schizophrenia in terms of the manifestations of the thought disorder and preservation of the sensorium.

Although we associate thiamine deficiency with ethanol abuse, any patient who is nutritionally deprived due to anorexia, vomiting, malabsorption, or even dieting is at a risk of thiamine deficiency.

It is important to recognize that the neuropsychiatric effects of vitamin B_{12} deficiency frequently appear prior to the development of suggestive hematologic manifestations such as macrocytosis and anemia.

These include, but are not limited to, corticosteroids, dopaminergic and sympathetic agents, non-steroidal anti-inflammatory drugs, and antiarrhythmics.[8,9,29–31] Sympathetic stimulant drugs of abuse such as cocaine or amphetamine and its congeners acutely cause psychomotor agitation, elation, grandiosity, and hypervigilance in association with physical manifestations of sympathetic stimulation such as mydriasis, fever, tachycardia, hypertension, diaphoresis, and vomiting.[7] Phencyclidine and its congeners cause variable and less predictable signs of autonomic stimulation. The most consistent finding in the patient with phencyclidine toxicity is the presence of nystagmus, usually in all fields of gaze.[32] Commonly abused hallucinogens such as lysergic acid diethylamide (LSD), psilocybin, and tetrahydrocannabinol (marijuana) may cause paranoia, agitation, impairment of judgment, and visual hallucinations in an otherwise alert and oriented patient.[33] While drug-related psychosis is usually short-lived and resolves as the signs of autonomic stimulation resolve, cocaine, phencyclidine, and amphetamines may lead to a delusional state that persists beyond the acute effects of the drug. The delusions are persecutory and manifested by ideas of reference, aggressiveness and hostility against perceived enemies, extreme anxiety, and psychomotor agitation.[7] These characteristic delusions have been attributed to the dopaminergic effects of these agents.[34] Angrist showed that persistent psychoses clinically identical to schizophrenic psychosis could be induced by amphetamines in nonschizophrenic volunteers. The signs of thought disorder were reversed by the (presumably) dopaminergic blocking effects of haloperidol.[9] Acute psychotic episodes indistinguishable from functional psychoses have recently been associated with HIV infection in patients without organic central nervous system disease demonstrable at the time of presentation. In most cases, these episodes responded to drug therapy and did not persist.[6,10]

Frightening tactile illusions or hallucinations leading to a sensation of "bugs crawling under the skin" occur characteristically in patients who abuse cocaine or amphetamines. This may result in dermal injury caused by the patient's attempt to rid himself or herself of the parasites.[9,35] Sensory illusions occur in "alcoholic hallucinosis," a rare form of ethanol withdrawal. These patients have a clear sensorium, intact memory, and no other evidence of thought disorder. Although the illusions are usually auditory and of a perverse sexual or persecutory nature, they may also be visual.[36–38]

Organic affective disturbances may be clinically indistinguishable from those that have a functional etiology. Al-

The most consistent finding in the patient with phencyclidine toxicity is the presence of nystagmus, usually in all fields of gaze.

Organic affective disturbances may be clinically indistinguishable from those that have a functional etiology.

though depression has been most widely associated with reserpine administration, many drugs including cimetidine, propranolol, and methyldopa also cause depression, as do disturbances of thyroid, parathyroid, and adrenal function.[7,11,39–42] Recently, severe depression has been reported as a manifestation of central nervous system infection with *Borrelia burgdorferi*, the spirochete that causes Lyme Disease.[43] Acute mania has been reported with insults to the right hemisphere associated with metastatic tumors, cerebral infarction, and subarachnoid hemorrhage.[44–46] Other drugs including central nervous system stimulants, levodopa, and monoamine oxidase inhibitors have been associated with acute manic episodes.[8,11,30,44] Thyrotoxicosis has been mistaken for and treated as mania.[47]

ETIOLOGIES OF DELIRIUM

The differential diagnosis of delirium is extensive and includes many infectious, metabolic, toxic, and structural etiologies.[2,3,11] The etiologies are readily grouped into four classes: (1) processes that directly affect the brain, such as brain tumors, cerebrovascular accidents, central nervous system infections and head trauma; (2) systemic diseases or metabolic disturbances that affect the brain, such as hypoglycemia, renal failure with uremia, chronic obstructive pulmonary disease with hypercapnia, hepatic failure, vasculitis, and other metabolic and endocrine disorders; (3) exogenous toxins; and (4) drug withdrawal syndromes.[2] Structural neurologic lesions that may present as delirium include cerebral frontal lobe contusion, subdural hematoma, subarachnoid hemorrhage, and rare focal central nervous system lesions.[18,48] In the elderly, systemic illness is more frequently implicated in the etiology of delirium.[49] However, it is essential to exclude structural or infectious brain disease as the cause of delirium in these patients. Other processes such as myocardial infarction, abdominal catastrophe, localized infection, malignancy, or dehydration should also be carefully sought.[49] In cases where the diagnosis of delirium appears most certainly related to drug intoxication or withdrawal from a sedative hypnotic agent such as ethanol, a barbiturate, or a benzodiazepine, complicating structural or infectious etiologies must obligatorily be considered. In a study by Baden of causes of death in methadone users, approximately 50% died of drug overdose, 25% of trauma, and 25% of infection.[50] The chronic intravenous substance abuser and the chronic alcoholic patient are at high risk for infectious or traumatic etiologies of the altered mental state.

In cases where the diagnosis of delirium appears most certainly related to drug intoxication or withdrawal from a sedative hypnotic agent such as ethanol, a barbiturate, or a benzodiazepine, complicating structural or infectious etiologies must obligatorily be considered.

The elderly are especially susceptible to the central nervous system effects of drugs, and almost any medication may be suspected. The 1989 Medical Letter lists over 100 drugs that have been associated with psychiatric symptoms.[51] These include albuterol, levodopa, amiodarone, cimetidine, ephedrine, digoxin, amantidine, non-steroidal antiinflammatory agents, and corticosteroids. Patients with Parkinson's disease or patients with psychiatric disorders who are chronically treated with anticholinergic drugs are particularly at risk for medication-related organic brain dysfunction.[2,49,52,53]

The elderly are especially susceptible to the central nervous system effects of drugs, and almost any medication may be suspected.

HISTORY

The history provides important clues to the diagnosis of organic etiologies of apparent psychiatric illness and will confirm the presence of an acute global organic brain disorder. Reports from family or friends of an acute or recent change from a previously normal state of neuropsychiatric functioning should suggest an underlying organic etiology. Since most functional psychiatric disorders present before the age of 40, older patients with apparent psychiatric presentations should be carefully screened for organic etiologies.[2,3,11] Conversely, a previous history of psychiatric illness supports that diagnosis when the mental status examination is consistent with a functional disorder. A history of problems with attention or memory, difficulty with previously mastered cognitive tasks, deterioration of functioning in the workplace, or apathy also supports the possibility of organic illness. Recent head injury, headaches, incontinence, clumsiness, difficulty in walking, or seizures strongly suggest an organic etiology of the mental status change.[11] The clinician should record a detailed examination of drug or alcohol use, including all prescribed and over-the-counter medications, and medications available to other family members. Particular attention should be given to the practice of self-medication with vitamins or herbal preparations, antihistamines, and salicylate-containing products. Any significant current or past illnesses and any recent unexplained symptoms such as fever or weight loss may also be important clues. The possibility of HIV infection should be considered in at-risk patients who present with psychotic symptoms without previous history of psychiatric illness.[6,10]

PHYSICAL EXAMINATION

The physical examination of the delirious or agitated patient provides important diagnostic information regarding the etiology of the behavioral disturbance. Vital sign abnormalities are especially useful. Hypothermia is associated with sepsis, liver disease, hypoglycemia, or drug overdose. Fever, tachycardia, and mydriasis with tremor and diaphoresis suggest poisoning with a sympathomimetic agent, thyrotoxicosis, or the intense sympathetic stimulation of sedative hypnotic withdrawal.[54] Fever, tachycardia, and mydriasis associated with dry, flushed skin, absent bowel sounds, and urinary retention provide evidence for poisoning with an anticholinergic agent.[55] Patients with chronic anticholinergic poisoning may have no such diagnostic findings.[52,53] Fever, of course, also indicates the possibility of infection.

Signs characteristic of poisoning with cholinergic agents, such as organophosphate insecticides, include miotic pupils, increased salivation, lacrimation, bronchorrhea, diaphoresis, and diarrhea. The heart rate is often unexpectedly increased in these patients. This may be a consequence of hypoxia secondary to increased bronchial secretions or related to acetylcholinesterase blockade in cholinergic sympathetic ganglia.[56]

Metabolic causes of delirium are readily suspected on the basis of the physical examination. Cyanosis suggests hypoxia or methemoglobinemia. Cachexia, alopecia, thyromegaly, and lid lag or proptosis support a clinical diagnosis of thyrotoxicosis. The presence of spider angiomata, abdominal venous distension, icterus, and ascites characterizes hepatic encephalopathy. Funduscopic evidence of high-grade hypertensive retinopathy associated with a diastolic pressure greater than 130 mmHg suggests the diagnosis of hypertensive encephalopathy.[57] Abnormal intracorneal pigmentation (a Kayser-Fleischer ring) will be present in patients with mental status abnormality secondary to Wilson's disease.[58]

Physical evidence of drug abuse such as nasal septum perforation or track marks should be sought. Odors characteristic of uremia, hepatic failure, or ketoacidosis may be apparent. In addition, the odors of ethanol, hydrocarbons, insecticides, and cyanide provide important clues to an underlying toxic diagnosis.

The neurologic examination contributes substantially to the diagnosis of delirium. Asterixis and myoclonus are relatively nonspecific neurologic signs associated with toxic disturbances, such as poisoning with lithium or an anticholinergic agent, or with metabolic disturbances including hepatic or uremic encephalopathy or hypercapnea. These signs are not seen in uncomplicated psychiatric illness and are virtually pathognomonic of delirium.[3] Muscular rigidity has many etiologies and often precedes the development of life-threatening hyperthermia. Rigidity may ac-

Asterixis and myoclonus are relatively nonspecific neurologic signs associated with toxic disturbances, such as poisoning with lithium or an anticholinergic agent, or with metabolic disturbances including hepatic or uremic encephalopathy or hypercapnea. These signs are not seen in uncomplicated psychiatric illness and are virtually pathognomonic of delirium.

company an exacerbation of parkinsonism,[59,60] poisoning with a monoamine oxidase inhibitor,[61] or a severe extrapyramidal reaction to neuroleptic agents (the so-called neuroleptic malignant syndrome).[62,63] The presence of focal findings on the neurological examination is usually indicative of structural abnormalities, but transient focality may be associated with diffuse metabolic injury, including hypoxia, uremia, hypertensive or hepatic encephalopathy, and hypoglycemia.[18,57] Prominent nystagmus is a nonspecific sign of organic central nervous system disturbance. It is commonly seen in patients with phencyclidine poisoning, ethanol intoxication and withdrawal, and various structural lesions.[18,32]

Changes that occur in the physical examination during a period of observation also provide useful diagnostic information. Signs of sympathetic stimulation seen in the agitated psychotic patient usually resolve early in the course of treatment, as do vital sign and mental status abnormalities in the postictal state or in the patient with low-dose exposure to a short-acting sympathetic stimulant such as cocaine. Patients with more life-threatening problems such as severe sedative hypnotic withdrawal, space-occupying intercranial lesions, or central nervous system infection show persistence or deterioration of mental status and vital sign abnormalities.[18]

The presence of focal findings on the neurological examination is usually indicative of structural abnormalities, but transient focality may be associated with diffuse metabolic injury, including hypoxia, uremia, hypertensive or hepatic encephalopathy, and hypoglycemia.

LABORATORY INVESTIGATION

Initial laboratory studies should include an arterial blood gas and electrocardiogram, complete blood count, electrolytes, blood urea nitrogen, glucose, magnesium, and calcium. These studies will quickly diagnose hypoxia, hypercapnea, uremia, hyperglycemia, hypoglycemia, high anion gap acidosis, and sodium or calcium abnormalities. Hypernatremia, hyponatremia, and hypercalcemia of any etiology may be primary causes of delirium.[3,18] Hypomagnesemia is noted in one-third of patients with ethanol withdrawal.[37] In addition to an association with cardiac arrhythmias, hypomagnesemia may also cause persistent hypocalcemia.[64,65] Hypocalcemia and hyperkalemia may be secondary to acute rhabdomyolysis, which is commonly seen as a consequence of agitation, seizures, or neuromuscular rigidity.[66] Hypokalemia may also be a clue to the diagnosis of Cushings syndrome or hyperaldosteronism,[18] and the combination of hyperkalemia and hyponatremia suggests Addison's disease. Adrenal insufficiency has been reported as a complication of adrenal infection in patients with acquired immunodeficiency syndrome.[67]

A respiratory alkalosis noted on the arterial blood gas suggests the presence of cardiopulmonary disease, sepsis, hepatic failure, increased intracranial pressure or salicylism.

Thrombocytopenia is a common manifestation of the acquired immunodeficiency syndrome, and its presence suggests a patient at risk of AIDS-related central nervous system infection. Investigation of the cause of a low platelet count in a patient with acute psychosis has also led to the diagnosis of lupus cerebritis.[3] A respiratory alkalosis noted on the arterial blood gas suggests the presence of cardiopulmonary disease, sepsis, hepatic failure, increased intracranial pressure or salicylism.[18] Although metabolic acidosis does not in itself cause mental status alteration,[18] its presence indicates the possibility of toxic alcohol ingestion, ketoacidosis, uremia, cyanide, carbon monoxide, salicylate, or iron poisoning, sepsis, or a postictal state.[68] The demonstration of an elevated anion gap suggests accumulation of an endogenously or exogenously derived acid as the etiology of metabolic acidosis. An abnormally low anion gap is seen in patients poisoned with bromides or in patients with abnormal elevation of positively charged serum proteins such as myeloma proteins.[68,69] Rhythm abnormalities or QRS widening on the electrocardiogram supports a clinical diagnosis of poisoning with a tricyclic antidepressant,[70] certain phenothiazines (particularly mesoridazine or thioridazine), digoxin, a calcium channel, or a beta-adrenergic blocking agent.[71]

Broad toxicololgic screening may be useful to confirm a suspicion of poisoning. It should be recalled however, that: (1) screens rarely provide information at the time of most urgent need and cannot replace a thoughtful and thorough history and physical examination, (2) a positive screen for a commonly abused substance does not exclude the presence of an infectious or trauma etiology of the mental status change, nor the presence of an uncommonly abused substance not screened for by the lab, and (3) a negative screen means only that the drugs that the laboratory tests for are not present; it does not exclude a toxic etiology.[72] Screens for most drugs provide only qualitative information regarding the presence or absence of the drug. Quantitative determination of serum drug levels in the delirious patient is useful in the case of poisoning with phenobarbital, carbamazepine, lithium, phenytoin, aminophylline, and salicylates.[72] In addition, although elevated serum acetaminophen levels do not commonly lead to mental status abnormalities, early quantitative determination of acetaminophen in the suicidal patient will detect this commonly ingested concomitant agent at a time when hepatic injury is preventable. Most labs require that these quantitative studies be considered and requested separately.

A computerized axial tomographic study of the brain and lumbar puncture will identify many acute structural and infectious disorders. A magnetic resonance imaging or contrast-enhanced computerized axial tomography scan may be required for the demonstration of abscesses, tumors, or old collections of subdural or epidural blood.

INITIAL MANAGEMENT

Initial management of the agitated delirious patient involves stabilization of the airway and vital signs, empirical treatment of possible hypoglycemia, hypoxia and thiamine deficiency, and establishment of control of the patient.

In addition to stabilization of the airway and treatment of shock, it is critically important to determine the patient's temperature. Many deaths in agitated patients are associated with undetected or inadequately treated hyperthermia.[73–76] In addition, delirium may be a primary manifestation of hyperthermia-related cerebral injury. Temperatures of 106°F or greater are associated with tissue injury.[77,78] Hyperthermia must be treated aggressively by immersion in an iced bath and/or evaporative cooling with water spray and fans. Temperatures should be continuously monitored with a flexible rectal probe. Standard cooling blankets do not provide adequate treatment of life-threatening elevations of temperature. Antipyretic agents lower temperature by decreasing the hypothalamic set point for temperature regulation, which is usually normal in patients with heatstroke, therefore they have no role in the management of severe temperature elevations.[79] Heatstroke occurs more readily during environmental heat exposure in patients taking therapeutic amounts of drugs that interfere with thermoregulation such as beta-adrenergic blockers and diuretics (lower cardiac output), alpha-agonists (vasoconstriction), neuroleptic agents (central hypothalamic effects), and anticholinergic agents (decreased sweating).[79] Utilization of sedating agents with anticholinergic effects, such as phenothiazines or antihistamines, may predispose the agitated patient to hyperthermia.[79–81]

Careful attention to volume status and replacement of fluid deficits is particularly important in the delirious patient. The adequacy of fluid therapy should be determined by monitoring vital signs and urine output. Significant fluid deficits are common in patients with delirium tremens[37,82,83] and in patients with nonexertional heatstroke.[84–86] In addition to treatment of hypotension, maintenance of adequate volume status has an important role in the prevention of myoglobinuric renal failure, a common complication of rhabdomyolysis in the agitated and hyperthermic patient.[66,87–90]

The administration of oxygen will initiate treatment for undetected hypoxia or carbon monoxide poisoning. Fol-

Many deaths in agitated patients are associated with undetected or inadequately treated hyperthermia.

In addition to treatment of hypotension, maintenance of adequate volume status has an important role in the prevention of myoglobinuric renal failure, a common complication of rhabdomyolysis in the agitated and hyperthermic patient.

lowing placement of an intravenous line and withdrawal of laboratory blood samples, possible thiamine deficiency and hypoglycemia are treated empirically with administration of 100 mg of intravenous thiamine and 50 ml of 50% dextrose in water. It is important to recall that administration of glucose alone to the nutritionally depleted patient has been reported to precipitate acute Wernicke's encephalopathy.[91] In the nutritionally deprived patient, repletion of all the B complex vitamins should be considered, as replacement of thiamine and pyridoxine alone has been reported to result in worsening of encephalopathy (pellagra) related to acute niacin deficiency.[25]

Severe hypertension in agitated patients usually responds to sedation. An extensive discussion of the management of hypertension unresponsive to sedation is beyond the scope of this chapter, however, several caveats apply. Patients with hypertension secondary to high levels of circulating catecholamines (eg, cocaine poisoning, tyramine reactions in patients on monoamine oxidase inhibitors, pheochromocytoma) should be treated initially with a short-acting, easily titrated intravenous agent such as sodium nitroprusside. A growing body of clinical evidence shows that the use of beta-adrenergic blockers for blood pressure control in high catecholamine states may cause further elevated blood pressure due to blockade of beta$_2$-adrenergic (vasodilating) receptors in association with unopposed alpha-adrenergic receptor stimulation. Significant paradoxical hypertension has been described following therapy with both propranolol and labetolol, a beta-adrenergic blocker with limited alpha-adrenergic blocking capability.[92–95] Use of a selective alpha blocker such as phentolamine is also a reasonable choice for blood pressure lowering in high-catecholamine states.[96] In any patient with chronic long-standing hypertension, even if it results in hypertensive encephalopathy, the blood pressure should initially be reduced to no lower than 25% of the initial mean arterial pressure to avoid relative hypotension and cerebral infarction. Patients with mental status changes secondary to acute elevations of blood pressure (usually patients with catecholamine excess states, acute glomerulonephritis, or preeclampsia) may have their pressures safely normalized.[57,97,98]

It may be difficult to clinically distinguish the patient who is agitated due to an intoxication from the patient who is agitated from other etiologies. In cases where poisoning is considered, it is reasonable to administer 1 g/kg of activated charcoal through a nasogastric tube as an initial intervention. Activated charcoal is particularly useful in the management of phencyclidine toxicity. Phencyclidine is a weak base that is secreted into the acidic lumen of the stom-

A growing body of clinical evidence shows that the use of beta-adrenergic blockers for blood pressure control in high catecholamine states may cause further elevated blood pressure due to blockade of beta$_2$-adrenergic (vasodilating) receptors in association with unopposed alpha-adrenergic receptor stimulation.

ach and trapped there in its ionized form where it is readily bound by activated charcoal. Because most phencyclidine is metabolized by the liver, there is no rationale for urinary acidification, which had been recommended by many authors. Urinary acidification may enhance renal tubular precipitation of myoglobin.[32] Most central nervous system stimulants that lead to agitation are not usually ingested in large quantities. Unless there is reason to suspect a massive toxic ingestion, routine gastric emptying in the agitated patient is hazardous and not indicated.[99] Complications of this procedure include esophageal, pharyngeal, and airway injury, aspiration, increased blood pressure, and increased intracranial pressure in the patient with an undetected structural brain lesion. Most drug-related psychoses respond to conservative management with attention to the protection of the patient from harm. Significant morbidity or death from toxic psychoses results most often from complications of agitated behaviour: self-induced trauma or trauma brought on by the patient's aggressive behavior, hyperthermia, and myoglobinuric renal failure. A rare exception is the patient who is a "body-stuffer" (usually a prisoner caught off of his or her guard) who swallows the evidence of cocaine or phencyclidine dealing and has a large gastrointestinal source of drug that may lead to ongoing and possibly fatal intoxication.[100] A similar event occurs in the more professional "body-packer," usually a young person recently arrived from South America who has swallowed carefully double- or triple-wrapped latex packets containing cocaine. The patient may seek medical attention when symptoms of cocaine effect indicate a leaking packet or, more commonly, the patient may be found in status epilepticus at an airport or in a hotel room, unable to give a history.[101] Routine gastric emptying procedures are of little use in these patients. The problem must be suspected clinically, diagnosed, and a management plan formulated that may involve aggressive whole bowel irrigation with a polyethylene glycol-electrolyte solution irrigant, and/or endoscopic and/or surgical removal of packets.[101,102]

Naloxone is routinely administered as an empirical therapeutic and diagnostic intervention in patients with altered mental status.[103] It is not uncommon to unmask an agitated, delirious state following the administration of naloxone to a depressed patient. Failure of the mental status to normalize completely following administration of naloxone to an opioid-depressed patient suggests another underlying problem, such as a mixed-drug overdose, head injury, hypoxia, or infection. Opioid withdrawal does not cause mental status alteration or fever and should not be considered in the differential diagnosis of these condi-

Because most phencyclidine is metabolized by the liver, there is no rationale for urinary acidification, which had been recommended by many authors. Urinary acidification may enhance renal tubular precipitation of myoglobin.

Failure of the mental status to normalize completely following administration of naloxone to an opioid-depressed patient suggests another underlying problem, such as a mixed-drug overdose, head injury, hypoxia, or infection.

tions.[103] Signs of opioid withdrawal following the administration of naloxone (rhinorrhea, yawning, vomiting and diarrhea, piloerection) indicate adequate reversal of opioid effect. Further administration of naloxone will only aggravate the withdrawal effects and will not further improve the mental status. There are clinical settings in the management of the agitated patient where it is prudent to administer naloxone very cautiously or not at all. Already agitated patients who chronically use opioids, such as certain patients with cancer, those on methadone maintenance, and patients who inject heroin several times daily should be considered to be opioid-dependent. Precipitation of acute opioid withdrawal in these patients may complicate the patient's condition. Caution in the use of naloxone is also justified in the management of the delirious patient who chronically ingests meperidine. Accumulation of the meperidine metabolite, normeperidine, may cause agitated delirium and seizures.[103] Seizures in these patients have been reported to be precipitated by the administration of naloxone.[104] Naloxone should not be withheld in the treatment of any patient who develops characteristic signs of opioid poisoning: miosis, hypoventilation, hypotension, lethargy, or coma.[54] Very large doses may be required to reverse toxicity secondary to synthetic opioids such as propoxyphene, fentanyl, or pentazocine.[103]

The third step of initial management involves establishing control so that adequate evaluation and therapy can proceed. Physical, and if indicated, chemical restraints may be necessary to protect the delirious patient. Sedating agents have a potential to increase disorientation and should sometimes be avoided. Many patients will respond to frequent and consistent orienting contact with ICU staff. Simple actions such as the placement of a familiar photograph, clock and calendar in the room, adequate lighting, and leaving the curtains drawn back so that the patient can see his or her surroundings can be very helpful.[49] Diminished sensory input may contribute to the well-recognized increase in nocturnal disorientation noted in the delirious patient.[49] Problems associated with agitation include accidental extubation or disruption of other life-sustaining catheters, injury to the patient or staff, and inability to cooperate with care.[105–107] While physical restraints alone are useful in keeping an otherwise physically calm patient from falling out of bed, the agitated patient should never be left to struggle in physical restraints, as this significantly increases the risk of hyperthermia and rhabdomyolysis.[88] The patient whose agitated behavior represents a risk to him- or herself or to the staff requires chemical sedation.[4,49]

No adequate controlled studies have been done to determine the most efficacious agent for control of agitation

While physical restraints alone are useful in keeping an otherwise physically calm patient from falling out of bed, the agitated patient should never be left to struggle in physical restraints, as this significantly increases the risk of hyperthermia and rhabdomyolysis.

in the ICU patient. Many regimens have been tried, including butyrophenones, opioids, benzodiazepines, and phenothiazines.[105–111] Benzodiazepines have been shown to be safe and effective in management of critically ill ICU patients with all etiologies of behavioral disturbance[110,111]; they are the agents of choice for the management of alcohol withdrawal.[37,112,113] Apnea and hypotension have occurred with rapid intravenous administration,[105,114] and excessive sedation may occur.[108,111] In one study that compared high-dose intravenous haloperidol with diazepam in the management of acute functional psychosis in otherwise healthy patients, no difference could be demonstrated between treatment groups at 4 or 24 hours. There were no significant hemodynamic side effects in either group. The authors suggested that the early effects of neuroleptics on thought disorder are related to their anxiolytic actions and not to any specific effect on thought disorder.[115] Intravenous lorazepam or diazepam given in small doses and titrated to sedation is safe, even though large doses may be required. When adequate sedation is achieved with diazepam, the effects last for a long period of time because of the prolonged half-lives of the metabolites.[37,116,117]

The use of phenothiazines in the management of delirium was studied extensively in patients with alcohol withdrawal. They were associated with significant hypotension, hyperthermia, an increased frequency of seizures, and failure to prevent progression of withdrawal.[118,119] Phenothiazines have also been associated with heatstroke syndromes due to their effects on hypothalamic thermoregulatory mechanisms and to their anticholinergic effects.[120–122] Since agitated patients are at risk of hyperthermia, phenothiazines should be avoided in the management of delirium.

Many clinicians prefer to use low doses of haloperidol to control agitation in hospitalized patients, particularly in the elderly, citing the drug's relative lack of sedative and autonomic effects.[49,123] However, hypotension following administration of haloperidol may complicate the management of critically ill patients, and extrapyramidal reactions occur in 20–33% of patients receiving the drug.[107,115,123,124] Exacerbation of extrapyramidal symptoms by neuroleptic therapy is an especially significant problem in patients with Parkinson's disease.[125] Large intravenous doses of haloperidol alone or in combination with lorazepam have been reported to be safe and effective in the management of hemodynamically unstable, agitated ICU patients, although data consist primarily of anecdotal experience and limited case series.[107–109] (It should be noted that haloperidol has not received FDA approval for intravenous use.) Combining haloperidol with lorazepam may decrease the

Benzodiazepines have been shown to be safe and effective in management of critically ill ICU patients with all etiologies of behavioral disturbance; they are the agents of choice for the management of alcohol withdrawal.

incidence of extrapyramidal reactions.[126] Haloperidol has been demonstrated to aggravate seizures during alcohol withdrawal in mice,[127] however, this effect has not been substantiated in humans.[124] Haloperidol has also been associated with severe hyperthermia when used as a single agent to treat alcohol withdrawal.[76] Concern about the administration of haloperidol to patients with high catecholamine states was raised by the demonstration that administration of dopamine-2 receptor blocking agents to exercising subjects resulted in increased hypertension and tachycardia and increased levels of norepinephrine and epinephrine. This effect was attributed to blockade of pre-synaptic dopamine-2 receptor effects on regulation of catecholamine release in sympathetic neurons.[128] In studies of animals given lethal doses of cocaine, hyperthermia associated with convulsions was the leading single cause of death. Muscle paralysis with pancuronium, sedation and seizure control with diazepam, external cooling, and chlorpromazine led to improved survival. Animals treated with propranolol alone were not protected from the lethal effects. Chlorpromazine did not prevent seizures.[129]

SEDATIVE-HYPNOTIC WITHDRAWAL

Withdrawal from sedative-hypnotic agents, particularly ethanol, is a common cause of delirium.

Withdrawal from sedative-hypnotic agents, particularly ethanol, is a common cause of delirium. The pathophysiology of sedative hypnotic withdrawal has some important clinical implications. Prolonged exposure to sedative-hypnotic agents produces physical dependence manifest as tolerance to the depressant effects of these substances. Animal research has shown that those areas of neurologic function that are chronically depressed show greater tolerance to increasing doses (eg, gait and arousal), while other functions not chronically depressed, such as breathing, do not develop tolerance. This finding may explain the commonly accepted observation that there is little increase in the lethal dose of barbiturates despite tolerance to the sedative effects. When animals are repeatedly challenged with doses of barbiturates or ethanol sufficient to depress respiration, the lethal dose is increased.[130–132] Proposed biochemical mechanisms of tolerance include "stiffening" of cell membranes, which produces resistance to the effects of ethanol, compensatory adaptation of neurotransmitter response and receptor number and sensitivity, changes in the flow of chloride through channels controlled by γ-aminobutyric acid receptors, and compensatory changes in ethanol-stimulated calcium fluxes.[23,133,134]

The tolerance that develops to repeated doses of sedative-hypnotics relates directly to physical dependence on those substances. As the substance is withdrawn or the dose is decreased, signs and symptoms of withdrawal begin to occur. Despite the very different chemical structures of ethanol, the barbiturates, nonbarbiturate sedative hypnotics, and benzodiazepines, acute abstinence or decreased use of these agents results in a remarkably similar withdrawal syndrome in both human and animal models. The time of onset and duration of symptoms are related to the half-life of the agent. Agents with short half-lives (ethanol, pentobarbital) have rapid onset of symptoms following abstinence, while agents with long half-lives (ethchlorvynol) or agents with active metabolites (diazepam) have delayed onset of symptoms, presumably due to persistence of the substance or its metabolites. The severity of withdrawal symptoms is related to the dose, duration, and frequency of administration. Shorter-acting agents produce more severe withdrawal symptoms than longer-acting agents when equivalent levels of neurological dysfunction are induced during habituation.[135–141]

These concepts have important clinical significance. The patient who is dependent on a short-acting sedative-hypnotic agent who is forced by illness or hospitalization to abstain develops rapid and severe symptoms of withdrawal. Signs of withdrawal in patients dependent on long-acting sedative-hypnotic agents develop slowly, and recognition may be delayed until progression to a severe state of withdrawal occurs. The similarity of the withdrawal syndromes caused by abstinence from these drugs suggests similar areas of neurological tolerance/dependence. This principle of cross-tolerance/dependence allows the physician to substitue one agent for another in the management of the withdrawal syndrome.

DELIRIUM TREMENS

Delirium tremens related to ethanol withdrawal is an extreme manifestation of the abstinence syndrome that follows chronic sedative-hypnotic depression of the central nervous system. Delirium tremens is characterized by marked hyperadrenergic stimulation (mydriasis, diaphoresis, severe tremor, tachycardia, hypertension, and fever), terrifying visual hallucinations, and global cognitive impairment. Milder early signs of withdrawal such as tachycardia, hypertension, low-grade fever, tremor, and irritability precede the development of more serious signs[83,142] and indicate a point at which therapeutic intervention can completely halt progression of withdrawal.[37,119] These signs of withdrawal are rarely missed in the indigent alcoholic patient but may be overlooked in the patient ad-

Signs of withdrawal in patients dependent on long-acting sedative-hypnotic agents develop slowly, and recognition may be delayed until progression to a severe state of withdrawal occurs.

Signs of withdrawal are rarely missed in the indigent alcoholic patient but may be overlooked in the patient admitted for acute medical or surgical illness where there is no history or suspicion of ethanol abuse, or in the affluent patient when the appropriate questions are not asked.

Any patient experiencing ethanol withdrawal who develops status epilepticus should be suspected of having a structural neurological lesion, as should any patient who manifests focality or whose seizures follow the onset of delirium tremens.

mitted for acute medical or surgical illness where there is no history or suspicion of ethanol abuse, or in the affluent patient when the appropriate questions are not asked.

Seizures may herald or follow the onset of signs of withdrawal. The majority of alcohol withdrawal seizures occur within 36 hours of the cessation of drinking. The seizures are short-lived, do not require specific anticonvulsive therapy, and rarely lead to status epilepticus.[23,142] Any patient experiencing ethanol withdrawal who develops status epilepticus should be suspected of having a structural neurological lesion, as should any patient who manifests focality or whose seizures follow the onset of delirium tremens. In Victor and Brausch's classic 1967 study, one-third of the patients with alcohol withdrawal seizures went on to develop delirium tremens.[142]

Physicians are occasionally confused by the presence of an elevated ethanol level in a patient with signs of alcohol withdrawal. Chronic heavy drinkers develop tolerance to the depressant effects of ethanol and may have a normal mental status at blood ethanol levels that could be lethal for a novice. These patients manifest signs of withdrawal as the blood ethanol level falls. It was this observation that long prevented the medical community from accepting that ethanol withdrawal syndromes were caused by withdrawal of ethanol and were not a manifestation of its toxic effects. Two hundred years passed between the recognition of delirium tremens as a specific entity associated with the abuse of ethanol and the classic 1953 paper of Victor and Adams that demonstrated that "rum fits," hallucinosis, and delirium tremens were a consequence of decreased levels of ethanol in the tolerant patient.[83]

Specific Management of Delirium Tremens

Prior to routine admission to ICUs and the use of modern therapeutics in patients with severe alcohol withdrawal, mortalities as high as 35% were reported for uncomplicated delirium tremens, and a rate as high as 72% was reported when delirium tremens was associated with other recognized illness such as pancreatitis, gastrointestinal hemorrhage, pneumonia, and hepatitis. Historically, deaths attributable to delirium tremens alone have been difficult to distinguish from those caused by complicating illnesses.[143,144] Mortality reviews of deaths associated with delirium tremens suggest that severe hyperthermia with coma and vascular collapse is commonly associated with death. Pulmonary emboli, arrhythmias, and inadvertent sedative-hypnotic overdose in inadequately monitored patients have all been cited as possible causes of unexpected sudden death.[34,74] Several authors have documented serious cardiac arrhythmias in patients with delirium tremens.[145,146]

The mortality of delirium tremens is low when appropriate management is instituted. Stabilization requires adequate sedation with a cross-tolerant, long-acting sedative-hypnotic agent, adequate fluid and nutrient replacement, correction of electrolyte and acid–base abnormalities, diagnosis and treatment of underlying complicating disorders, and intensive care monitoring. It was recognized many years ago that treatment of an alcoholic patient with a sedative-hypnotic agent would prevent the development of delirium tremens.[143] However, until Victor and Adams' paper in 1953 and the work of Isbell and Fraser that demonstrated the effects of chronic barbiturate administration and abstinence in volunteers, the utility of sedative-hypnotics in the treatment of the delirious patient was widely debated.[83,138,139] Many authors advocated, instead, the use of bromides, antihistamines, and ergotamine preparations. During the 1960s, trials of the new phenothiazines demonstrated a lack of efficacy in treating alcohol withdrawal. Thomas and Freedman treated 39 patients with advanced delirium tremens with paraldehyde or promazine and reported a 35% mortality in the promazine-treated group, compared to a 4.5% mortality in the paraldehyde-treated group.[119] Sereny and Kalant compared chlordiazepoxide and promazine in the management of patients with mild alcohol withdrawal and demonstrated the efficacy of both agents in suppressing the earliest manifestations of withdrawal. The group treated with the benzodiazepine had no serious consequences of withdrawal, while five patients in the promazine-treated group went on to develop seizures or delirium tremens.[118]

For many years paraldehyde was a popular sedative-hypnotic for the therapy of alcohol withdrawal. The major difficulties associated with delivering reliable amounts, however, made both overdosage and underdosage equally probable.[113] Paraldehyde is no longer used for the management of withdrawal due to the development of benzodiazepines. Many studies demonstrate the safety and efficacy of intravenous benzodiazepines in management of alcohol withdrawal.[112,113,116,117]

Cross-tolerant sedative-hypnotic agents blunt the major manifestations of delirium tremens and prevent the most lethal consequences, however, they do not completely reverse all signs of delirium. The ability of a cross-tolerant agent such as diazepam or phenobarital to prevent the onset of delirium tremens and the failure to completely suppress all signs of withdrawal may be related to the irreversibility of these signs once full-blown delirium tremens develops. A more interesting explanation of the incomplete reversal of withdrawal signs by cross-tolerant agents is that cross-tolerance is not complete. That is, that ethanol specifically affects areas of the nervous system that diazepam or the barbiturates do not affect.[133,147] In support of this proposal, Ellis et al. demonstrated that intravenous ethanol could reverse all signs of even much advanced withdrawal in ethanol-dependent cats.[149]

The toxicity of ethanol is well documented and precludes its safe use in the management of withdrawal.

While these findings have great pharmacologic interest, the toxicity of ethanol is well documented and precludes its safe use in the management of withdrawal. The half-life is too short to allow easy titration of signs of withdrawal, and the toxic/therapeutic ratio is limited; that is, the difference between levels causing toxic central nervous system depression and adequate sedation is very narrow. Other direct toxic effects of alcohol on the liver and hematologic and nervous systems also make it a poor choice. The cross-tolerant effects of the long-acting benzodiazepines allow gradual decrease in blood levels and safe titration of symptoms, with adequate suppression of the lethal manifestations of withdrawal.

The tremendous sympathetic stimulation seen in sedative-hypnotic withdrawal and the documented increased levels of catecholamines have led to trials of adrenergic receptor blockers in the management regimens of ethanol and other sedative-hypnotic withdrawal.[112,150,151] Clinical investigations of lofexidine (a clonidine analog with central alpha-2 agonist effects) in patients with mild withdrawal demonstrated its ability to attenuate the autonomic effects of withdrawal.[152] In a recent well-controlled study, Kraus et al. demonstrated the efficacy of atenolol in contributing to earlier normalization of vital signs, decreased requirement for sedation, and decreased length of hospital stay in patients with mild to moderate alcohol withdrawal. None of their patients were critically ill.[153] Abernethy et al. used propranolol exclusively to relieve symptoms of withdrawal in patients chronically taking a benzodiazepine. Ten to 40 mg of propranolol every 6 hours controlled tachycardia and hypertension, however, anxiety and dysphoria worsened.[154]

Because adrenergic receptor blockers do not prevent the serious neuropsychological manifestations of alcohol withdrawal, a strong argument can be made against their routine use in the critically ill patient. The sympathetic signs that accompany withdrawal from ethanol are a readily accessible measure of the severity of illness. In the patient with delirium tremens, blocking these signs with sympatholytic agents affects this important means of assessing the adequacy of sedation, a critical component of therapy.

In the patient with signs of early ethanol withdrawal, progression to a more critical state may be masked by treatment with adrenergic receptor blockers. This problem has been reported in the clinical setting.[155]

CONCLUSION

Acute psychiatric disturbances are common in the ICU. They may be a manifestation of functional psychiatric illness that has been precipitated or exacerbated by the acute illness. More often, they are organic in etiology, related to the systemic effects of metabolic disturbances or toxins or to direct brain impairment caused by infection, vascular, or structural lesions. Certain organically based cognitive disturbances may be clinically indistinguishable from functional psychiatric illness. A thorough history, basic laboratory assessment, mental status examination, and physical examination are important, and may reveal the etiology of organic disturbances. Management includes general resuscitative interventions such as stabilization of vital signs, administration of glucose and thiamine, oxygenation, and correction of electrolyte and acid–base abnormalities. The patient must be protected from injuries caused by agitation, which include trauma from falls, disruption of catheters and endotracheal tubes, hyperthermia, and rhabdomyolysis. Physical restraints are appropriate to prevent falls. Chemical restraints are necessary when agitation is significant. Benzodiazepines are safe and effective for this purpose and are the drugs of choice for management of sedative-hypnotic withdrawal. Further management involves identification of the cause of the disorder so that specific therapies can be instituted.

In the patient with signs of early ethanol withdrawal, progression to a more critical state may be masked by treatment with adrenergic receptor blockers.

References

1. Koranyi EK: Morbidity and rate of undiagnosed physical illnesses in a psychiatric clinic population. Arch Gen Psychiatry 36:414, 1979

2. Lipowski ZJ: Delirium (acute confusional states). JAMA 258:1789, 1987

3. Daniel DG, Rabin PL: Disguises of delirium. South Med J 78:666, 1985

4. Francis J, Martin D, Kapoor WN: A prospective study of delirium in hospitalized elderly. JAMA 263:1097, 1990

5. Massie MJ, Holland JC, Glass E: Delirium in terminally ill cancer patients. Am J Psychiatry 140:1048, 1983

6. Buhrich N, Cooper DA, Freed E: HIV infection associated with symptoms indistinguishable from functional psychosis. Br J Psychiatry 152:649, 1988

7. Diagnostic and statistical manual of mental disorders. 3rd ed. American Psychiatric Association, Washington, 1980

8. Ellison JM: DSM-III and the diagnosis of organic mental disorders. Ann Emerg Med 13:521, 1984

9. Angrist BG, Wilk SS, Gershon S: Amphetamine psychosis: behavioral and biochemical aspects. J Psychiatr Res 11:13, 1974

10. Halstead S, Riccio M, Harlow P et al: Psychosis associated with HIV infection. Br J Psychiatry 153:618, 1988

11. McEvoy JP: Organic brain syndromes. Ann Intern Med 95:212, 1981

12. Guze SB, Daengsurisri S: Organic brain syndromes: prognostic significance in general medical patients. Arch Gen Psychiatry 17:365, 1967

13. Rabins PV, Folstein MF: Delirium and dementia: diagnostic criteria and fatality rates. Br J Psychiatry 140:149, 1982

14. Henker FO: Acute brain syndromes. J Clin Psychiatry 40:117, 1979

15. Fauman MA: The emergency psychiatric evaluation of organic mental disorders. Psychiatr Clin North Am 6:233, 1983

16. Gillick MR, Serrell NA, Gillick LS: Adverse consequences of hospitalization in the elderly. Soc Sci Med 16:1033, 1982

17. Warshaw GA, Moore JT, Friedman SW et al: Functional disability in the hospitalized elderly. JAMA 248:847, 1982

18. Plum F, Posner JB: The diagnosis of stupor and coma. FA Davis, Philadelphia, 1980

19. Folstein MF, Folstein SE, McHugh PR: "Mini-mental state": a practical method for grading the cognitive state of patients for the clinician. J Psychiatr Res 12:189, 1975

20. Jacobs JW, Bernhard MR, Delgado A, Strain JJ: Screening for organic mental syndromes in the medically ill. Ann Intern Med 86:40, 1977

21. Strub RL, Black FW: The mental status examination in neurology. FA Davis, Philadelphia, 1977

22. Leigh D: Psychiatric aspects of head injury. J Contin Ed Psychiatry 40:21, 1979

23. Charness ME, Simon RP, Greenberg DA: Ethanol and the nervous system. N Engl J Med 321:442, 1989

24. Lopez RI, Collins GH: Wernicke's encephalopathy: a complication of chronic hemodialysis. Arch Neurol 18:248, 1968

25. Serdaru M, Hausser-Hauw C, Laplane D et al: The clinical spectrum of alcoholic pellagra encephalopathy: a retrospective analysis of 22 cases studied pathologically. Brain 111:829, 1988

26. Perez MM, Trimble MR: Epileptic psychosis: diagnostic comparison with process schizophrenia. Br J Psychiatry 137:245, 1980

27. Logsdail SJ, Toone BK: Post-ictal psychoses: a clinical and phenomenological description. Br J Psychiatry 152:246, 1988

28. Lindenbaum J, Healton EB, Savage DG et al: Neuropsychiatric disorders caused by cobalamin deficiency in the absence of anemia or macrocytosis. N Engl J Med 318:1720, 1988

29. Hollister LE: Drug-induced psychiatric disorders and their management. Med Toxicol Adverse Drug Exp 1:428, 1986

30. Snoey ER: Acute psychosis afer amantadine overdose. Ann Emerg Med 19:668, 1990

31. The Boston Collaborative Drug Surveillance Program: acute adverse reactions to prednisone in relation to dosage. Clin Pharmacol Ther 13:694, 1972

32. Goldfrank LR, Lewin NA, Osborn H: Phencyclidine. p. 517. In Goldfrank LR (ed): Goldfrank's toxicologic emergencies. 4th ed. Appleton & Lange, Norwalk, 1990

33. Aaron CK: Lysergic acid diethylamide and other psychedelics. p. 523. In Goldfrank LR (ed): Goldfrank's toxicologic emergencies. 4th ed. Appleton & Lange, Norwalk, 1990

34. Lieberman JA, Kinon BJ, Loebel AD: Dopaminergic mechanisms in idiopathic and drug-induced psychoses. Schizophr Bull 16:97, 1990

35. Elpern DJ: Cocaine abuse and delusions of parasitosis. Cutis 42:273, 1988

36. Victor M, Hope JM: The phenomenon of auditory hallucinations in chronic alcoholism. J Nerv Ment Dis 126:451, 1958

37. Thompson WL: Management of alcohol withdrawal syndromes. Arch Intern Med 138:278, 1978

38. Khantzian EJ, McKenna GJ: Acute toxic and withdrawal reactions associated with drug use and abuse. Ann Intern Med 90:361, 1979

39. McKinney WT, Kane Jr: Depression with the use of alpha-methyldopa. Am J Psychiatry 124:90, 1967

40. Fitzgerald JD: Propranolol-induced depression. (letter) Br Med J 2:372, 1967

41. Goodwin FK, Bunney WE: Depressions following reserpine: a reevaluation. Semin Psychiatry 3:435, 1971

42. Whelan TB, Schteingart DE, Starkman MN, Smith A: Neuropsychological deficits in Cushing's syndrome. J Nerv Ment Dis 168:753, 1980

43. Logigian EL, Kaplan RF, Steere AC: Chronic neurologic manifestations of Lyme Disease. N Engl J Med 323:1438, 1990

44. Krauthammer C, Dlerman GL: Secondary mania: manic syndromes associated with antecedent physical illness or drugs. Arch Gen Psychiatry 35:1333, 1978

45. Jamieson RC, Wells CE: Manic Psychosis in a patient with multiple metastatic brain tumors. J Clin Psychiatry 40:280, 1979

46. Cohen MR, Niska RW: Localized right cerebral hemisphere dysfunction and recurrent mania. Am J Psychiatry 137:847, 1980

47. Wharton RN: Accidental lithium carbonate treatment of thyrotoxicosis as mania. Am J Psychiatry 137:747, 1980

48. Medina JL, Rubino FA, Ross E: Agitated delirium caused by infarctions of the hippocampal formation and fusiform and lingual gyri. Neurology 24:1181, 1974

49. Lipowski ZJ: Transient cognitive disorders (delirium, acute confusional states) in the elderly. Am J Psychiatry 140:1426, 1983

50. Baden MM: Pathology of addictive states. p. 189. In Richter RW (ed): Medical aspects of drug abuse. Harper & Row, New York, 1975

51. Drugs that cause psychiatric symptoms. Med Lett Drugs Ther 31:113, 1989

52. Moreau A, Jones BD, Banno V: Chronic central anticholinergic toxicity in manic depressive illness mimicking dementia. Can J Psychiatry 31:339, 1986

53. Katz IR, Greenberg WJ, Barr GA et al: Screening for cognitive toxicity of anticholinergic drugs. J Clin Psychiatry 46:323, 1985

54. Goldfrank LR, Flomenbaum NE, Weisman RS et al: Vital signs and toxic syndromes. p. 65 In Goldfrank LR (ed): Goldfrank's toxicologic emergencies. Appleton & Lange, Norwalk, 1990

55. Delaney KA: Anticholinergics. In Rosen (ed): Rosen's textbook of emergency medicine. CV Mosby, St. Louis (In press)

56. Tafuri J, Roberts J: Organophosphate poisoning. Ann Emerg Med 16:193, 1987

57. Healton EB, John CB, Brust et al: Hypertensive encephalopathy and the neurologic manifestations of malignant hypertension. Neurology 32:127, 1982

58. Menkes JH: Disorders of metal metabolism. p. 426. In Rowland L (ed): Merritt's textbook of neurology. 7th ed. Lea & Febiger, Philadelphia, 1984

59. Figa-Talamanca L, Gualandi C, Domeo L et al: Hyperthermia after discontinuance of levodopa and bromocriptine therapy: impaired dopamine receptors a possible cause. Neurology 35:258, 1985

60. Sechi GP, Tanda F, Mutani R: Fatal hyperpyrexia after withdrawal of levodopa. Neurology 34:249, 1984

61. Linden CH, Rumack BH, Strehlke C: Monoamine oxidase inhibitor overdose. Ann Emerg Med 13:1377, 1984

62. Levinson DR, Simpson GM: Neuroleptic-induced extrapyramidal symptoms with fever. Arch Gen Psychiatry 43:839, 1986

63. Guze BH, Baxter LR: Current concepts: neuroleptic malignant syndrome. N Engl J Med 313:163, 1985

64. Frankushen D, Raskin D, Dimich A et al: The significance of hypomagnesemia in alcoholic patients. Am J Med 37:802, 1964

65. Rude RK: Hypocalcemia due to magnesium deficiency. p. 134 In Favus MJ (ed): Primer on the metabolic bone diseases and disorders of mineral metabolism. 1st ed. ASBMR, Kelseyville, 1990

66. Gabow PA, Kaehny WD, Kelleher SP: The spectrum of rhabdomyolysis. Medicine 61:141, 1982

67. Green LW, Cole W, Greene JB et al: Adrenal insufficiency as a complication of the acquired immunodeficiency syndrome. Ann Intern Med 101:497, 1984

68. Delaney KA, Goldfrank LR: Metabolic acidosis and metabolic alkalosis. In Callaham M (ed): The current practice of emergency medicine. BC Decker, Philadelphia (In press)

69. Oh MS, Carroll HJ: The anion gap. N Engl J Med 297:814, 1977

70. Boehnert MT, Lovejoy FH: Value of the QRS duration versus the serum drug level in prediction of seizures and ventricular arrhythmias after an acute overdose of tricyclic antidepressants. N Engl J Med 313:474, 1985

71. Benowitz NL, Rosenberg J, Becker CE: Cardiopulmonary catastrophes in drug-overdosed
patients. Med Clin North Am 63:267, 1979

72. Weisman RS, Howland MA, Flomenbaum NE: The toxicology Laboratory. p. 39. In Goldfrank
LR: Goldfrank's toxicologic emergencies. 4th ed. Appleton & Lange, Norwalk, 1990

73. Ginsberg MD, Hertzman M, Schmidt-Nowara WW: Amphetamine intoxication with coagulopathy, hyperthermia, and reversible renal failure: a syndrome resembling heatstroke.
Ann Intern Med 73:81, 1970

74. Tavel ME, Davidson W, Batterton TD: A critical analysis of mortality associated with delirium
tremens: review of 39 fatalities in a 9-year period. Am J Med Sci 242:18, 1961

75. Shulack NR: Sudden "exhaustive" death in excited patients. Psychiatr Q 18:3, 1944

76. Greenblatt DJ, Gross PL, Harris J et al: Fatal hyperthermia following haloperidol therapy of
sedative hypnotic withdrawal. J Clin Psychiatry 39:673, 1978

77. Shibolet S, Coll R, Gilat T, Sohar E: Heatstroke: its clinical picture and mechanism in 36
cases. Q J Med 36:525, 1967

78. Knochel JP: Environmental heat illness: an eclectic review. Arch Intern Med 133:841, 1974

79. Vassallo SU, Delaney KA: Pharmacologic effects on thermoregulation: mechanisms of drug-
related heatstroke. J Toxicol Clin Toxicol 27:199, 1989

80. Kollias J, Bullard RW: The influence of chlorpromazine on physical and chemical mechanisms
of temperature regulation in the rat. J Pharmac Exp Ther 145:373, 1984

81. Maickel RP: Interaction of drugs with autonomic nervous function and thermoregulation.
Fed Proc 29:1973, 1970

82. Victor M: The alcohol withdrawal syndrome, theory and practice. Postgrad Med. p. 69, April,
1970

83. Victor M, Adams RD: The effect of alcohol on the nervous system. Res Publ Assoc Res Nerv
Ment Dis 32:526, 1953

84. Graham GS, Lichtenstein MJ, Hinson JM, Theil GB: Nonexertional heatstroke: physiologic
management and cooling in 14 patients. Arch Intern Med 146:87, 1986

85. Sprung CL: Hemodynamic alterations of heatstroke in the elderly. Chest 75:362, 1979

86. O'Donnel TF, Clowes GHA: The circulatory abnormalities of heatstroke. N Engl J Med
287:734, 1972

87. Ron D, Taitelman U, Michaelson M et al: Prevention of acute renal failure in traumatic
rhabdomyolysis. Arch Intern Med 144:277, 1984

88. Brody SL, Wrenn KD, Wilber MM, Slovis CM: Predicting the severity of cocaine-associated
rhabdomyolysis. Ann Emerg Med 19:1137, 1990

89. Roth D, Alarcon FJ, Fernandez JA et al: Acute rhabdomyolysis associated with cocaine intoxication. N Engl J Med 319:673, 1988

90. Akmal M, Valdin JR, McCarron MM, Massry SG: Rhabdomyolysis with and without acute renal failure in patients with phenyclidine intoxication. Am J Nephrol 1:91, 1981

91. Victor M, Adams RD, Collins GH: The Wernicke-Korsakoff syndrome. FA Davis, Philadelphia, 1971

92. McMurtry RJ: Propranolol, hypoglycemia, and hypertensive crisis. Ann Intern Med 80:669, 1974

93. Briggs RS: Hypertensive response to labetolol in pheochromocytoma. Lancet 1:1045, 1978

94. Feek CM: Hypertensive response to labetolol in pheochromocytoma. Br Med J 281:387, 1980

95. Ramoska E: Propranolol induced hypertension in treatment of cocaine intoxication. Ann Emerg Med 14:1112, 1985

96. Olson KR, Pentel PR: Management of cocaine poisoning (letter). Ann Emerg Med 12:655, 1983

97. Ledingham JGG, Rajapololan B: Cerebral complications in the treatment of accelerated hypertension. Q J Med 189:25, 1979

98. Strandgaard S: Autoregulation of cerebral blood flow in hypertensive patients. Circulation 53:720, 1976

99. Smilkstein MJ, Price D, Flomembaum NE: Gastrointestinal principles. p. 119. In Goldfrank LR (ed): Goldfrank's toxicologic emergencies. 4th ed. Appleton & Lange, Norwalk, 1990

100. Roberts JR, Price D, Goldfrank L, Hartnett L: The body stuffer syndrome: a clandestine form of drug overdose. Am J Emerg Med 4:24, 1986

101. McCarron MM, Wood JD: The cocaine body packer syndrome. JAMA 250:1417, 1983

102. Hoffman R, Smilkstein M, Goldfrank LR: Bowel irrigation and the cocaine body packer: a new approach to a common problem. Am J Emerg Med 8:523, 1990

103. Goldfrank LR, Bresnitz EA: Opioids. p. 443. In Goldfrank LR (ed): Goldfrank's toxicologic emergencies. 4th ed. Appleton & Lange, Norwalk, 1990

104. Kaiko RF, Foley KM, Grabinski PY et al: Central nervous system excitatory effects of meperidine in cancer patients. Ann Neurol 13:180, 1983

105. Shapiro JM, Westphal LM, White PF et al: Midazolam infusion for sedation in the intensive care unit: effect on adrenal function. Anesthesiology 64:394, 1986

106. Sos J, Cassem NH: Managing postoperative agitation. Drug Ther Bull 3:103, 1980

107. Tesar GE, Murray GB, Cassem NH: Use of high-dose intravenous haloperidol in the treatment of agitated cardiac patients. J Clin Psychopharmacol 5:344, 1985

108. Adams F: Emergency intravenous sedation of the delirious, medically ill patient. J Clin Psychiatry 49(Suppl):22, 1988

109. Adams F: Neuropsychiatric evaluation and treatment of delirium in the critically ill cancer patient. Cancer Bulletin 36.3:156, 1984

110. McClish A: Intravenous diazepam for psychiatric reactions following open heart surgery. Can J Anaesth 15:63, 1968

111. Abel RM, Reis RL: Intravenous diazapam for sedation following cardiac operations: clinical and hemodymanic assessments. Anesth Analg 50:244, 1971

112. Baumgartner GR, Rowen RC: Clonidine vs chlordiazepoxide in the management of acute alcohol withdrawal syndrome. Arch Intern Med 147:1223, 1987

113. Thompson WL, Johnson AD, Maddrey WL et al: Diazepam and paraldehyde for treatment of severe delirium tremens: a controlled trial. Ann Intern Med 82:175, 1975

114. Hall SC, Ovassapian A: Apnea after intravenous diazepam therapy. JAMA 238:1052, 1977

115. Lerner Y, Lwow E, Levitin A, Belmaker RH: Acute high-dose parenteral haloperidol treatment of psychosis. Am J Psychiatry 136:1061, 1979

116. Nolop KB, Natow A: Unprecedented sedative requirements during delirium tremens. Crit Care Med 14:246, 1985

117. Sellers EM, Naranjo CA, Harrison M et al: Diazepam loading: simplified treatment of alcohol withdrawal. Clin Pharmacol Ther 34:822, 1983

118. Sereny G, Kalant H: Comparative clinical evaluation of chlordiazepoxide and promazine in treatment of alcohol-withdrawal syndrome. Br Med J 1:92, 1967

119. Thomas DW, Freedman DX: Treatment of the alcohol withdrawal syndrome. JAMA 188:244, 1964

120. Standyk AN, Glezo JD: Drug-induced heat stroke. Can Med Assoc J 128:957, 1983

121. Zelman S, Guillin R: Heatstroke in phenothiazine-treated patients: a report of three fatalities. Am J Psychiatry 126:1787, 1970

122. Sarnquist F, Larson CP: Drug-induced heatstroke. Anesthesiology 39:348, 1973

123. Steinhart MJ: The use of haloperidol in geriatric patients with organic mental disorder. Curr Ther Res 33:132, 1983

124. Clinton JE, Sterner S, Stelmachers Z et al: Haloperidol for sedation of disruptive emergency patients. Ann Emerg Med 16:319, 1987

125. Wolters EC, Hurwitz TA, Mak E et al: Clozapine in the treatment of parkinsonian patients with dopaminomemetic psychosis. Neurology 40:832, 1990

126. Menza MA, Murray GB, Holmes VF et al: Controlled study of extrapyramidal reactions in the management of delirious, medically ill patients: inravenous haloperidol versus intravenous haloperidol plus benzodiazepines. J Crit Care 17:238, 1988

127. Blum K, Eubanks ID, Wallace IE et al: Enhancement of alcohol withdrawal convulsions in mice by haloperidol. J Toxicol Clin Toxicol 9:427, 1976

128. Mercuro G, Gianluigi G, Rivano C et al: Evidence for a dopaminergic control of sympathoadrenal catecholamine release. Am J Cardiol 62:827, 1988

129. Catravas JD, Waters IW: Acute cocaine intoxication in the conscious dog: studies on the mechanism of lethality. J Pharmacol Exp Ther 217:350, 1981

130. Okamoto M, Rosenberg HC, Boisse NR: Tolerance characteristics produced during the maximally tolerable chronic pentobarbital dosing in the cat. J Pharmacol Exp Ther 192:555, 1975

131. Okamoto M, Boisse NR, Rosenberg HC, Rosen R: Characteristics of functional tolerance during barbiturate physical dependency production. J Pharmacol Exp Ther 207:906, 1978

132. Boisse NR, Okamoto M: Physical dependence to barbital compared to pentobarbital. III. Withdrawal characteristics. J Pharmacol Exp Ther 204:514, 1978

133. Tabakoff B, Cornell N, Hoffman PL: Alcohol tolerance. Ann Emerg Med 15:1005, 1986

134. Goldstein DB: Effect of alcohol on cellular membranes. Ann Emerg Med 15:1013, 1986

135. Okamoto M, Jinman DJ, Aaronson LM: Comparison of ethanol and barbiturate physical dependence. J Pharmacol Exp Ther 218:701, 1981

136. Fraser HF: Tolerance to physical dependence on opiates, barbiturates and alcohol. Annu Rev Med 8:427, 1987

137. Fraser HF, Wikler A, Essig CF, Isbell H: Degree of physical dependence induced by secobarbital or phenobarbital. JAMA 166:126, 1958

138. Isbell H: Abuse of bariturates. JAMA 162:660, 1956

139. Isbell H, Fraser HF, Wikler A et al: An Experimental study of the etiology of "rum fits" and delirium tremens. Q J Stud Alcohol 16:1, 1955

140. Busto U, Sellers EM, Naranjo CA et al: Withdrawal reaction after long-term therapeutic use of Benzodiazepines. N Engl J Med 315:854, 1986

141. Vyas I, Carney MWP: Diazepam withdrawal fits. Br Med J 4:44, 1975

142. Victor M, Brausch C: The role of abstinence in the genesis of alcoholic epilepsy. Epilepsia 8:1, 1967

143. Ransom SW, Scott GD: The results of medicinal treatment in eleven hundred and six cases of delirium tremens. Am J Med Sci 141:673, 1911

144. Moore M, Gray MG: Delirium tremens: a study of cases at the Boston City Hospital 1915–1936. N Engl J Med 220:953, 1939

145. Fisher J, Abrams J: Life threatening ventricular tachyarrhythmias in delirium tremens. Arch Intern Med 137:1238, 1977

146. Smile DH: Acute alcohol withdrawal complicated by sypraventricular tachycardia: treatment with intravenous propranolol. Ann Emerg Med 13:1395 1984

147. Aaronson LM, Hinman DJ, Okamoto M: Effects of diazepam on ethanol withdrawal. J Pharmacol Exp Ther 22:319, 1982

148. Solomon J, Rouck LA, Koepke HH: Double-blind comparison of lorazepam and chlordiazepoxide in the treatment of the acute alcohol abstinence syndrome. Clin Ther 6:52, 1983

149. Ellis FW, Pick JR: Experimentally induced ethanol dependence in Rhesus monkeys. J Pharmacol Exp Ther 175:88, 1970

150. Carlsson C, Haggendal J: Arterial noradrenaline levels after ethanol withdrawal. Lancet 2:889, 1967

151. Linnoila M, Mefford I, Nutt D, Adinoff B: Alcohol withdrawal and noradrenergic function. Ann Intern Med 107:875, 1987

152. Cushman P, Forbes R, Lerner W, Stewart M: Alcohol withdrawal syndromes: clinical management with lofexidine. Alcoholism 9:103, 1985

153. Kraus ML, Gottlieb LD, Horwitz RI, Anscher M: Randomized clinical trial of atenolol in patients with alcohol withdrawal. N Engl J Med 313:905, 1985

154. Abernathy DR, Greenblatt DJ, Shader RI: Treatment of diazepam withdrawal syndrome with propranolol. Ann Intern Med 94:354, 1981

155. Hughes PL, Morse RM: Use of clonidine in a mixed drug detoxification regimen: possibility of masking of clinical signs of sedative withdrawal. Mayo Clin Proc 60:47, 1985

MANAGEMENT OF HEMODYNAMIC COMPROMISE IN THE POISONED PATIENT

THEODORE C. BANIA, MD[†]
DIANE SAUTER, MD, FACEP, ABMT[††]
ROBERT S. HOFFMAN, MD, ABMT[†††]

Overt hypotension, or the potential for cardiovascular instability, accounts for a large percentage of admissions to the critical care unit. As such, the intensivist is generally adept at the initial stabilization, assessment, and long-term management of this situation. In typical medical or surgical patients, the etiology for cardiovascular compromise may often be assessed by evaluation of simple parameters such as vital signs, skin turgor, capillary refill, and urine output and concentration. Occasionally, more precise assessment will be required, and measurement of central venous pressures, cardiac filling pressures, or cardiac output and systemic vascular resistance will be indicated. Frequently a single etiology for the patient's hypotension exists, which can be determined from the history and physical examination, thus obviating the need for invasive monitoring. Hemodynamic compromise may complicate the clinical presentation of any poisoned patient. In the poisoned patient, however, hemodynamic compromise typically results from the simultaneous occurrence of multiple stresses on the cardiovascular system. Some of these events are often quite distinct from the usual etiologies for hypotension and may require specific pharmacologic intervention. Furthermore, many commonly used agents such as dopamine may have little efficacy in toxin-induced hypotension.

In the poisoned patient hemodynamic compromise typically results from the simultaneous occurrence of multiple stresses on the cardiovascular system.

[†] Chief Resident, Department of Emergency Medicine, Metropolitan Hospital Center, New York, New York

[††] Director, Emergency Medicine Residency Training Program, Metropolitan Hospital Center, New York, New York

[†††] Associate Medical Director, New York City Poison Control Center, Instructor Clinical Surgery/Emergency Medicine, New York University School of Medicine, New York, New York

Poor tissue perfusion may result from a variety of mechanisms. Hypovolemia, decreased peripheral vascular resistance, myocardial depression, catecholamine depletion, prevention of catecholamine synthesis, the generation of unstable tachy- and bradyarrhythmias, and hypertension may result from poisoning. Rational treatment of each of these complications requires an understanding of the pathophysiology of the toxic ingestion. This paper will review the pathophysiology of hemodynamic compromise as it relates to common and prototypic poisonings and provide specific guidelines for management. Only drug- or toxin-related etiologies of these cardiovascular problems will be discussed. The term toxin will be used to include all drugs (whether prescription, over-the-counter, or illicit), as well as all chemicals with known adverse effects in humans.

BASIC PRINCIPLES: PATHOPHYSIOLOGY

HYPOTENSION

Intravascular Volume Depletion

In the poisoned patient, intravascular volume depletion may result from gastrointestinal losses, urinary losses, increased insensible losses, and/or the redistribution of intravascular volume in the third space. Other manifestations of toxicity such as myocardial depression, cardiac arrhythmias, and relative hypovolemia (from massive vasodilation) may complicate intravascular volume depletion. The net result is either the production or exacerbation of hypotension.

Poisoning may exist in the setting of other illness, such as a motor vehicle accident that occurs as the result of an impaired driver, or carbon monoxide poisoning in a fire victim who may also have significant burns or trauma. In such instances, the first objective is always to exclude the possibility that significant blood loss is contributing to intravascular volume depletion. The most common cause, however, of intravascular volume depletion in the poisoned patient involves the loss of fluid from the gastrointestinal tract. The persistent vomiting and/or diarrhea that is characteristic of so many toxins may produce substantial loss of intravascular fluid volume resulting in cardiovascular collapse. Vomiting may occur as a result of local gastric irritation or an increase in gastric secretions, or may be of central origin (through stimulation of the chemotactic trigger zone). This is particularly true of a variety of plant toxins. The toxins abrin (found in the rosary pea) and ricin (produced by the castor bean plant) both inhibit protein synthesis and result in gastrointestinal mucosal sloughing and hemorrhage.[1] Abrin and ricin bind to cell surface glycoproteins on the gastrointestinal mucosa and become internalized by endocytosis. Once inside the cells, abrin and ricin inhibit protein synthesis by modifying the 60S ribosomal subunit, making it unable to react with elongation factor 2.[1-3] The inhibition of protein synthesis results in severe gastroenteritis followed by the development of bloody diarrhea. Pokeweed contains the glycoprotein saponin, which is an irritant when applied to the gastrointestinal mucosa. The ingestion of this plant also results in a severe hemorrhagic gastroenteritis.[4] In addition, syrup of ipecac, a plant-derived product used to produce emesis as a means of gastrointestinal decontamination, has been implicated as a common cause of excessive fluid loss in the overdose setting. Other toxins, such as arsenic, frequently produce such severe gastrointestinal fluid losses[5,6] that the term "rice-water stools" (often used to describe cholera) has been applied. A list of toxins that commonly result in consequential gastrointestinal fluid losses and significant volume depletion appears in Table 1.

Cathartics are frequently employed in standard overdose management protocols. A variety of agents including magnesium salts (citrate and sulfate), sorbitol, and polyethylene glycol electrolyte lavage solutions are used. Their expressed purpose is to hasten the elimination of toxin, which is either free or adsorbed to activated charcoal, from the gastrointestinal tract. While gentle catharsis seems advantageous,[7] excessive catharsis with magnesium or sorbitol agents is potentially harmful. Hypermagnesemia may result from multiple doses of magnesium salts, even in patients with normal renal function.[8] Similarly, excessive sorbitol has produced life-threatening hypernatremic dehydration.[9]

An increase in insensible losses may result from excessive diaphoresis or respiratory losses from centrally mediated hyperpnea. Table 2 lists toxins commonly associated with volume depletion resulting from insensible losses. Within this group, cocaine, sympathomimetics, and organophosphate insecticides are the most frequently encountered causes of massive diaphoresis. In addition, the uncoupling of oxidative phosphorylation that results from the effects of toxins such as salicylate and dinitrophenol may produce hyperthermia and diaphoresis with subsequent volume loss.

Loss of intravascular volume into the interstitial space is often referred to as 'third spacing." This typically results from a disruption of capillary membranes and increased

TABLE 1   Toxins Associated With Significant GI Losses

Antibiotics
Arsenic salts
Castor bean (ricin)
Colchicine
Cyclopeptide mushroom
  poisoning
Disulfiram reaction
Iodine
Iron
Laxatives
Lithium
Mercury salts
Non-steroidal
  antiinflammatory drugs
Opioid withdrawal
Organophosphate and
  carbamate insecticides
Podophylline
Pokeweed (saponins)
Rosary pea (abrin)
Theophylline
Zinc phosphide

TABLE 2   Toxins Associated With Significant Insensible Losses

Amphetamines
Carbamates
Chlorphenoxy herbicides
  (such as 2-4 D)
Cocaine
Dinitrophenol
Organophosphates and
  carbamate insecticides
Salicylates

capillary permeability. Third spacing is commonly associated with tissue injury from corrosive or caustic agents such as strong acids or alkalis, phenol, iron, and iodine, or as a direct manifestation of capillary instability as seen with severe salicylate toxicity or crotalid (pit viper) envenomation.

Increased urinary losses may result from a variety of toxic mechanisms such as altered resorption of solute in the renal tubules resulting in an osmotic diuresis. This may occur as the result of intoxication with ethanol, salicylates, theophylline, or diuretics. Certain toxins, such as Vacor (a rodenticide) are known to produce severe hyperglycemia, which can lead to significant osmotic renal losses.[10] Use of outdated tetracycline was formerly associated with the production of a Fanconi syndrome that can not only lead to volume loss, but also produce electrolyte abnormalities.[11] Chronic utilization of the antidepressant lithium may result in hypovolemia secondary to nephrogenic diabetes insipidus. The renal tubules become unresponsive to antidiuretic hormone[12] through the interference with hormone-activated adenyl cyclase.[13] Volume depletion and shock may result. In general, however, urinary losses have minor effects on overall hemodynamics.

Relative Hypovolemia

Relative hypovolemia may result from the toxicity of agents with either central or peripheral actions. Clonidine, for example, has central α_2-adrenergic agonist activity in both the medulla oblongata and locus ceruleus. This effect inhibits sympathetic discharge, decreasing both peripheral vascular resistance and cardiac output, thus producing hypotension. Hypotension as a result of peripherally acting agents may be secondary to the blockade of α-adrenergic receptors, the stimulation of β_2-adrenergic receptors, or the decreased availability of catecholamines. A decrease in presynaptic stores of catecholamine occurs as the result of the interference with normal synthesis, release, or reuptake mechanisms of catecholamines. Multiple antihypertensive agents, tricyclic antidepressants, phenothiazines, theophylline, and cocaine may act through these mechanisms (Table 3). In addition, the interference by toxins with the normal activity of calcium or sodium channels may result in vasodilation and relative hypovolemia. Agents that act as direct vasodilators such as nitrites and nitrates will have a similar effect. Direct vasodilation may apply to intoxications with ethanol and other simple alcohols, and those agents associated with cutaneous flushing, such as antihistamines and other anticholinergic agents.

TABLE 3   Toxins Associated With Relative Intravascular Volume Depletion

Alcohols
Angiotensin-converting enzyme inhibitors
Anticholinergic agents
Calcium channel blockers
Disulfiram reaction
Hydralazine
Iron
Nitrates
Nitrites
Phenothiazines
Reserpine
Theophylline
Tricyclic antidepressants

CARDIOGENIC SHOCK AND ARRHYTHMIAS

Myocardial depression and overt pump failure are common manifestations of life-threatening toxicologic exposures. Decreased myocardial contractility may result from the antagonism of catecholamines, membrane stabilization (mediated largely through sodium channel effects), or the blockade of calcium ion channels. Table 4 lists toxins associated with significant myocardial depression. Quinidine, phenothiazines, tricyclic antidepressants, and high doses of some β-adrenergic blockers produce membrane-stabilizing effects that may increase the risk of various ventricular arrhythmias and further exacerbate myocardial depression.

TABLE 4	Toxins Associated With Myocardial Depression
Alcohols	
Barbiturates	
β-adrenergic blockers	
Calcium channel blockers	
Cocaine	
Iron	
Tricyclic antidepressants	

Membrane Stabilization or Quinidine-like Effects

In the myocardium, phase 0 depolarization is caused by an increase in conduction of Na^+ ions through specific Na^+ ion channels. This results in a local membrane circuit that increases the conduction of Na^+ ions in the adjacent membrane. "Quinidine-like" compounds block these Na^+ ion channels. Thus, the rate of depolarization during phase 0 (measured by Vmax or the maximal conduction velocity) is decreased and the conduction of the action potential along the myocardium is slowed.[14,15] This decrease in conduction velocity is responsible for the widened QRS and QT intervals commonly seen as toxic manifestations of drugs with quinidine-like activity.[16] In addition, these effects on sodium channels decrease the rate and force of contraction in the myocardial cells outside the conduction system, further decreasing cardiac output. In addition to the type IA antiarrhythmic agents (such as procainamide, quinidine, and disopyramide),[17] this effect has also been described with type IC antiarrhythmics (such as flecainide encainide),[18,19] tricyclic antidepressants,[14,15] certain phenothiazines (thioridiazine and mesoridazine),[20] carbamazepine,[22] propoxyphene,[23] amantadine,[24] cocaine,[25] and possibly cyclobenzaprine.[21]

Arrhythmogenesis

Supraventricular and ventricular arrhythmias may be related to electrolyte abnormalities, acidemia, alkalemia, hypoxia, and catecholamine excess, or may be a direct effect

Of arrhythmias that may require specific intervention, supraventricular tachycardia is the arrhythmia most often seen in toxicology.

of the toxin. Clearly, sinus tachycardia is the most common abnormal rhythm seen in the poisoned patient. This may result from fever, stress or anxiety, pain, hypovolemia or hypotension, or catecholamine excess. Of arrhythmias that may require specific intervention, supraventricular tachycardia is the arrhythmia most often seen in toxicology. This is usually produced by agents with anticholinergic effects (antihistamines, tricyclic antidepressants, and phenothiazines), type IA antiarrhythmics, agents with sympathomimetic effect (pseudoephedrine, cocaine, and theophylline). Tricyclic antidepressants and antihistamines have similar effects through the antagonism of H1 receptors. Unopposed sympathetic stimulation and tachyarrhythmias may result. Severe hemodynamic compromise may result, especially if the myocardium is already compromised due to coronary artery disease or if myocardial contractility is depressed as an additional effect of the toxin.

Supraventricular and ventricular tachycardias frequently complicate the toxicity of the sympathomimetic agents. Sympathomimetics may stimulate ventricular arrhythmias by the generation of ectopic foci of ventricular activity. Frequently, toxins without intrinsic sympathomimetic effects may produce "sympathomimetic-like" arrhythmias through modulation of endogenous catecholamines or their effects. Theophylline indirectly elevates the systemic levels of norepinephrine and epinephrine through direct effects on the adrenal medulla.[26] Chlorinated hydrocarbons sensitize the myocardium to endogenous catecholamines and frequently result in arrhythmias. The term "sudden sniffing death" has been used to describe the fatal events (presumed to be ventricular arrhythmias) associated with the abuse of halogenated hydrocarbons.[27,28] These events occur when endogenous catecholamine levels are high (patients are involved in physical activity) but insufficient to produce arrhythmias in patients with normal myocardial tissue. Similar arrhythmias have been noted in chloral hydrate overdose (another halogenated hydrocarbon).[29] Table 5 lists toxins commonly associated with the production of arrhythmias.

For many toxins, it is readily apparent that the cause for cardiovascular compromise is multifactorial. Iron toxicity specifically illustrates this point. Iron has a direct corrosive effect on the gastrointestinal mucosa. Significant amounts of intravascular volume may be lost through gastrointestinal hemorrhage and the third spacing of fluid into the mucosa of the small bowel.[30,31] In addition, as high iron concentrations overwhelm the mechanisms that regulate its gastrointestinal absorption, free iron levels may exceed the iron-binding capacity of transferrin. The absorbed free

TABLE 5 Toxins Associated With Arrhythmias

Quinidine-like	Bradyarrhythmias	Tachyarrhythmias
Amantadine	Alpha agonists	Amphetamines
Carbamazepine	β-adrenergic blockers	Anticholinergics
Cocaine	Calcium channel blockers	Antihistamines
Cyclobenzaprine	Central-acting antihypertensives	Catecholamines
Phenothiazines	Digoxin	Cocaine
Tricyclic antidepressants		Phencyclidine
Type IA and IC antiarrhythmics		Theophylline
		Thyroid preparations

iron subsequently disrupts capillary membranes and results in an increased capillary permeability. This effect may further contribute to third spacing of intravascular volume into the interstitium. Free iron may potentiate gastrointestinal hemorrhage by producing a coagulopathy through inhibition of the action of thrombin and fibrinogen.[32] Also, high serum ferritin levels may result in massive post arteriolar vasodilation exacerbating the hypovolemic state.[31,33] Finally, the multifactorial systemic acidosis associated with life-threatening iron toxicity further compounds the above mechanisms by producing myocardial depression.

A similar multifactorial process can be described with salicylate toxicity. While salicylate toxicity is complicated by insensible losses that result from tachypnea, fever, and diaphoresis, increased urinary losses may also contribute to volume depletion. The latter result from renal excretion of an increased solute and organic acid load.[34–36]

Hypertension

Hypertensive emergencies may result from the ingestion or administration of the direct-acting sympathomimetic agents such as norepinephrine. These agents directly combine with and activate postsynaptic α-adrenergic receptors. Alternatively, the indirect-acting agents such as amphetamines may produce hypertension by causing the release of norepinephrine that has been stored in the presynaptic sympathetic nerve terminal. Pseudoephedrine, ephedrine, and phenylpropanolamine are commonly available over-the-counter preparations that potentiate presynaptic norepinephrine release and directly activate the α-adrenergic receptor.[37,38] Cocaine produces sympathetic stimulation, both through central nervous system stimulation and through blockade of the presynaptic reuptake of norepinephrine and dopamine. This results in an excess of cate-

TABLE 6   Common Toxins That Produce Hypertension

Amphetamines
Anticholinergics
Cocaine
Monoamine oxidase
  inhibitor food and drug
  interactions
Phencyclidine
Phenylpropanolamine
Pseudoephedrine

Hypotension resulting from relative or absolute hypovolemia, with or without signs of hypoperfusion, is most appropriately initially managed with intravascular volume replacement. For the majority of patients, adequate tissue perfusion will be achieved with volume replacement alone.

cholamines at the postsynaptic receptor site.[39,40] Ergot alkaloids and other vasoactive compounds may produce vasospasm with resultant hypertension and peripheral ischemia.[41,42] Finally, food-drug interactions (such as the ingestion of tyramine-containing foods by patients taking therapeutic doses of monoamine oxidase inhibitors) or drug-drug interactions (such as the administration of meperidine to a patient receiving a monoamine oxidase inhibitor) have also been implicated as causes of life-threatening hypertension (see Table 6).[43,44]

TREATMENT

For information regarding the management of a variety of individual toxic agents, the reader is referred to one of the standard reference toxicology texts.[45–47] General principles as well as some specific illustrative examples are given below. The discussion will focus on the management of hypotension and finish with a few brief statements regarding drug-induced hypertension.

Hypotension resulting from relative or absolute hypovolemia, with or without signs of hypoperfusion, is most appropriately initially managed with intravascular volume replacement. For the majority of patients, adequate tissue perfusion will be achieved with volume replacement alone. Care must always be taken to avoid volume overload. The administration of 100–200 ml boluses of normal saline to adults until 1,000–2,000 ml has been infused or signs of volume overload develop has been recommended.[48] Children should receive boluses of 10–20 ml/kg. When greater than 20 ml/kg (in either adults or children) is needed within the first 2 hours, or when signs of pulmonary congestion or decreased oxygenation develop, invasive hemodynamic monitoring through the placement of a pulmonary artery catheter should be used to guide further fluid management.[48] As long as the pulmonary capillary wedge pressure remains low, additional volume replacement may be given safely. It should be noted, however, that in cases of noncardiogenic pulmonary edema (that commonly complicate toxin exposures such as opioid overdose, salicylate toxicity, smoke inhalation, etc.), filling pressures correlate poorly with the presence or absence of pulmonary congestion and clinical criteria must be utilized. In any individual patient it may become necessary to adjust the pulmonary capillary wedge up or down to determine the pressure that results in the optimal cardiac output.[49]

If hypotension persists despite a maximal cardiac output, another mechanism such as postarteriolar vasodilation is operating and pharmacologic agents may be required for the reversal of shock. Although dopamine is the pressor agent employed most frequently for the management of shock that is unresponsive to volume replacement, this agent may fail in the poisoned patient. The pharmacologic pressor effect of dopamine results from a combination of direct and indirect α-adrenergic agonism. The efficacy of this agent depends upon the normal metabolism of catecholamines at the presynaptic sympathetic nerve terminal. The monoamine pump that takes up catecholamines for repackaging or degradation must be functional. In addition, the normal metabolism of dopamine to norepinephrine through the action of dopamine β-monooxygenase must remain intact. Adequate presynaptic stores of norepinephrine must be present to assure that the administration of dopamine will produce the desired pharmacologic effect. Patients who have ingested drugs that impair the functioning of the monoamine pump, such as tricyclic antidepressants, cocaine, or phenothiazines, may be unable to respond to the administration of dopamine as its uptake into the presynaptic terminal may be inhibited. In addition, disulfiram inhibits the enzymatic activity of dopamine β-monooxygenase and dopamine metabolism to norepinephrine is impaired, thus limiting its pressor activity. Similarly, patients who have inadequate presynaptic stores of norepinephrine such as those who chronically abuse cocaine will be unlikely to respond to dopamine administration.

Patients who are maintained on therapeutic doses of monoamine oxidase inhibitors will have an expanded pool of presynaptic norepinephrine. The administration of an indirect-acting pressor agent may result in the release of this expanded pool and a hypertensive crisis. Thus, many toxins that result in hypotension and are unresponsive to fluid resuscitation may also be unresponsive to dopamine. Agents such as norepinephrine or phenylephrine with direct α-adrenergic agonist activity will be safer and more effective.

Many toxins that result in hypotension and are unresponsive to fluid resuscitation may also be unresponsive to dopamine.

SPECIFIC EXAMPLES OF COMMON TOXINS AND THEIR THERAPY

CALCIUM CHANNEL BLOCKERS

Overdose of calcium channel blocking agents is a common toxicologic cause of hypotension, which may progress to cardiogenic shock. These agents produce varying degrees of negative inotropy, conduction blockade, and vasodilation. Management of calcium channel blocker toxicity is based on a specific understanding of the mechanism of action of these drugs, and those of the "antidotal agents."

The force of myocardial contractility and vascular tone is proportional to the available intracellular calcium. When activated, the sarcolemma releases its store of calcium that binds to troponin, a regulatory protein. Troponin interacts with myosin and actin to produce cross-bridging and myocardial contraction. Calcium enters the myocardial or vascular smooth muscle cell through slow channels that are opened during phase 2 of the action potential. The slow channels are nonspecific channels and are 100 times more permeable to Na^+ than calcium. Calcium channel blockers prevent the influx of calcium during phase 2 of the action potential, resulting in a decrease in available calcium, which decreases myocardial contractility and vascular tone.[50]

The initial management for hypotension resulting from intoxication with calcium channel blocking agents is the administration of fluid. Crystalloid will effectively correct the relative intravascular volume depletion that results from vasodilation and increase the contractility of a poorly inotropic ventricle by increasing its filling pressures. When fluid administration is insufficient to restore hemodynamic instability or profound bradycardia is present, the most effective treatment is the rapid infusion of calcium.[51,52] Excess intravascular calcium may overcome some of the blockade at the level of the calcium channel. While the optimal dose of calcium is unknown, most authors recommend an initial dose of 10 ml of a 10% solution of calcium chloride (14.6 mEq/10 ml), which may be repeated if necessary.[53] Alternatively, a 10% solution of calcium gluconate may be used, although it should be remembered that this contains about one-third the available calcium per gram (4.3 mEq/10 ml) as the chloride salt. Care must be taken to exclude the possibility of digoxin poisoning in the patient with bradycardia of unknown etiology, as the administration of calcium may result in systolic tetany and asystolic cardiac arrest.[54,55] Glucagon has also been used successfully in calcium channel blocker overdose in animal models[56-58] and human case reports.[59] Glucagon acts by increasing intracellular cyclic adenosine monophosphate (cAMP). This effect increases intracellular calcium concentration by releasing calcium from its stores in the sarcoplasmic reticulum.[60,61] The combined use of amrinone (a phosphodiesterase inhibitor) and isoproterenol or glucagon may also have theoretical advantages by synergistically increasing intracellular cAMP and therefore myocardial

When fluid administration is insufficient to restore hemodynamic instability or profound bradycardia is present, the most effective treatment is the rapid infusion of calcium.

Care must be taken to exclude the possibility of digoxin poisoning in the patient with bradycardia of unknown etiology, as the administration of calcium may result in systolic tetany and asystolic cardiac arrest.

contractility.[62] While standard pressor agents (epineph-rine, norepinephrine, and dopamine) may be used, it should be remembered that any increase in afterload to a poorly inotropic ventricle may further decrease cardiac out-put. Also, while atropine and isoproterenol have been used for bradycardia, results have been somewhat disappoint-ing. Finally, in cases of refractory hypotension and/or brad-ycardia, the use of a pacemaker and/or an intraaortic bal-loon pump or cardiac bypass is strongly recommended.[63]

BETA BLOCKERS

Toxicity from overdose with β-adrenergic receptor blocking agents may result in myocardial pump failure due to an-tagonism of the action of catecholamines at the level of the myocardium. Normally, when catecholamines bind to the β-adrenergic receptor, adenyl cyclase is activated and in-tracellular levels of cAMP are increased. Increased levels of cAMP will lead to the binding of actin to myosin and enhance myocardial contractility. Thus, by decreasing cAMP, β-adrenergic receptor blockade will lead to a de-crease in myocardial contractility.[64] In addition, β-adre-nergic blockade may decrease the stimulus to the sinus and AV nodes resulting in bradyarrhythmias and atrioventric-ular blockade.

Standard therapy for hypotension and bradycardia, in-cluding fluids, atropine, and cardiac pacemaker, should all be considered. Although atropine is the most frequently used agent for β-adrenergic blocker toxicity, its efficacy may be limited.[65] However, atropine is so frequently used for the treatment of bradycardia of unknown etiology that cases responding favorably may go unreported. Thus, the reported incidence of its efficacy may be deceptively low. If the blood pressure and heart rate do not increase after a trial of fluids and atropine, other therapeutic modalities are indicated.

Toxicity may be antagonized by agents that will directly elevate levels of intracellular cAMP. While β-adrenergic agonists are theoretically capable of increasing intracellular cAMP, their efficacy in the presence of β-adrenergic block-ade is limited. Furthermore, many β-adrenergic agonists have activity at both the β_1- and β_2-adrenergic receptors. Certain β-adrenergic blockers have a relative preference for the β_1-adrenergic receptor. If a mixed β_1- β_2-adrenergic ag-onist is given to a patient with relative β_1-adrenergic block-ade, then it might be expected that β_2-adrenergic effects would predominate. This might result in vasodilation with an exacerbation of the hypotensive state. Thus, when is-oproterenol is administered to the patient with a metopro-

Although atropine is the most frequently used agent for β-adrenergic blocker toxicity, its efficacy may be limited. However, atropine is so frequently used for the treatment of bradycardia of unknown etiology that cases responding favorably may go unreported. Thus, the reported incidence of its efficacy may be deceptively low.

Administration of glucagon has been shown to increase the force of myocardial contraction and cardiac output.

lol overdose and hypotension, the hypotension may be exacerbated.

Administration of glucagon has been shown to increase the force of myocardial contraction and cardiac output.[60] Glucagon's inotropic effect is also mediated through activation of adenyl cyclase, with a resultant increase in intracellular cAMP. This effect, however, is not mediated through β-adrenergic receptors and is therefore unaffected by the presence of β-adrenergic blockade.[66] As in the case of calcium channel blocker overdose, glucagon has been demonstrated to be effective when administered alone or in combination with other agents such as isoproterenol.[67–69] Glucagon is now considered the treatment of choice for circulatory failure due to a β-adrenergic blocker overdose when fluid resuscitation and atropine have failed.[45–47]

The recommended dose for glucagon is 3–10 mg intravenously followed by an infusion of 5 mg/h or 0.7 mg/kg/h.[65] Increased myocardial contractility lasts for approximately 10–15 minutes after a single dose and returns to normal within 25 minutes. Since the biological half-life of β-adrenergic blockers is very long, a continuous infusion of glucagon may be required. Common side effects of glucagon include nausea and vomiting, which are short-lived, and an increased myocardial oxygen demand, which may precipitate myocardial ischemia in patients with coronary artery disease. Even though glucagon mobilizes glycogen through glycogenolysis, there have been no reported cases of hyperglycemia requiring treatment. The administration of a single intravenous bolus of glucagon in most patients with symptomatic β-adrenergic blocker overdoses is without consequential risk and should be used.

If glucagon fails to improve the hemodynamic state of the patient, then a β-adrenergic agonist such as isoproterenol can be utilized with caution.

If glucagon fails to improve the hemodynamic state of the patient, then a β-adrenergic agonist such as isoproterenol can be utilized with caution. A phosphodiesterase inhibitor such as amrinone can increase levels of cAMP by preventing its degradation and thus theoretically may improve the hemodynamic status of the patient with β-adrenergic blocker toxicity. The theoretical use of the combination of amrinone and glucagon is attractive because glucagon may increase cAMP while amrinone may decrease destruction of cAMP, thereby working synergistically to improve myocardial function. Use of these agents in combination should be considered in all cases that fail to respond to fluids and atropine. As in the case of severe calcium channel blocker overdose, either cardiac bypass or the insertion of an intraaortic balloon pump should be considered in all refractory cases.[70]

DISULFIRAM

Disulfiram-induced hypotension is multifactorial in nature. When a patient who is maintained on disulfiram ingests ethanol, flushing and severe gastroenteritis combine to produce both significant volume loss and relative intravascular volume depletion. The reaction results from disulfiram's ability to inhibit aldehyde dehydrogenase, which leads to the accumulation of acetaldehyde (the first metabolic product of ethanol). The increased levels of acetaldehyde produce the characteristic flushing, nausea, and vomiting.[71,72] The direct vasodilatory effect of ethanol may further exacerbate toxicity. In addition, disulfiram is metabolized in the liver and red blood cells to diethyldithiocarbamate. This metabolite inhibits the enzyme dopamine β-monooxygenase, which blocks the conversion of dopamine to norepinephrine.[73] Thus, hypotension may also result from presynaptic norepinephrine depletion.

Most patients, even those with severe disulfiram-ethanol interactions, will respond to fluid resuscitation alone. If, however, hemodynamic support is required, dopamine should be expected to have little clinical utility in the face of catecholamine depletion. A direct-acting agent such as norepinephrine itself is preferred.

TRICYCLIC ANTIDEPRESSANTS

Overdose with one of the tricyclic antidepressants (such as amitriptyline, nortriptyline, desipramine, etc.) produces cardiovascular compromise through a combination of effects at multiple sites. Tricyclic antidepressants are potent blockers of postsynaptic α-adrenergic receptors. Evidence suggests that inhibition of presynaptic α_2-receptors may occur.[74] Thus, they interfere with the ability of sympathomimetic stimulation to maintain normal vascular tone. The ensuing vasodilation results in a relative intravascular volume depletion. Tricyclic antidepressants also work presynaptically to block neuronal catecholamine reuptake. In addition, these agents have a quinidine-like effect on the myocardium, reducing the myocardial contractility and conduction velocity. Finally, it should be noted that tricyclic antidepressants are potent antihistamines. The ability of some of these agents to inhibit the H1 receptor may be from 10- to 1,000-fold greater than diphenhydramine.[75] The tachycardia and flushing seen as manifestations of anticholinergic poisoning may contribute or exacerbate the patient's hemodynamic compromise.

The earliest manifestation of tricyclic antidepressant toxicity is a transient, mild elevation of blood pressure that results from the presynaptic blockade of catecholamine reuptake mechanisms. A more common, more persistent, and more significant effect is presynaptic catecholamine depletion with resultant hypotension.[76]

The treatment for tricyclic antidepressant-induced vasodilation and myocardial depression-associated hypotension begins with standard techniques of fluid resuscitation. In severe toxicity, however, this approach usually proves inadequate.

The treatment for tricyclic antidepressant-induced vasodilation and myocardial depression-associated hypotension begins with standard techniques of fluid resuscitation. In severe toxicity, however, this approach usually proves inadequate. The quinidine-like effect of tricyclic antidepressants may be reversed by the administration of sodium bicarbonate. Sasyniuck demonstrated *in vitro* that the decrease in conduction velocity (Vmax) and slowed conduction in Purkinje cells that are produced during tricyclic antidepressant poisoning can be reversed with the administration of sodium bicarbonate.[15] This effect can be reproduced in part by manipulation of the extracellular Na^+ ion concentration and the pH. An increase in extracellular sodium concentration (as would result from hypertonic saline administration) also improved conduction velocity, but less so than an equivalent dose of sodium bicarbonate. Similarly, increasing extracellular fluid pH (alkalinizing) while maintaining a normal sodium concentration (as would result from hyperventilation) was effective, but not as effective as a sodium bicarbonate infusion that produced a similar pH.[15] Sodium bicarbonate, however, has a limited duration of effect (up to 15 minutes) so repeated doses or continuous infusions are often needed.[14,15] If the patient fails to respond to sodium bicarbonate and fluid therapy, inotropic agents may be required. Evidence supports the use of direct-acting pressors (norepinephrine) over dopamine for these patients.[77] In addition, since catecholamine depletion may have a substantial contribution to tricyclic antidepressant-induced hypotension, indirect-acting agents can be expected to be of limited value.

A wide QRS complex produced by the sodium channel blockade may mimic ventricular tachycardia, and ventricular tachycardia may complicate a tricyclic antidepressant overdose. Ventricular arrhythmias precipitated by tricyclic antidepressant toxicity are often refractory to conventional therapy. Sasyniuck demonstrated that both ventricular and supraventricular arrhythmias accompanied by conduction delays secondary to tricyclic antidepressant poisoning reverted to a normal rhythm following the administration of sodium bicarbonate.[14,15] Therefore, initial therapy for either a ventricular arrhythmia or wide complex tachycardia of unclear origin associated with tricyclic antidepressant poisoning should include the infusion of sodium bi-

Ventricular arrhythmias precipitated by tricyclic antidepressant toxicity are often refractory to conventional therapy.

carbonate. Lidocaine is the antiarrhythmic agent of choice for controlling ventricular arrhythmias that fail to respond to the bicarbonate administration. Type IA and IC antiarrhythmic agents may exacerbate preexisting conduction abnormalities and complicate tricyclic antidepressant overdose. Drugs such as quinidine, procainamide, and flecainide should therefore be avoided.[48,78,79]

ORGANOPHOSPHATES

Organophosphate toxicity results in both gastrointestinal fluid losses and insensible fluid losses. Toxicity is characterized by excessive cholinergic stimulation secondary to the inactivation of acetylcholinesterase. This produces a syndrome consisting of diaphoresis, diarrhea, urination, lacrimation, emesis, and salivation, which can rapidly produce profound loss of intravascular volume.[80] Specific treatment with atropine (to antagonize muscarinic symptoms and thereby reduce volume losses) and 2-PAM (to regenerate acetylcholinesterase activity) is required to prevent further volume loss.

THEOPHYLLINE

As with many other toxins, theophylline-induced hypotension is multifactorial. It may result from volume loss associated with repetitive vomiting, tachycardia, and arrhythmias or occur as the result of an excess of β_2-adrenergic activity. In addition, although theophylline may produce a diuresis through a mechanism similar to the thiazide diuretics, this effect is rarely clinically relevant.[81] While it is unclear whether theophylline itself has direct vasoactive properties in either therapeutic or in overdose models, increased levels of circulating catecholamine (epinephrine and to a lesser extent norepinephrine) have been described.[26,82,83] In support of this concept is a strong body of animal evidence that suggests that β-adrenergic blockade will not only reverse the electrolyte abnormalities associated with theophylline toxicity, but will also correct the hemodynamic manifestations.[84,85] In humans, propranolol has been used successfully to treat the tachycardia and hypotension associated with theophylline toxicity in isolated case reports.[86,87] This therapy is obviously very dangerous, and we feel that it should be reserved for severely ill patients who have failed standard therapy and in whom invasive hemodynamic monitoring has confirmed a high cardiac index, vasodilated state. Extra caution should be observed in patients with asthma or chronic obstructive pulmonary disease, as β-adrenergic blockade may induce bronchospasm in these patients.

MONOAMINE OXIDASE INHIBITORS

The antidepressant, monoamine oxidase inhibitors have complex pharmacologic effects that may result in severe hypertension or shock. The enzyme monoamine oxidase regulates the intraneuronal oxidative deamination of epinephrine, norepinephrine, dopamine, and 5-hydroxytryptamine (5HT or serotonin) to inactive metabolites.[88,89] Monoamine oxidase inhibitors inhibit monoamine oxidase in all tissues. In the presence of monoamine oxidase inhibitors, the pool of stored catecholamines in the presynaptic nerve terminal will be enlarged. Hypotension following the overdose of monoamine oxidase inhibitors may follow a transient period of hypertension and results from the depletion of catecholamines from storage sites.[91] However, the ingestion or administration of any of the indirect-acting sympathomimetic agents will cause the release of this expanded pool of catecholamines.[92] Tyramine, an indirect-acting sympathomimetic agent found in many foods, is usually inactivated by gut monoamine oxidase. Following the use of monoamine oxidase inhibitors, tyramine will be absorbed from the gut unaltered, which results in the release of a large pool of neurotransmitter and may produce a hypertensive crisis.[93]

Hypertension associated with sympathomimetic excess or induced by sympathomimetic poisoning should be rigidly controlled. Indications for the treatment of hypertension in this setting include any manifestation of end-organ failure such as signs of encephalopathy, the onset of angina, renal failure or cerebrovascular hemorrhage. Other relative indications, such as an extreme elevation of blood pressure even in the absence of end-organ damage, may exist—especially in the presence of headache. The mechanism of action of the toxic agent involved is important in anticipating the need for treatment, since the duration of the hypertension may be transient, and may result in catecholamine depletion and ultimately profound hypotension. The hypertension produced by a monoamine oxidase inhibitor overdose, by phenylpropanolamine and monoamine oxidase inhibitor, or the tyramine and monoamine oxidase inhibitor interactions may have a longer duration of action, be more severe, and require more aggressive treatment.

Hypotension following the overdose of monoamine oxidase inhibitors may follow a transient period of hypertension and results from the depletion of catecholamines from storage sites. However, the ingestion or administration of any of the indirect-acting sympathomimetic agents will cause the release of this expanded pool of catecholamines.

Sedation may be the only treatment required for the anxious hypertensive patient and should be used early in the patient's management. Sedation itself may result in a significant reduction of the patient's blood pressure. Patients with signs of end-organ damage require intervention with agents that antagonize the sympathetic effect. The ideal agent to use is sodium nitroprusside because of its rapid onset and short duration of action. Phentolamine, a specific α-adrenergic blocking agent, may be effective, especially in states of catecholamine excess such as those that occur with monoamine oxidase inhibitors and tyramine interactions. The use of selective β-adrenergic antagonists (propranolol or esmolol) or mixed α- and β-adrenergic antagonists (such as labetalol) may result in the unopposed stimulation of α-adrenergic receptors and the exacerbation of the hypertension.

COCAINE

A comprehensive discussion of the cardiovascular effects of cocaine and their associated complications is beyond the scope of this paper and has been extensively reviewed elsewhere.[39,40] A brief discussion of the management of cocaine-induced hypertension and tachycardia, however, is warranted. Cocaine produces its effects largely through a combination of direct central nervous system stimulation and prevention of the presynaptic neuronal reuptake of catecholamines.[40] The net effect is the production of a "sympathetic storm."

Several animal models have evaluated the role of β-adrenergic blockers for the treatment of cocaine-induced hypertension and tachycardia.[94,95] A recent animal investigation has also demonstrated that mixed α- and β-adrenergic blockade with labetalol is ineffective as an antidote.[96] Despite this evidence, several authors continue to advocate the use of β and mixed α- and β-adrenergic blockade for cocaine toxicity.[97–100] Human evidence is beginning to mount that supports the fact that when administered to patients with either minor or major manifestations of cocaine toxicity, β-adrenergic blockers can exacerbate hypertension and coronary vasospasm.[101–103] Strong animal evidence and arguments have been given for the use of sedatives and cooling (if necessary) to reverse the effects of cocaine-induced catecholamine excess.[40,94–96] Should a specific antihypertensive agent be required, the use of sodium nitroprusside is preferred because of its short duration of effect and ease of titration. Alternatively, the use of phentolamine may be acceptable because of documented utility in the human cardiac catheterization study.[102]

TACHYCARDIAS INDUCED BY ANTICHOLINERGIC AGENTS

Acetylcholinesterase inhibitors have been used successfully to reverse the toxic manifestations of pure anticholinergic agents.

Significant tachycardia can complicate the toxicity of anticholinergic agents, such as the ingestion of anticholinergic plants (*Datura stramonium*), tricyclic antidepressants, and antihistamines, and may result in or exacerbate hypotension. Acetylcholinesterase inhibitors have been used successfully to reverse the toxic manifestations of pure anticholinergic agents. Acetylcholinesterase inhibitors allow for the accumulation of acetylcholine and increased parasympathetic stimulation. Physostigmine is a reversible acetylcholinesterase inhibitor and antagonizes both the central and peripheral toxicity of anticholinergic excess. It is recommended for the treatment of symptomatic hypotension, tachycardia, or extreme agitation in patients with anticholinergic poisoning that is refractory to the administration of sedative agents. Due to the risks associated with the use of physostigmine, the agent is recommended only when peripheral signs of anticholinergic poisoning are present and a history confirms an anticholinergic overdose. Its use is contraindicated in the presence of any cardiac conduction delays. In an animal model, physostigmine has been shown to exacerbate tricyclic antidepressant toxicity,[104] and, when given to humans with tricyclic antidepressant overdose, it has resulted in bradyarrhythmias and asystole.[105] Thus, prior to the administration of physostigmine in a patient with manifestations of severe anticholinergic poisoning, a 12-lead electrocardiogram should be obtained to exclude the possibility of conduction disturbances that are suggestive of tricyclic antidepressant poisoning. Because the effects of physostigmine are transient, the manifestations of tricyclic antidepressant overdose are multifactorial, and asystole has been reported with the use of physostigmine, the agent can no longer be recommended in this setting. The dose of physostigmine is 1–2 mg infused intravenously over 5 minutes. If physostigmine is given too rapidly, it may precipitate a seizure or cholinergic crisis. Repeated doses of physostigmine may be necessary. Relative contraindications to its use include underlying bronchospastic disease, peripheral vascular disease, intestinal or bladder obstruction, and previous treatment with choline esters or depolarizing neuromuscular blocking agents such as succinylcholine.[38]

CONCLUSIONS

The pathophysiology of hypotension that complicates most toxic ingestions is usually extremely complex, resulting from multiple mechanisms. While a standardized approach to hypotension (which begins with fluid administration) will often suffice, more specific therapy is indicated when cardiovascular insufficiency persists. Common therapeutic modalities such as the use of dopamine for hypotension frequently fail in the presence of toxin exposure. Similarly, common strategies such as the administration of β-adrenergic antagonists to patients with hypertension and tachycardia can actually exacerbate toxicity. A sound understanding of the special considerations in poisoned patients is essential to successful resuscitation. In addition, aggressive implementation of advanced cardiac life support principles and basic and advanced poison management will ensure the most positive outcome. Therapy in each case should be tailored by the clinical scenario and an understanding of toxicologic and pharmacologic factors.

References

1. Olsnes S, Refsnes K, Pihl A: Mechanism of action of the toxic lectins abrin and ricin. Nature 249:627, 1974

2. Wedin GP, Neal JS, Everson GW, Krenzelok EP: Castor bean poisoning. Am J Emerg Med 4:260, 1986

3. Montgomery H: Hazard to health Jequirity-bean poisoning. N Engl J Med 268:885, 1963

4. Roberge R, Brader E, Martin M et al: The root of evil-Pokeweed intoxication. Ann Emerg Med 15:470, 1986

5. Schoolmeester WL, White DR: Arsenic poisoning. S Med J 73:198, 1980

6. Fesmire FM, Schauben JL, Roberge RJ: Survival following massive arsenic ingestion. Am J Emerg Med 6:602, 1988

7. Keller RE, Schwab RA, Krenzelok EP: Contribution of sorbitol combined with activated charcoal in prevention of salicylate absorption. Ann Emerg Med 19:654, 1990.

8. Smilkstein MJ, Steedle D, Kulig KW et al: Magnesium levels after magnesium-containing cathartics. J Toxicol Clin Toxicol 26:51, 1988

9. Farley TA: Severe hypernatremic dehydration after use of an activated charcoal-sorbitol suspension. J Pediatr 109:719, 1986

10. LeWitt PA: The neurotoxicity of the rat poison Vacor: a clinical study of 12 cases. N Engl J Med 302;73, 1980

11. Frimpter GW, Timpanelli AE, Eisenmenger WJ et al: Reversible "Fanconi syndrome" caused by degraded tetracycline. JAMA 184:111, 1963

12. Padfield PL, Morton JJ, Lindop G, Timbury GC: Lithium induced nephrogenic diabetes insipidus: changes in plasma vasopressin and angiotensin. II. Clin Nephrol 3:220, 1975

13. Singer I, Rotenberg D: Mechanisms of lithium action. N Engl J Med 289:244, 1973

14. Sasyniuk B, Jhamandas V: Mechanism of reversal of toxic effects of amitriphtyline on cardiac Purkinje fibers by sodium bicarbonate. J Pharm Exp Ther 231:386, 1984

15. Sasyniuk BI, Jhamandas V, Valois M: Experimental amitriptyline intoxication: treatment of cardiac toxicity with sodium bicarbonate. Ann Emerg Med 15:1052, 1986

16. Niemann J, Bessen H, Rothstein R, Laks M: Electrocardiographic criteria of tricyclic antidepressant cardiotoxicity. Am J Cardiol 57:1154, 1986

17. Wasserman F, Brodsky L, Dick MM et al: Successful treatment of quinidine and procaine amide intoxication. N Engl J Med 259:797, 1958

18. Pentel P, Goldsmith SR, Salerno DM et al: Effect of hypertonic sodium bicarbonate on encainide overdose. Am J Cardiol 57:878, 1986

19. Bajaj AK, Woosley RL, Roden DM: Acute electrophysiologic effects of sodium administration in dogs treated with 0-desmethyl encainide. Circulation 80:994, 1989

20. Ellenhorn MJ, Barceloux DG: Neuroleptic drugs. p. 477. In Ellenhorn MJ, Barceloux DG (eds): Medical toxicology. Elsevier, New York, 1988

21. Linden CH, Mitchiner JC, Lindzon RD et al: Cyclobenzaprine overdose. J Toxicol Clin Toxicol 20:281, 1983

22. Seger D: Phenytoin and other anticonvulsants. p. 877. In Haddad LM, Winchester JF (eds): Clinical management of poisoning and drug overdose. 2nd ed. WB Saunders, Philadelphia, 1990

23. Whitcomb DC, Gilliam FR, Starmer CF, Grant AO: Marked QRS complex abnormalities and sodium channel blockade by propoxyphene reversed with lidocaine. J Clin Invest 84:1629, 1989

24. Spoerke DG: Amantidine. In: Poisindex. Vol. 66. Micromedex, Denver, 1990

25. Parker RB, Beckman KJ, Hariman RJI et al: The electrophysiologic and arrhythmogenic effects of cocaine (Abstr). Pharmacotherapy 9:176, 1989

26. Poisner AM: Direct stimulant effect of aminophylline on catecholamine release from the adrenal medulla. Biochem Pharmacol 22:469, 1973

27. Reinhardt CF et al: Cardiac arrhythmias in aerosol sniffing. Arch Environ Health 22:265, 1971

28. Bass M: Sudden sniffing death. JAMA 212:2075, 1970

29. Gustafson A, Svensson S, Ugander L: Cardiac arrhythmias in chloral hydrate poisoning. Acta Med Scand 201:227, 1977

30. Banner W, Tong TG: Iron poisoning. Pediatr Clin North Am 33:393, 1986

31. Robotham J, Lietman PS: Acute iron poisoning. Am J Dis Child 134:875, 1980

32. Rosenmund A, Haeberli A, Struab PW: Blood coagulation and acute iron toxicity. J Lab Clin Med 103:524, 1984

33. Whitten CF, Chen Y, Gibson GW: Studies in acute iron poisoning. II. Further observations on desferrioxamine in the treatment of acute experimental iron poisoning. Pediatrics 38:102, 1966

34. Smith MJH: The metabolic basis of the major symptoms in acute salicylate intoxication. Clin Toxicol 1:387, 1968

35. Temple AR: Acute and chronic effects of aspirin toxicity and their treatment. Arch Intern Med 141:364, 1981

36. Hill JB: Salicylate intoxication. N Engl J Med 286:1110, 1973

37. Mariani PJ: Pseudophedrine-induced hypertensive emergency: treatment with labetalol. Am J Emerg Med 4:141, 1986

38. Reidenberg MM: A review of reported adverse cardiovascular reactions to phenylpropanolamine. Presented at the conference Phenylpropanolamine: Examining Benefits and Risks, New York Academy of Medicine, New York, June 1984

39. Cregler LL, Herbert M: Medical complications of cocaine abuse. N Engl J Med 315:1495, 1986

40. Goldfrank LR, Hoffman RS: The cardiovascular effects of cocaine. Ann Emerg Med 20:165, 1991

41. Anderson PK, Christensen KN, Hole P et al: Sodium nitroprusside and epidural blockade in the treatment of ergotism. N Engl J Med 296:1271, 1977

42. Carliner NH, Denune DP, Finch CS, Goldberg LI: Sodium nitroprusside treatment of ergotamine-induced peripheral ischemia. JAMA 227:308, 1974

43. Horowitz D, Lovenberg W, Engelman K et al: Monoamine oxidase inhibitors, tyramine and cheese. JAMA 188:1108, 1964

44. Vigran IM: Dangerous potentiation of meperidine hydrochloride by pargyline hydrochloride. JAMA 187:953, 1964

45. Goldfrank LE, Flomenbaum NE, Lewin NA et al (eds): Goldfrank's toxicologic emergencies. 4th ed. Appleton and Lange, Norwalk, 1990

46. Ellenhorn MJ, Barceloux DG (eds): Medical toxicology: diagnosis and treatment of human poisoning. Elsevier, New York, 1988

47. Haddad LM, Winchester JF (eds): Clinical management of poisoning and drug overdose. 2nd ed. WB Saunders, Philadelphia, 1990

48. Benowitz NL, Rosenberg J, Becker CE: Cardiopulmonary catastrophes in drug-overdosed patients. Med Clin North Am 63:267, 1979

49. Houston M, Thompson L, Robertson D: Shock diagnosis and management. Arch Intern Med 144:1433, 1984

50. Braunwald E: Mechanism of action of calcium-channel-blocking agents. N Engl J Med 307:1618, 1982

51. Hariman R, Lucia MM, McAllister RG et al: Reversal of the cardiovascular effects of verapamil

by calcium and sodium: differences between electrophysiologic and hemodynamic responses. Circulation 59:797, 1979

52. Morris LD, Goldschlager N: Calcium infusion for reversal of adverse effects of intravenous verapamil. JAMA 249:3212, 1989

53. Lewin NA, Howland MA: Antihypertensive agents: including beta blockers and calcium channel blockers. p. 369. In Goldfrank LR, Flomenbaum NE, Lewin NA, Weisman RS, Howland MA (eds): Goldfrank's toxicologic emergencies. 4th ed. Appleton and Lange, Norwalk, 1990

54. Nola GT, Pope S, Harison DC: Assessment of the synergistic relationship between serum calcium and digitalis. Am Heart J 79:499, 1970

55. Hoffman BF, Bigger JT: Digitalis and allied cardiac glycosides. p. 814. In Gilman AG, Rall TW, Niew AS, Taylor P (eds): Goodman and Gillman's the pharmacologic basis of therapeutics. 8th ed. Pergamon Press, New York, 1990

56. Zaloga GP, Malcolm D, Holaday J, Chernow B: Glucagon reverses the hypotension and bradycardia of verapamil overdose in rats. Crit Care Med 13:273, 1985

57. Zaritsky AL, Horowitz M, Chernow B: Glucagon antagonism of calcium channel blocker-induced myocardial dysfunction. Crit Care Med 16:246, 1988

58. Jolly S, Kipnis J, Lucchesi B: Cardiovascular depression by verapamil: reversal by glucagon and interactions with propronol. Pharmacology 35:249, 1987

59. Horowitz BZ, Rhee K: Massive verapamil ingestion: a report of two cases and a review of the literature. Am J Emerg Med 7:624, 1989

60. Parmley WW, Glick G, Sonnenblick EH: Cardiovascular effects of glucagon in man. N Engl J Med 279:12, 1968

61. Hall-Boyer K, Zaloga GP, Chernow B: Glucagon: hormone of therapeutic agent? Crit Care Med 12:584, 1984

62. Goenen M, Col J, Compere A, Bonte J: Treatment of severe verapamil poisoning with combined amrinone-isoproterenol therapy. Am J Cardiol 58:1142, 1986

63. Hendren WG, Schieber RS, Garrettson LK: Extracorporeal bypass for the treatment of verapamil poisoning. Ann Emerg Med 18:948, 1989

64. Hoffman BB, Lefkowitz RJ: Adrenergic receptor antagonist. p. 221. In Gilman AG, Rall TW, Niew AS, Taylor P (eds): Goodman and Gilman's the pharmacological basis of therapeutics. 8th ed. Pergamon Press, New York, 1990

65. Weinstein RS: Recognition and management of poisoning with beta-adrenergic blocking agents. Ann Emerg Med 13:1123, 1984

66. Kosinski EJ, Malindzak GS: Glucagon and isoproternol in reversing propanolol toxicity. Arch Intern Med 132:840, 1973

67. Robson RH: Glucagon for beta-blocker poisoning. Lancet 1:1357, 1980

68. Illingsworth RN: Glucagon for beta-blocker poisoning. Practitioner 223:863, 1979

69. Agura ED, Wexler LF, Witzburg RA: Massive propranolol overdose: successful treatment with high-dose isoproterenol and glucagon. Am J Med 80:755, 1986

70. Lane AS, Woodward AC, Goldman MR: Massive propranolol overdose poorly responsive to pharmacologic therapy: use of the intra-aortic balloon pump. Ann Emerg Med 16:1381, 1987

71. Eneanya D, Bianchine J, Duran D, Andresen B: The actions and metabolic fate of disulfiram. Annu Rev Pharmacol Toxicol 21:575, 1981

72. Seixas F: Alcohol and its drug interactions. Ann Intern Med 83:86, 1975

73. Rogers WK, Benowitz NL, Wilson KM, Abbot JA: Effect of disulfiram on adrenergic function. Clin Pharmacol Ther 24:469, 1979

74. Collis MG, Shepherd JT: Antidepressant drug action at presynaptic alpha receptors. Mayo Clin Proc 55:567, 1980

75. Richelson E: Antimuscarinic and other receptor blocking properties of antidepressants. Mayo Clin Proc 58:40, 1983

76. Rosenbaum AH, Maruta T, Richelson E: Clinical pharmacology series on pharmacology in practice. 1. Drugs that alter mood: tricyclic agents and monoamine oxidase inhibitors. Mayo Clin Proc 54:335, 1979

77. Teba L, Schiebel F, Dedhia HV, Lazzell VA: Beneficial effect of norepinephrine in the treatment of circulatory shock caused by tricyclic antidepressant overdose. Am J Emerg Med 6:566, 1988

78. Biggs JT, Spiker D, Petit J, Ziegler V: Tricyclic antidepressant overdose incidence of symptoms. JAMA 238:135, 1977

79. Smilkstein MJ: Reviewing cyclic antidepressant cardiotoxicity: wheat and chaff. J Emerg Med 8:645, 1990

80. Taturi J, Roberts J: Organophosphate poisoning. Ann Emerg Med 16:193, 1987

81. Maren TH: The additive renal effect of oral aminophylline and trichlormethiazide in man. Clin Res 9:57, 1961

82. Atuk NO, Blaydes C, Westervelt FB, Wood JE: Effect of aminophylline on urinary excretion of epinephrine and norepinephrine in man. Circulation 35:745, 1967

83. Vestal RE, Eiriksson CE, Musser B et al: Effect of intravenous aminophylline on plasma levels of catecholamines and related cardiovascular and metabolic responses in man. Circulation 67:162, 1983

84. Kearney TE, Manoguerra AS, Curtis GP, Ziegler MG: Theophylline toxicity and the beta-adrenergic system. Ann Intern Med 102:766, 1985

85. Gaar GG, Banner W: The effects of esmolol on the hemodynamics of acute theophylline toxicity. Ann Emerg Med 16:1334, 1987

86. Biberstein MP, Ziegler MG, Ward DM: Use of B-Blockade and hemoperfusion for acute theophylline poisoning. West J Med 141:485, 1984

87. Amin DN, Henry JA: Propranolol administration in theophylline overdose. Lancet 1:520, 1985

88. Denny RM, Fritz RR, Patel NT, Abel CW: Human liver MAO-A and MAO-B reported by

immunoaffinity chromatography with MAO-B specific monoclonal antibody. Science 215:1400, 1982

89. Goldstein DS: Catecholamines in plasma and cerebrospinal fluid: sources and meanings. p. 15. In Buckley JP, Ferrario CM (eds): Brain peptides and catecholamines in cardiovascular regulation. Raven Press, New York, 1987

90. Murphy DL, Sunderland T, Cohen RM: Monoamine oxidase-inhibiting antidepressants. Psychiatr Clin North Am 7:549, 1984

91. Linden CH, Rumack BH, Strehike C: Monoamine oxidase inhibitor overdose. Ann Emerg Med 13:1137, 1984

92. Boakes AJ, Laurence DR, Teoh PC et al: Interactions between sympathomimetic amines and antidepressant agents in man. Brit Med J 1:311, 1977

93. Goldberg LI: Monoamine oxidase inhibitors: adverse reactions and possible mechanisms. JAMA 190:456, 1964

94. Guinn MM, Bedford JA, Wilson MC: Antagonism of intravenous cocaine lethality in non-human primates. Clin Toxicol 16:499, 1980

95. Catravas JD, Waters IW: Acute cocaine intoxication in the conscious dog: studies on the mechanism of lethality. J Pharmacol Exp Ther 217:350, 1981

96. Spivey WH, Schoffstall JM, Kirkpatrick R et al: Comparison of labetalol, diazepam and haloperidol for the treatment of cocaine toxicity in a swine model (Abstr). Ann Emerg Med 19:467, 1990

97. Rappolt TR, Gay G, Inaba DS, Rappolt NR: Propranolol in cocaine toxicity (Letter). Lancet 2:640, 1976

98. Gay GR: Clinical management of acute and chronic cocaine poisoning. Ann Emerg Med 11:562, 1982

99. Dusenberry SJ, Hicks MJ, Mariani PJ: Labetalol treatment of cocaine toxicity (Letter). Ann Emerg Med 16:235, 1987

100. Gay GR, Loper KA: The use of labetalol in the management of cocaine crisis. Ann Emerg Med 17:282, 1988

101. Ramoska E, Sacchetti AD: Propranolol-induced hypertension in treatment of cocaine intoxication. Ann Emerg Med 14:112, 1985

102. Lange RA, Cigarroa RG, Flores ED et al: Potentiation of cocaine-induced coronary vasoconstriction by beta-adrenergic blockade. Ann Intern Med 112:897, 1990

103. Sand IC, Brody SL, Wrenn KD, Slovis CM: Experience with esmolol for the treatment of cocaine-associated cardiovascular complications. Am J Emerg Med 9:161, 1991

104. Vance MA, Ross SM, Millington WR, Blumberg JB: Potentiation of tricyclic antidepressant toxicity by physostigmine in mice. J Toxicol Clin Toxicol 11:413, 1977

105. Pentel P, Peterson CD: Asystole complicating physostigmine treatment of tricyclic antidepressant overdose. Ann Emerg Med 9:588, 1980

SMOKE INHALATION

DIANE LIU, MD, MPH[†]
KENT R. OLSON, MD, FACEP, ABMT[††]

Smoke inhalation is a well-known cause of airway injury in fire victims and firefighters.[1] It contributes significantly to the acute mortality and morbidity of burn victims. Approximately 8,000 deaths from fire-related injuries occur in the United States each year, and of these, more than 50% can be attributed to inhalational injuries.[2,3] It has been demonstrated that burn victims who also suffer from smoke inhalation have a greater mortality risk than those with only cutaneous burns.[4,5] One author reports a 20% increased risk of mortality in smoke inhalation victims compared to those who suffer only from burn injuries.[6]

Carbon monoxide poisoning and oxygen deprivation are often implicated as primary problems in the early treatment of fire victims. Hydrogen cyanide gas, liberated when certain polymers and nitrogen-containing compounds are burned, has become increasingly recognized as a major cause of death due to smoke inhalation.[3]

Smoke consists of a mixture of combustion products depending on the temperature and the composition of the materials that are being burned.[7] The toxic inhalants are chemicals in the form of gases, vapors, aerosols, particulates, and fumes. Many substances only become toxic when burned, liberating toxic pyrolysis products (Table 1).

The health effects from smoke inhalation can best be described by mechanism of injury. Several irritant gases are formed when natural and synthetic building materials and furnishings are burned. These gases include ammonia, acrolein, and sulfur dioxide. Their mechanism of injury is a direct cytotoxic effect on the epithelium of the oropharynx and airways.

The second class of chemical intoxicants liberated from fires are the asphyxiants. Hydrogen cyanide and carbon

Approximately 8,000 deaths from fire-related injuries occur in the United States each year, and of these, more than 50% can be attributed to inhalational injuries.

[†] San Francisco Bay Area Regional Poison Control Center, San Francisco General Hospital, Center for Municipal Occupational Safety and Health, San Francisco, California

[††] Medical Director, San Francisco Bay Area Regional Poison Control Center, Associate Clinical Professor of Medicine, Lecturer in Pharmacy, University of California, San Francisco, San Francisco General Hospital, San Francisco, California

TABLE 1   Toxic Gases and Vapors Encountered in Fires

Toxic Gas	Source	ACGIH TLV*	IDLH†
Acrolein	Cellulose, acrylic	0.1 ppm	5 ppm
Ammonia	Nylon, silk, wool	25 ppm	500 ppm
Hydrogen chloride	Polyvinyl chloride, retardant-treated materials	5 ppm	100 ppm
Chlorine	Operations using chlorine: paper manufacturing, sewage treatment	0.5 ppm	25 ppm
Sulfur dioxide	Sulfur-containing materials	2 ppm	100 ppm
Nitrogen dioxide	Cellulose nitrate, fabrics, celluloid	3 ppm	50 ppm
Phosgene	Polyvinyl chloride, chlorine-containing materials	0.1 ppm	2 ppm
Carbon monoxide	Incomplete combustion of wood, cotton, polyvinyl chloride, petroleum products	50 ppm	1500 ppm
Hydrogen cyanide	Polyurethane, melamine resins, nylon	10 ppm	50 ppm

* Threshold limit values (TLV) and biological exposure indices. 8th ed. American council of governmental industrial hygeinists (ACGIH), 1989.
† NIOSH/OSHA: Pocket guide to chemical hazards. NIOSH Publication No. 78-210. US Department of Health and Human Services, 1985.
IDLH = Immediately dangerous to life and health.

monoxide are chemical asphyxiants that interrupt oxygen utilization at the cellular level. Carbon dioxide is an example of a simple asphyxiant that can displace available oxygen, usually in a closed environment, preventing the victim from aerating the lungs with oxygen.

Fire victims also suffer from thermal injury to the upper respiratory tract. However, this diagnosis can be overlooked because the classical signs of smoke or thermal injury, carbonaceous sputum, singed nasal hairs, and oropharyngeal burns, may be absent. In one study, up to 85% of patients with upper respiratory tract burns have no facial burns. Only 50% of these patients had carbonaceous sputum.[8]

PATHOPHYSIOLOGY

IRRITANT GASES

The physical and chemical properties of the irritant gas determine the extent of injury to the respiratory tract. Those substances that are water soluble are irritating to the mucous membranes of the conjunctiva and upper airway, including the mouth, nose, throat, and bronchi.

Irritant gases have a direct cytotoxic effect on the epithelium of the oropharynx and respiratory tract. These irritants are capable of causing extensive damage to the airways and parenchyma. The physical and chemical properties of the irritant gas determine the extent of injury to the respiratory tract. Those substances that are water soluble are irritating to the mucous membranes of the conjunctiva and upper airway, including the mouth, nose, throat, and bronchi. Highly water-soluble compounds dissolve in the mucous along the upper respiratory tract and relatively little reaches the lower airways and gas-exchanging alveoli. Some examples of these substances include ammonia, hydrogen chloride, and sulfur dioxide (Table 1).[9] Substances that are less water soluble do not dissolve as readily in the mucous of the upper airway and can reach the distal airways; significant exposure can cause delayed pulmonary edema. An example of this is the chemical phosgene, a product of pyrolysis of chlorine-containing compounds. If the victim is exposed to extremely high levels of irritant gas, or is unable to escape from exposure, the ability of the upper airway to "scrub out" the irritant gas from the inhaled air may be overwhelmed, allowing the distal airway and alveoli to be exposed. In these instances, even highly water soluble gases may cause pulmonary edema.

Substances that are less water soluble do not dissolve as readily in the mucous of the upper airway and can reach the distal airways; significant exposure can cause delayed pulmonary edema.

Acrolein

Acrolein is a three-carbon aldehyde that is generated from the incomplete combustion of organic materials (eg, wood and cotton), tobacco, polymers, and plastics. It is an intense irritant to the eyes and upper respiratory tract. Patients who are exposed to high concentrations may develop bronchitis and pulmonary edema.[10] Exposure to 0.25 parts per million (ppm) can cause eye and skin irritation; 10 ppm may produce pulmonary edema.[11,12]

Acrolein is toxic by all routes of exposure (dermal, oral, inhalational), but is primarily absorbed by inhalation. The respiratory tract is the primary target of injury. It has been shown to cause a reflex decrease in respiratory rate, ciliastasis (paralysis of the bronchial cilia), pulmonary hypersensitivity, and pulmonary edema. Pulmonary edema can be delayed in onset.[9] Symptoms of exposure include nasal irritation, cough, and dyspnea. Eye irritation is also prominent, but eye injury has not been demonstrated clinically.

Eye and mucous membrane irritation occurs at 0.25 ppm, the level immediately dangerous to life and health (IDLH) is 5 ppm, and the rapid onset of pulmonary edema has been reported at 10 ppm. It should be noted that exposure to 10 ppm for 10 minutes has led to fatalities.[13] In a survey of 200 fires that occurred in Boston, 10% of fires were noted to have a level of acrolein that exceeded 3 ppm.[12] Acrolein has been implicated as a major cause of fatalities due to smoke inhalation.[9]

Ammonia

Ammonia is a colorless, highly water-soluble alkaline gas that is highly irritating when in contact with the skin and mucous membranes. It is liberated during the combustion of nylon, silk, wool, and melamine.[9] Melamine is commonly used in the construction of office and household furnishings, for example, desks, bookshelves, and cupboards.

Symptoms of exposure include immediate irritation of the eyes, skin, and upper respiratory contact. Upon contact with moist mucosa, ammonia reacts with water and forms ammonium hydroxide, a strong corrosive agent. The extent of injury depends on the concentration of the ammonium hydroxide and the duration of exposure. Because ammonia is highly water-soluble, injury is generally limited to the upper airway.

Most reported incidences of ammonia gas exposure are related to industrial accidental exposure.[14] Signs and symptoms include irritation of mucous membranes; edema of the trachea; extensive burns of the eyes, skin, nose oropharynx, and tracheobroncheal tree; and death.

Hydrogen Chloride and Chlorine

Hydrogen chloride, chlorine, and multiple other chemicals are produced when polyvinyl chloride (PVC) is burned in a process known as thermal degradation. Typical symptoms reported by firefighters after exposure to a PVC fire include tachypnea, cough, hoarseness, dyspnea, chest tightness, and wheezing.

Hydrogen chloride, chlorine, and multiple other chemicals are produced when polyvinyl chloride (PVC) is burned in a process known as thermal degradation.[15] Furniture and building fixtures often consist of PVC components. Typical symptoms reported by firefighters after exposure to a PVC fire include tachypnea, cough, hoarseness, dyspnea, chest tightness, and wheezing.[16]

Hydrogen chloride gas is a highly water-soluble acid that forms hydrochloric acid (HCl) when it comes in contact with moist mucosal surfaces. Brand-Rauf et al.[17] reported levels of hydrogen chloride to be 13.3 ppm at one fire. This level corresponds to symptoms of irritation of the mucous membranes and throat.[11] If escape from exposure is impossible, then high exposure (1,000 ppm) can cause pulmonary edema.[11,18] The irritative property of HCl leads to early warning of its presence. Most people can detect a level of 5 ppm.[9] The threshold limit value (TLV) averaged over 8 hours is 5 ppm[19]; the IDLH is 100 ppm.[20]

Chlorine gas causes injury by a direct oxidative effect of an oxygen-free radical liberated when it is in the presence of water. Chlorine is a chemical of intermediate water solubility. Therefore, the gas can reach the distal airways and alveoli and may cause injury throughout the entire respiratory tract. Chlorine also combines with water to produce hydrochloric acid, which may add to the damage caused by the oxygen-free radicals. The gas also has early warning properties. Symptoms of mucous membrane irritation occur near the TLV of 0.5 ppm. Chlorine gas is immediately dangerous to life and health at 25 ppm.

Sulfur Dioxide

Sulfur dioxide can be liberated when some sulfur-containing natural and synthetic materials are exposed to heat or fire.[11] When in contact with moisture of the mucous membranes, sulfur dioxide produces highly water-soluble sulfuric acid, which is an intense irritant to the eyes and respiratory tract. Injury is generally limited to the upper respiratory tract.

Sulfur dioxide was detected in greater than 50% of fires examined in one study.[17] The concentrations ranged from 0.2 ppm to 42 ppm with 40% of the values above the TLV of 2 ppm. Exposure to 6–10 ppm causes immediate irritation. Most of the gas dissolves into the mucous of the nasopharynx and oropharynx at low concentrations (1–50 ppm) and only reaches the more distal airways when exposures exceed this level.[9]

Oxides of Nitrogen

Combustion of celluloid, cellulose nitrate, and nitrogen-containing fabrics (wool) can produce oxides of nitrogen (NO_x), such as nitric oxide (NO) and nitrogen dioxide (NO_2).[7,9] The oxides of nitrogen are respiratory tract irritants that have relatively low solubility in water. Therefore, they may not be as irritating to the upper respiratory tract as a water-soluble compound. A person may be exposed to potentially hazardous levels of NO_x without adequate warning. This may allow the NO_x to be inhaled deeply, where it combines with water in the distal airways and alveoli to produce nitric acid. Nitrites and nitrates are formed when nitric acid dissociates causing local inflammation and tissue destruction.[21] The NO_x have been shown to impair lung surfactant activity,[22] increase sensitivity to bronchoconstrictors, and possibly initiate tissue destruction through lipid peroxidation.[21]

Acute symptoms are related to irritation of the distal airways and lung parenchyma. Symptoms include cough and dyspnea that occur at approximately 250 ppm for a brief exposure.[13] Pulmonary edema may develop within the next 1–2 hours, associated with tachypnea, cyanosis, and rales and rhonchi on auscultation. Severe exposure can lead to bronchiolitis obliterans.[23] It is unclear whether exposure to NO_x causes persistent severe respiratory impairment.

Exposure to the oxides of nitrogen during a fire may also cause methemoglobinemia.[24] Inhalation of 20 ppm of NO in human volunteers has been shown to cause a rise in methemoglobin levels. Normal hemoglobin is converted to methemoglobin when the iron molecule is oxidized from Fe^{2+} (ferrous state) to the Fe^{3+} (ferric state) by a variety of compounds including the oxides of nitrogen. Hemoglobin that contains Fe^{3+} cannot bind oxygen. Also, methemoglobin shifts the oxyhemoglobin dissociation curve to the left, thereby increasing the affinity of normal hemoglobin for oxygen. These two effects of methemoglobinemia inhibit oxygen delivery to the tissues. This can be devastating in a victim that may already be suffering from CO poisoning and oxygen deprivation.

Phosgene

Phosgene causes local irritation to the skin, eyes, and upper respiratory tract. It is an extremely toxic compound formed during the combustion of chlorinated hydrocarbons, such as polyvinyl chloride. The lungs are its major target organ.

Exposure to less than 25 ppm in a single acute exposure is relatively nontoxic.[25] Exposure to 25–50 ppm can lead to pulmonary inflammation, which usually resolves in 2–3 weeks. However, exposure to 50–150 ppm may initially result in pulmonary inflammation, which often precedes pulmonary edema. Pulmonary edema and its associated complications are usually the cause of death except in the case of extremely high exposure. In this instance, the irritative nature of the compound can cause severe bronchoconstriction.

Pulmonary edema occurs after a clinically latent period that can vary depending on the dose of exposure but rarely extends beyond 24 hours, although some authors state that the onset can be delayed up to 72 hours.[26] No reliable predictors as to who will develop pulmonary edema when phosgene inhalation is suspected are known.

ASPHYXIANT GASES

Carbon Monoxide

Carbon monoxide (CO) is produced from incomplete combustion of organic materials, which occurs in virtually every fire.[7] Smoke from fires may contain from 0.1% to 10% CO (1,000 ppm to 100,000 ppm).[27] Poisoning from CO is the most common cause of death in fires.[28] Carbon monoxide is a colorless, odorless gas that has a reversible affinity for hemoglobin 210 times that of oxygen, forming carboxyhemoglobin. Carbon monoxide causes a shift in the oxyhemoglobin dissociation curve to the left[29] and binds numerous other heme-containing proteins.

The hemoglobin molecule can bind up to four oxygen or

Carbon monoxide is a colorless, odorless gas that has a reversible affinity for hemoglobin 210 times that of oxygen, forming carboxyhemoglobin. Carbon monoxide causes a shift in the oxyhemoglobin dissociation curve to the left and binds numerous other heme-containing proteins.

CO molecules to its heme groups. Because CO has a higher affinity for hemoglobin than oxygen, CO competes successfully for the binding sites, thus reducing the carrying capacity of blood for oxygen and ultimately resulting in tissue hypoxia.[30] The binding of carbon monoxide to the heme groups also appears to increase the bond strength of the remaining heme groups in the molecule for oxygen, therefore shifting the oxyhemoglobin dissociation curve to the left. This binding of CO to hemoglobin is reversible, therefore high concentrations of administered O_2 can effectively remove CO from the heme groups.

Carbon monoxide also binds with other heme-containing molecules such as the cytochromes, myoglobin, and the peroxidases. Carbon monoxide reversibly binds to and inhibits cytochrome oxidase in mitochondria, which blocks cellular respiration. However, oxygen has a higher affinity for cytochrome oxidase than CO. Adequate oxygenation prevents this binding from occurring. Myoglobin is also a large storage depot for oxygen, second only to hemoglobin. It may facilitate in the transport of oxygen to mitochondria. Carbon monoxide blocks these functions of myoglobin, thereby decreasing delivery of oxygen to the myocardium and other muscle tissue.[31]

Carbon monoxide is present at all times in the air we breathe. Humans can tolerate up to 100 ppm for up to 8 hours. It is dangerous to be exposed to 1,500 ppm for 1 hour, which corresponds to the IDLH, and levels of 4,000 ppm can be fatal in less than 1 hour.[11] Investigators have reported levels from 0 to 15,000 ppm at fire sites. Brandt-Rauf et al.[17] measured CO at 14/14 fire sites (ranging from 11.4 to 1,087 ppm). The Permissible Exposure Limit (PEL), an 8-hour time-weighted exposure limit established by the Occupational Safety and Health Administration, is 35 ppm. At a level of 500 ppm, it takes 90 minutes for humans to attain a carboxyhemoglobin (COHb) level of 20%; symptoms and signs at this level include headache and dilation of cutaneous vessels.[11] A COHb level of 50% can be reached in 300 minutes at 500 ppm and in 60 minutes at 1,000 ppm.[11] The CO-poisoned victim begins to have serious cardiovascular and central nervous system compromise at this level of carboxyhemoglobin, which can lead to coma, convulsions, and death.[13] Twenty percent of those individuals who die from CO poisoning, however, do so with COHb levels less than 50%.[7]

Hydrogen Cyanide

Hydrogen cyanide gas is generated when some nitrogen-containing materials, such as polyurethane, wool and silk,

Hydrogen cyanide gas is generated when some nitrogen-containing materials, such as polyurethane, wool and silk, are burned.

are burned. Because upholstery, plastic furnishings, and these fabrics are ubiquitous, hydrogen cyanide can be expected to be present in most fires.[3]

Cyanide (CN) is rapidly absorbed through bronchial mucosa and alveoli. It is an intracellular toxin and works by inhibiting the final step of oxidative phosphorylation by binding to the ferric state (Fe^{3+}) of the cytochrome a-a_3 complex. This prevents both the transfer of electrons to oxygen and the formation of adenosine triphosphate. Cellular respiration is therefore interrupted, which is the cause of death in CN poisoning. However, since the binding of CN to cytochrome a-a_3 is reversible, though very stable, the cyano-cytochrome complex can be dissociated. This allows the mitochondrial enzyme, sulfurtransferase (rhodenese), to transfer a sulfur to the CN ion in the presence of thiosulfate, thereby forming the less toxic compound, thiocyanate. Thus cellular respiration can be restored. Thiocyanate is excreted by the kidneys.

Hydrogen cyanide has been measured at fire sites. One investigator[17] recorded levels between 0 and 10 ppm in 13 of 14 fires, and a level of 75 ppm in the 14th fire. Other investigators have also demonstrated CN levels at fires, generally lower than the IDLH (50 ppm). Measured blood CN levels have been reported to be as high as 1.62 µg/ml.[32] Cyanide levels greater than 0.2 µg/ml are associated with toxicity and levels greater than 2–3 µg/ml are usually fatal.

Cyanide is an intracellular toxin and works by inhibiting the final step of oxidative phosphorylation by binding to the ferric state (Fe^{3+}) of the cytochrome a-a_3 complex. This prevents both the transfer of electrons to oxygen and the formation of adenosine triphosphate.

THERMAL INJURY

Although intense amounts of heat are generated during a fire, lung parenchymal burns are rare.[9,28,33] The temperature on the top floor of a burning building may reach 900°–1,000°F, but because the nasopharyngeal passages are so efficient at cooling air, temperatures of inhaled air are essentially cooled.[28,33] Generally, inhaled smoke is approximately 260°F and dry. Steam, on the other hand, has 4,000 times the heat-carrying capacity of dry air and can cause extensive damage.[34] Moritz and coworkers[35] observed mucosal injury as far as the major bronchioles, but thermal injury is usually limited to the supraglottic region.[9] In conscious patients, a reflex closure of the larynx in response to heated air protects the distal airways.

Pharyngeal edema, laryngeal edema, and laryngospasm are classic signs of thermal injury to the upper airway. These events can lead to life-threatening obstruction at the level of the vocal cords, usually within the first 24 hours of presentation.[28] Fluid resuscitation initiated for burn therapy may exacerbate pharyngeal/laryngeal edema leading to acute obstruction.[36]

Pharyngeal edema, laryngeal edema, and laryngospasm are classic signs of thermal injury to the upper airway.

DIAGNOSIS AND TREATMENT
GENERAL CONSIDERATIONS
Setting of Exposure

The circumstances of the exposure may provide some clues to the nature of the potential injury or systemic intoxication. It should be determined whether the exposure occurred in the open or in a confined space, such as being trapped in a small room or the cab of a car. The duration of potential exposure should also be assessed. With regard to the patient, clues to prognosis may include the presence or absence of concomitant thermal burns or intoxications such as ethanol. The toxicity of the chemical exposure in question may be gathered from information about other victims with regard to severity of symptoms, number of victims, and number of deaths. These variables are associated with an increased risk for smoke inhalation.[5]

Symptoms and Current History

Symptoms such as coughing, sore throat, or hoarseness suggest injury to the upper airway and the potential for developing airway obstruction. Shortness of breath or dyspnea suggests parenchymal injury. Systemic symptoms include headache, dizziness, nausea, vomiting, confusion, and syncope, and may occur as a result of poisoning by CO, CN, or other asphyxiants.[4,28,37] It is also important to determine if the firefighters, emergency response personnel, or paramedics have symptoms.

Past Medical History

The age and past medical history of the patient should be determined. Asthma or other chronic lung disease may be exacerbated by irritant gas inhalation. A history of coronary disease should prompt concern about possible aggravation of ischemia secondary to hypoxia induced by bronchoconstriction, CO, or parenchymal injury.[38]

AIRWAY INJURY
Clinical Presentation

The onset of airway edema and obstruction may be very rapid or delayed for several hours. History of prolonged exposure to smoke or highly irritant chemicals increases the likelihood of airway injury. The presence of stridor suggests impending obstruction. Facial burns, carbona-ceous sputum, soot in the nose and mouth, singed nasal hairs, and corneal burns are also commonly associated with smoke inhalation but do not necessarily predict the severity of airway injury.[5,28,37]

Special Studies

Most authorities recommend direct visualization of the lar-ynx as the most reliable method of determining presence of airway injury. This is usually accomplished with a flex-ible bronchoscope or laryngoscope[5,34,39]; immediate intu-bation over the endoscope can be performed if needed. In stable patients with mild symptoms, an alternate approach is to visualize the larynx by indirect laryngoscopy or simply admit and closely observe the patient,[28] being careful to follow clinical status and arterial oxygen saturation.

Treatment

For patients with mild injury characterized by slight sore throat or hoarseness, humidified oxygen and observation are recommended. More severe cases should be intubated, preferably early in the course, before progressive airway obstruction obscures visualization of anatomic landmarks and prevents passage of an endotracheal tube of sufficient size.

For patients with mild injury characterized by slight sore throat or hoarseness, humidified oxygen and observation are recommended. More severe cases should be intubated, preferably early in the course, before progressive airway obstruction obscures visualization of anatomic landmarks and prevents passage of an endotracheal tube of sufficient size. Tracheostomy or cricothyrotomy is rarely necessary. Maximal laryngeal edema usually occurs within 24 hours of the insult and resolution occurs within 2–5 days.[28] The use of steroids has been recommended but is not well doc-umented and remains controversial.[34]

PARENCHYMAL INJURY

Clinical Presentation

Injury to the lower respiratory tract may accompany upper airway injury or occur without significant upper airway findings. Patients may present with wheezing due to bron-chospasm. This is most common with injury involving ex-posures to very hot smoke, steam, or highly soluble gases such as ammonia or hydrogen chloride. Injury to the al-veoli with transudation of fluid and inflammatory exudate may lead to chemical pneumonia or noncardiogenic pul-monary edema.[28,37] This can be aggravated if excessive in-travenous fluid has been administered during burn resus-citation.[4] Focal atelectasis secondary to surfactant degra-dation or destruction may be visible on chest radiographs.

The onset of chemical pneumonitis may be very rapid, as with heavy exposures to highly irritant gases such as ammonia, acrolein, and hydrogen chloride, or delayed several hours, as with less soluble gases such as phosgene or oxides of nitrogen. Patients with less soluble gas exposure may have relatively little upper airway injury and their initial presentation may be misleadingly benign.[40] The onset of respiratory failure may be delayed by 8–36 hours after smoke inhalation. Patients without thermal skin burns are less likely to develop respiratory failure compared to those with serious burns.[4]

Special Studies

Pulse oximetry can be used to monitor oxygen saturation; however, pulse oximetry may be falsely normal in patients with carbon monoxide poisoning or methemoglobinemia. Arterial blood gases allow monitoring of oxygenation and ventilatory status and may indicate presence of metabolic acidosis. Arterial blood gases usually show hypoxemia with increased arterial alveolar gradient.[5,28,37] Tachypnea and metabolic acidosis may be caused by hypoxemia or may be secondary to other mechanisms such as hypovolemia secondary to burns, or carbon monoxide or other poisoning. Chest radiograph findings may lag behind clinical deterioration; a negative radiograph does not rule out subsequent worsening.[5,28]

Xenon-133 ventilation scanning has been used to assess ventilation defects associated with parenchymal injury.[41] Extravascular lung water has also been reported in animal experiments to correlate with the degree of injury. Computed tomography of the chest is more sensitive than chest radiography for locating focal atelectasis. However, these adjunctive techniques have a significant false negative rate, and they have not been found to be more useful than routine clinical evaluation in determining the course of therapy.[5,28]

Fiberoptic bronchoscopy has been recommended for determining the severity of injury and also for removal of debris from the bronchi.[39] However, others have argued that findings at bronchoscopy do not predict mortality or duration of intubation.[5]

Treatment

High-flow supplemental oxygen should be administered initially and the FIO_2 should be adjusted based on subsequent arterial oxygen content measurements as well as

Pulse oximetry can be used to monitor oxygen saturation; however, pulse oximetry may be falsely normal in patients with carbon monoxide poisoning or methemoglobinemia. Arterial blood gases allow monitoring of oxygenation and ventilatory status and may indicate presence of metabolic acidosis.

presence or suspicion of CO poisoning. If intubation is not required because there is no evidence of airway edema, it may still be necessary to assist ventilation or enhance oxygenation in patients with progressive parenchymal damage. Positive end-expiratory pressure assisted ventilation may be required for patients with severe parenchymal injury.

The use of steroids has been recommended for the treatment of smoke inhalation, but there are no convincing studies indicating that their use improves outcome.[5,28,37] On the other hand, their use may promote the development of an infection, which is a common cause of death in patients with inhalational injury. Antibiotics should be used for specific documented pathogens based on Gram stain results, and ultimately confirmed by cultures.

Pulmonary edema associated with chemical pneumonia and smoke inhalation results from alteration of lung permeability. Therefore, diuretic agents such as furosemide are not recommended for treatment, unless specific evidence for myocardial failure or hypervolemia is present (by pulmonary artery catheter monitoring). Excessive fluid administration should be avoided during burn resuscitation.[5]

SYSTEMIC ILLNESS OR INJURY
Carbon Monoxide Poisoning

Carbon monoxide poisoning is the single most common cause of poisoning in patients with smoke inhalation, and it is the leading cause of death.

Clinical Presentation Carbon monoxide poisoning is the single most common cause of poisoning in patients with smoke inhalation, and it is the leading cause of death. The majority of persons found dead in a fire have toxic levels of CO and/or CN in their blood.[28,42,43]

Patients with mild to moderate CO poisoning may have vague or nonspecific symptoms such as headache, nausea, vomiting, dizziness, and confusion. Persons with coronary artery disease may experience angina pectoris. With more serious intoxication, patients may experience syncope, seizures, hypotension, myocardial infarction, coma, and death.[42,44] Although there is considerable interindividual variability, symptoms and signs of CO poisoning correlate generally with CO blood levels (COHb saturation) (Table 2). In some patients, the COHb saturation may not appear to correlate with the severity of poisoning because the patients have received high-flow oxygen at the scene and during prehospital transport before COHb levels were obtained, leading to deceptively low results. This is particularly true for patients with severe poisoning who have suffered a major hypoxic insult. It has been argued that

TABLE 2   Signs and Symptoms of CO Poisoning at Various Concentrations of COHb

COHb Level (%)	Signs and Symptoms
0 to 10	Usually none.
10 to 20	Mild headache; mild dyspnea with exertion; patients with coronary disease may experience angina.
20 to 30	Throbbing headache; dyspnea with moderate exertion.
30 to 40	Throbbing headache; dizziness; nausea; vomiting; fatigue; poor judgment; dimness of vision.
40 to 50	Confusion; possible syncope; tachypnea; tachycardia.
50 to 60	Syncope; seizures; coma.
60 to 70	Coma; hypotension; respiratory failure, death.
>70	Rapidly fatal.

From Olson KR: Carbon monoxide poisoning: mechanisms, presentation and controversies in management. J Emerg Med 1:233, 1984. With permission.

CO may poison intracellular cytochrome oxidase or myoglobin and that such effects would not be reflected by the COHb.[44] However, it is unclear if such intracellular poisoning plays a significant role in CO poisoning. Some patients with CO poisoning will have flushed skin ("cherry red coloration") and bright red venous blood owing to the bright red color of the carboxyhemoglobin complex; however, these findings are not reliable and may be absent in patients with serious intoxication.[45]

Patients with severe CO poisoning (eg, those who present comatose or with seizures) are at risk for developing permanent neurologic or neuropsychiatric sequelae. One study reports the incidence of subtle memory loss and personality changes to be as high as 40%,[46] although others have reported these subtle neurological changes in 10–12% of patients.[47]

Laboratory Studies   The arterial oxygen saturation as reported on routine arterial blood gas testing is falsely normal because it is calculated from the arterial pO_2. The pO_2 is unaffected by CO poisoning because it reflects only oxygen dissolved in the plasma.[44] In addition, the oxygen saturation as measured by pulse oximetry is falsely normal because the pulse oximeter is incapable of distinguishing between COHb and oxyhemoglobin.[48] Thus, if CO poisoning is suspected it is necessary to obtain a specific measure of COHb using a cooximeter. However, the COHb level may not correlate with the severity of intoxication, particularly if it is obtained after significant time has elapsed since exposure, or if treatment with high-flow oxygen has been administered.[49]

Other findings in patients with CO poisoning may include metabolic acidosis (with or without respiratory compensation), and primary hyperventilation resulting from cellular hypoxia. The electrocardiogram may reveal nonspecific ST-T wave changes, arrhythmias, or evidence of myocardial ischemia or infarction.[50]

Computed tomographic scanning has been reported to predict brain damage in patients with severe poisoning; findings include loss of density in the central white matter and globus pallidus and cerebral edema.[49,51] In patients with less severe poisoning, neuropsychiatric testing has been reported to predict which patients have subtle neurologic deficits and who might develop neuropsychiatric sequelae.[47]

Treatment Carbon monoxide can be competitively removed from the hemoglobin complex by administration of oxygen. Although the elimination of COHb does not follow first-order kinetics, it is usually expressed as a "half-life." The half-life of COHb in room air is approximately 4–5 hours; however, with administration of 100% oxygen only, this can be shortened to 30–40 minutes. With administration of 100% oxygen in a hyperbaric chamber in which the ambient pressure is raised from the normal atmospheric pressure of 1 atmosphere (atm) to 2.5–3.0 atm, the half-life has been reported to be 15–20 minutes.[52]

Patients should initially be treated with the highest available oxygen concentration by a tight-fitting mask with high-flow oxygen and an oxygen reservoir, or via endotracheal tube. Selection of patients for hyperbaric oxygen (HBO) treatment remains unclear.[53,54] No controlled, randomized, prospective studies demonstrate improved outcome with HBO, although one nonrandomized study involving 629 adults found no benefit from HBO at 2 atm pressure compared with 100% oxygen at normal pressure (1 atm).[55] Proponents of HBO argue that their anecdotal experience justifies liberal use of HBO, particularly in patients with coma or other evidence of severe intoxication.[44,56,57] Also, because the fetus is much more sensitive to the effects of CO, a more liberal use of HBO for pregnant victims has been recommended.[58] Reported indications for use of HBO are listed below.[40,59,69]

1. Coma or other evidence of serious central nervous system dysfunction
2. COHb > 25%
3. Pregnancy

The half-life of COHb in room air is approximately 4–5 hours; however, with administration of 100% oxygen only, this can be shortened to 30–40 minutes.

If a chamber is readily available, then HBO may be appropriate for the patient with severe intoxication who does not respond to initial therapy. On the other hand, most hospitals do not have an HBO chamber and the patient may require transport to a distant facility that may not have intensive care monitoring equipment or personnel. Many chambers are small cylinders that can accommodate only the patient and not their caregivers. Thus, the potential risks and benefits should be carefully considered in patients with complications such as seizures, hypotension, or cardiac arrhythmias who may decompensate during transport to a distant or poorly equipped facility.[59]

Patients with mild to moderate metabolic acidosis should not receive sodium bicarbonate because acidemia promotes oxygen delivery to cells. All seriously symptomatic patients (chest pain, history of syncope, seizures, or coma) should be admitted for intensive cardiac and neurologic monitoring. A 12-lead electrocardiogram and cardiac enzymes should be obtained in all seriously symptomatic patients. Occasional delayed neurologic deterioration (leukoencephalopathy) has been reported after serious poisoning and usually occurs after 4–10 days; however, it is also reported in patients with hypoxic ischemic injury from other causes and is not specific for CO poisoning.[60–62]

Cyanide Poisoning

Clinical Presentation Cyanide poisoning also occurs frequently in victims of smoke inhalation. Many natural and synthetic materials release CN when burned. Victims of smoke inhalation with elevated COHb levels nearly always also have elevated CN levels, regardless of the type or location of the fire. In one study, all patients with significant smoke inhalation had elevated CN levels[43]; in another study, four of six house fire fatalities had toxic CN levels.[3]

Cyanide poisoning also produces cellular hypoxia, and therefore symptoms and signs of intoxication are very similar to those seen with CO poisoning. At low CN levels, patients experience headache, dizziness, nausea, and anxiety or confusion. At higher levels, syncope, hypotension, cardiac arrhythmias, seizures, coma, and death may occur.[63] Cyanide may have an additive or even synergistic effect with CO.[64]

Patients with CN poisoning may have an odor of "bitter almonds" although this is an unreliable finding, particularly since only about one-half of the population has the ability to detect the odor. The venous blood may appear to be bright red because oxygen is not being given up to the tissues, but red venous blood may also be a feature of CO poisoning.[63]

Laboratory Studies Blood CN levels are not readily available in most hospital laboratories but can be used for retrospective analysis and forensic documentation; CN levels greater than 0.2 μg/ml are associated with toxicity and levels greater than 2–3 μg/ml are usually fatal.[63]

Patients with serious CN poisoning usually have severe metabolic acidosis. The electrocardiogram may reveal evidence of myocardial ischemia or cardiac arrhythmias.

The measured venous oxygen content or oxygen saturation may be elevated (greater than 90% oxyhemoglobin saturation) in seriously poisoned patients because of lack of oxygen uptake by tissues.[63,65]

Treatment Although oxygen is relatively ineffective for treatment of CN poisoning, it may theoretically promote removal of CN from cytochrome oxidase and should be administered for treatment of simultaneous CO intoxication.

Several antidotal treatments for CN poisoning are available. In the United States, the only available approved treatment is the Lilly Cyanide Antidote kit (Table 3). Nitrites are thought to act by creating methemoglobin, which binds free CN.[63] Recently, it has been suggested that nitrites may also act by inducing vasodilation, which may increase the endothelial surface area for enzymatic intravascular degradation of CN, or by other undetermined means. Although nitrites appear to be very effective, they are potentially very toxic. Fatal methemoglobinemia and serious hypotension can occur after excessive or rapid administration.[66] Sodium thiosulfate acts as a substrate to promote the conversion of CN to the less toxic thiocyanate by the enzyme rhodanese, which is found in the liver and in the endothelium.

TABLE 3   Cyanide Antidote Kit

Antidote	Form	Dose
Amyl nitrite	12 aspirols (0.3 ml)	Crush 1–2 aspirols under patient's nose or over ET tube
Sodium nitrite	2 amps (300 mg each in 10 ml)	10 ml IV (children: 0.3 ml/kg or 9 mg/kg)
Sodium thiosulfate	2 amps (12.5 gm in 50 ml)	50 ml IV (children 1.6 ml/kg or 400 mg/kg)

Other antidotes include cobalt EDTA and hydroxocobalamin.[63,67] Hydroxocobalamin, used in France for CN poisoning, is a synthetic precursor of vitamin B_{12}, which combines with CN to form cyanocobalamin (vitamin B_{12}). It appears to be safe and effective, and is undergoing early clinical testing in the United States.[67]

Methemoglobinemia

Agents that induce methemoglobinemia are common combustion products (e.g., nitrogen oxides), and some patients with smoke inhalation from house and other fires have been reported to have elevated methemoglobin levels.[24]

Clinical Presentation
Patients with methemoglobinemia also experience the nonspecific symptoms and signs of cellular hypoxia, such as headache, dizziness, confusion, and nausea. With methemoglobin concentrations above 15–20% of hemoglobin saturation, patients may appear deeply cyanotic because of the dark color of the methemoglobin (MetHb) complex. Arterial and venous blood may appear a "chocolate brown" color. With more severe poisoning, patients may experience syncope, chest pain, seizures, coma, or death.[66]

Laboratory Studies
Methemoglobin saturation is performed using a co-oximeter to directly measure different hemoglobin complexes (oxyhemoglobin, methemoglobin, carboxyhemoglobin). The routine arterial blood gas machine measures the pO_2 of oxygen dissolved in plasma and will calculate a falsely normal oxygen saturation in methemoglobinemia. As with CO poisoning, using a pulse oximeter to measure oxygen saturation is unreliable because currently used pulse oximeters cannot distinguish the MetHb complex and falsely measure it as oxyhemoglobin.[68]

The routine arterial blood gas machine measures the pO_2 of oxygen dissolved in plasma and will calculate a falsely normal oxygen saturation in methemoglobinemia.

Treatment
Although it does not restore the MetHb complex to normal hemoglobin, oxygen therapy is usually administered due to the probability of simultaneous CO poisoning. Hyperbaric oxygen can deliver enough oxygen dissolved in plasma to provide all cellular needs and may be of some theoretical benefit for patients with dysfunctional hemoglobin, although it will probably not be readily available to most clinicians.

Antidotal treatment with methylene blue is very effective for most patients with methemoglobinemia. Methylene blue enhances the reduction of the oxidized ferric atom in the hemoglobin molecule. One to 2 mg/kg (0.1–0.2 cc/kg of a 1% solution) should be slowly administered intravenously; the dose may be repeated after 30 minutes. Methylene blue is not an effective treatment in persons with glucose-6-phosphate dehydrogenase deficiency or methemoglobin reductase deficiency.[66]

Overadministration of methylene blue can cause hemolysis and may induce methemoglobinemia. In addition, any use of methylene blue in patients who are suspected of also having CN poisoning may be counterproductive because it will reduce the availability of MetHb to bind free CN.[63,66]

SUMMARY OF TREATMENT AND DISPOSITION

Patients with a history of smoke inhalation should be evaluated in an emergency department and observed for at least several hours before discharge. Those patients with obvious evidence of airway compromise should be intubated early before laryngeal swelling makes anatomic visualization difficult. Patients with mild symptoms should undergo direct or indirect laryngoscopy in an attempt to document the presence of airway injury.

Patients with hypoxemia, tachypnea, and other signs of parenchymal injury (wheezing, rales, abnormal chest radiograph) should be admitted for intensive respiratory care. This may include endotracheal intubation and positive end-expiratory pressure if necessary. The clinician should remember that respiratory failure may be delayed 8–36 hours, particularly after inhalation of less-soluble gases.

Patients with the following clinical findings should be admitted or at least receive an extended period of observation: history of a closed space exposure, especially greater than 10 minutes; pO_2 less than 60 mm; serum bicarbonate less than 15 mmol/l; COHb > 10%; $[A - a]O_2$ difference on 100% O_2 greater than 100 mmHg[4]; abnormal chest radiography.

Several important systemic intoxications may exist simultaneously, with similar nonspecific symptoms and signs. Immediate treatment is desirable if the patient has severe intoxication by any of these poisons. However, it may not be possible to immediately identify which specific poison or combination of poisons is responsible for the patient's condition. Empiric treatment with oxygen may be helpful. However, the cyanide antidote kit or methylene blue may be dangerous or counterproductive and should be selectively used with caution.

For the patient with smoke inhalation who has signs of serious systemic intoxication (e.g., coma, seizures) the following approach is recommended: administer the highest-flow oxygen available and administer the sodium thiosulfate portion of the CN antidote kit. In contrast to nitrites, sodium thiosulfate is not harmful. In case of evidence of methemoglobinemia, it is probably best not to treat it unless it is severe (i.e., MetHb greater than 30–40%) because it may provide some protection against concomitant CN poisoning.

ACKNOWLEDGMENTS

Supported in part by a grant to the Center for Injury Research and Prevention. SFGH, CDC#R49/CCR 903697-02.

Dr. Liu was supported by a clinical fellowship from the Agency for Toxic Substances and Disease Registry (ATSDR).

References

1. Musk AW, Smith TJ, Peters JM, McLaughlin E: Pulmonary function in firefighters: acute changes in ventilatory capacity and their correlates. Br Med J 36:29, 1979

2. DiVincenti FC, Pruitt BA, Reckler JM: Inhalational injuries. J Trauma 11:109, 1971

3. Jones J, McMullen J, Dougherty J: Toxic smoke inhalation: cyanide poisoning in fire victims. Am J Emerg Med 5:318, 1987

4. Clark WR, Nieman GF: Smoke inhalation. Burns 14:473, 1988

5. Clark WR, Bonaventura M, Myers W: Smoke inhalation and airway management at a regional burn unit: 1974–1983. Part I. Diagnosis and consequences of smoke inhalation. J Burn Care Rehabil 10:52, 1989

6. Shirani KZ, Pruitt BA, Mason AD: The influence of inhalational injury and pneumonia on burn mortality. Ann Surg 250:82,1987

7. Nelson GL: Regulatory aspects of fire toxicology. Toxicology 47:181, 1987

8. Hunt JL, Agee RN, Pruitt BA: Fiberoptic bronchoscopy in acute inhalational injury. J Trauma 15:641, 1975

9. Schwartz DA: Acute inhalational injury. p. 297. In Rosenstock L (ed): Occupational medicine, state of the art reviews. Vol. 2. Hanley & Belfus, Philadelphia, 1987

10. Beauchamp RO: A critical review of the literature on acrolein toxicity. CRC Crit Rev Toxicol 14:309, 1985

11. Einhorn IN: Physiological and toxicological aspects of smoke produced during the combustion of polymeric materials. Environ Health Perspect June:163, 1975

12. Treitman RD, Burgess WA, Gold Avram: Air contaminants encountered by firefighters. Am Ind Hyg Assoc J 41(11):796, 1980

13. Proctor NH, Hughes JP, Fischman ML: Chemical hazards of the workplace. 2nd ed. JB Lippincott, Philadelphia, 1988

14. Close LG, Catlin FI, Cohn AM: Acute and chronic effects of ammonia burns to the respiratory tract. Arch Otolaryngol Head Neck Surg 106:151, 1980

15. Witten ML, Quan SF, Sobonya RE, Lemen RJ: New developments in the pathogenesis of smoke inhalation-induced pulmonary edema. West J Med 148:33, 1988

16. Markowitz JS: Self-reported short- and long-term respiratory effects among PVC-exposed firefighters. Arch Environ Health 44(1):30, 1989

17. Brandt-Rauf PW, Fallon LF, Tarantini T et al: Health hazards of firefighters: exposure assessment. Br J Ind Med 45:606, 1988

18. Charan NB, Lakshminarayan S, Myers GC, Smith DD: Effects of accidental chlorine inhalation on pulmonary function. West J Med 143:333, 1985

19. Threshold limit values and biological exposure indices. 8th ed. American Council of Governmental Industrial Hygienists, 1989

20. NIOSH/OSHA: Pocket guide to chemical hazards. NIOSH Publication No. 78-210. US Department of Health and Human Services, 1985

21. Goldstein IF, Lieber K, Andrews LR et al: Acute respiratory effects of short-term exposures to nitrogen dioxide. Arch Environ Health 43(2):138, 1988

22. Dowell AR, Kilburn KH: Ultrastructural effects of nitrogen dioxide on the lung. Am Rev Resp Dis 101:197, 1979

23. Scott EG, Hunt WB: Silo fillers disease. Chest 63:701, 1973

24. Hoffman RS, Sauter D: Methemoglobinemia resulting from smoke inhalation. Vet Hum Toxicol 31:168, 1989

25. Currie S: Pulmonary alteration in rats due to acute phosgene inhalation. Fundam Appl Toxicol 8:107, 1987

26. Diller WF: Medical phosgene problems and their possible solution. J Occup Med 20:189, 1978

27. Dolan M: Carbon monoxide poisoning. Can Med Assoc J 133:329, 1985

28. Heimbach DM, Waeckerle JF: Inhalation injuries. Ann Emerg Med 17:1316, 1988

29. Blinn L, Miller RH: Smoke inhalation injuries. Am J Otolaryngol 7:375, 1986

30. Mofenson H, Caracio T, Brody G: Carbon monoxide poisoning. Am J Emerg Med 2:254, 1984

31. Aronow W, Isbell M: Carbon monoxide effect on exercise induced angina pectoris. Ann Intern Med 79:392, 1973

32. Gonzales J, Sabatini S: Cyanide poisoning. Int J Artif Org 12:347, 1989

33. Wang CZ, Li A, Yang ZC: The pathophysiology of carbon monoxide poisoning and acute respiratory failure in a sheep model with smoke inhalation injury. Chest 97:736, 1990

34. Robinson L, Miller RH: Smoke inhalation injuries. Am J Otolaryngol 7:375, 1986

35. Moritz AR, Henriquez FC, Mclean R: The effects of inhaled heat on the air passages and lungs: an experimental investigation. Am J Pathol 21:311, 1945

36. Haponik FH, Meyers DA, Munster AM et al: Acute upper airway injury in burn patients: serial changes of flow-volume curves and nasopharyngoscopy. Am Rev Resp Dis 135:360, 1987

37. Desai MH, Rutan RL, Herndon DN: Managing smoke inhalation injuries. Postgrad Med 86:69, 1989

38. Marius-Nunez AL: Myocardial infarction with normal coronary arteries after acute exposure to carbon monoxide. Chest 97:491, 1990

39. Clark CJ, Reid WH, Telfer AB et al: Respiratory injury in the burned patient: the role of flexible bronchoscopy. Anaesthesia 38:35, 1983

40. Wald P, Becker CE: Toxic gases used in the microelectronics industry. p. 105. In La Dou J (ed): State of the art reviews: occupational medicine. Vol 1. Hanley & Belfus, Philadelphia, 1986

41. Moylan JA, Wilmore DW, Mouton DE et al: Early diagnosis of inhalation injury using Xenon-133 lung scan. Ann Surg 176:477, 1972

42. Olson KR: Carbon monoxide poisoning: mechanisms, presentation, and controversies in management. J Emerg Med 1:233, 1984

43. Clark CJ, Campbell D, Reid WH: Blood carboxyhemoglobin and cyanide levels in fire survivors. Lancet 1:1332, 1981

44. Thom SR, Keim LW: Carbon monoxide poisoning: a review of epidemiology, pathophysiology, clinical findings, and treatment options including hyperbaric oxygen therapy. J Toxicol Clin Toxicol 27:141, 1989

45. Meigs JW, Hughes JPW: Acute carbon monoxide poisoning: an analysis of 105 cases. Arch Ind Hyg Occup Med 6:344, 1952

46. Smith JS, Brandon S: Morbidity from acute carbon monoxide poisoning at three-year follow-up. Br Med J 1:318, 1973

47. Myers RA, Britten JS: Are arterial blood gases of value in treatment decisions for carbon monoxide poisoning? Crit Care Med 17:139, 1989

48. Barker SJ, Tremper KK: The effect of carbon monoxide inhalation on pulse oximetry and transcutaneous pO_2. Anesthesiology 66:677, 1987

49. Sawada Y, Takahashi M, Ohashi N et al: Computerized tomography as an indication of long-term outcome after acute carbon monoxide poisoning. Q J Med 36(144):445, 1967

50. Anderson RF, Allensworth DC, DeGroot WJ: Myocardial toxicity from carbon monoxide poisoning. Ann Intern Med 67:1172, 1967

51. Vieregge P, Klostermann W, Blumm RG, Borgis KJ: Carbon monoxide poisoning: clinical, neurophysiological, and brain imaging observations in acute disease and follow-up. J Neurol 236:478, 1989

52. Sasaki T: On half-clearance time of CO-hemoglobin in blood during hyperbaric oxygen therapy. Bull Tokyo Med Dent Univ 22:63, 1975

53. Grim PS, Gottlieb LJ, Boddie A, Batson E: Hyperbaric oxygen therapy. JAMA 263:2216, 1990

54. Ilano AL, Raffin TA: Management of carbon monoxide poisoning. Chest 97:165, 1990

55. Raphael UC, Elkharrat D, Jars-Guincestre MC et al: Trial of normobaric and hyperbaric oxygen for acute carbon monoxide intoxication. Lancet 2:414, 1989

56. Myers RA, Snyder SK, Emhoff TA: Subacute sequelae of carbon monoxide poisoning. Ann Emerg Med 14:1163, 1985

57. Norkool DM, Kirkpatrick JN: Treatment of acute carbon monoxide poisoning with hyperbaric oxygen: a review of 115 cases. Ann Emerg Med 14:1168, 1985

58. Van Hoesen KB, Camporesi EM, Moon RE et al: Should hyperbaric oxygen be used to treat the pregnant patient for acute carbon monoxide poisoning? A case report and literature. JAMA 261:1039, 1989

59. Sloan EP, Murphy DG, Hart R et al: Complications and protocol considerations in carbon monoxide-poisoned patients who require hyperbaric oxygen therapy: report from a ten-year experience. Ann Emerg Med 18:629, 1989

60. Myers RAM, Linberg SE, Cowley RA: Carbon monoxide poisoning: the injury and its treatment. JACEP 8:479, 1979

61. Ginsberg MD, Hedley-Whyte ET, Richardson EP: Hypoxic-ischemic leukoenceplopathy in Man. Arch Neurol 33:5, 1976

62. Plum F, Posner JB, Hain RF: Delayed neurological deterioration after anoxia. Arch Intern Med 110:56, 1962

63. Hall AH, Rumack BH, Karkal SS: Increasing survival in acute cyanide poisoning. Emerg Med Rep 9:129, 1988

64. Pitt BR, Radford EP, Gurtner GH et al: Interaction of carbon monoxide and cyanide on cerebral circulation and metabolism, Arch Environ Health Sep/Oct:354, 1979

65. Johnson RP, Mellors JW: Arteriolarization of venous blood gases: a clue to the diagnosis of cyanide poisoning. J Emerg Med 6:401, 1988

66. Hall AH, Kulig KW, Rumack BH: Drug- and chemical-induced methemoglobinemia: clinical features and management. Med Toxicol 1:253, 1986

67. Hall AH, Rumack BH: Hydroxocobalamin/sodium thiosulfate as a cyanide antidote. J Emerg Med 5:115, 1987

68. Watcha MF, Connor MT, Hing AV: Pulse oximetry in methemoglobinemia. Am J Dis Child 143:845, 1989

69. Hyperbaric center advisory committee emergency medical service: A registry for carbon monoxide poisoning in New York City. J Toxicol Clin Toxicol 26:419, 1988

ALKALI AND ACID INJURIES OF THE UPPER GASTROINTESTINAL TRACT

MARSHA FORD, MD, FACEP, ABMT[†]

Patients who ingest caustic materials, either alkali or acid, can present the clinician with two perplexing management questions: Who should undergo diagnostic endoscopy? What therapeutic measures can be used to limit the damage to the upper gastrointestinal tract, thereby decreasing the risk of morbidity and improving mortality? Patients who present with stridor or evidence of upper gastrointestinal tract perforation do not pose diagnostic dilemmas. The case of a small child, who otherwise appears healthy, with a history of caustic ingestion and perhaps an isolated oropharyngeal burn does raise the question as to whether or not endoscopy is indicated. The therapeutic role of corticosteroids remains debatable. Multiple studies in the literature address these questions, but few are adequately comparable or sufficiently rigorous to allow for interstudy comparison. The following shortcomings are often revealed in a survey of the literature: a lack of documentation of the quantity and concentration of acid or alkali ingested; a combination of acid, alkali and other caustic ingestions in the same study; the simultaneous analysis of adult and pediatric populations in spite of significant recognized differences in the amount of caustic material ingested and the potential for differences in healing characteristics; different classifications for staging the degree of mucosal burn, or, in many of the older studies, no classification of burn severity; and varying regimens for administering antibiotic, corticosteroid, or esophageal dilation therapies. This review will examine the alkali and acid caustic studies available in the literature in an attempt to answer the critical diagnostic and therapeutic questions raised above. Man-

Patients who ingest caustic materials, either alkali or acid, can present the clinician with two perplexing management questions: Who should undergo diagnostic endoscopy? What therapeutic measures can be used to limit the damage to the upper gastrointestinal tract, thereby decreasing the risk of morbidity and improving mortality?

[†] Director, Division of Toxicology, Assistant Chairman, Department of Emergency Medicine, Carolinas Medical Center, Charlotte, North Carolina

agement of injuries induced by agents that produce oxidation or reduction, desiccation, vesication, or protoplasmic poisoning of tissues will not be discussed.

ALKALI INGESTIONS

Alkali injuries are produced by bases that release hydroxide (OH$^-$) ions on dissociation in water. Sodium hydroxide (NaOH) is responsible for the majority of serious gastrointestinal alkali burns.[1-3] Lists of other potential alkali materials can be found in standard references.[4,5] Liquid preparations are more likely than solid preparations to produce deep, circumferential esophageal burns and serious gastric and small intestinal lesions.[6-9] The solid preparations tend to adhere to the oropharyngeal and proximal esophageal mucosa and produce burns in patches or linear streaks rather than in a circumferential manner.[9] In 1967, liquid NaOH became commercially available and the severity of alkali ingestions increased.[9] Responding to this problem, in 1973, the Food and Drug Administration (FDA) required safety packaging for all nonindustrial, commercially available strong alkalis with concentrations greater than 2% (and strong acids with concentrations greater than 10%).[5] Significant burns can occur, however, from compounds with lesser concentrations than those requiring safety packaging.[5] Burns can also result when packaging safeguards are circumvented by the transfer of a preparation into alternative containers or when an older child or adult ingests the agent with suicidal intent or subsequent to intellectual or psychiatric impairment. Additionally, many agricultural and industrial agents that are highly concentrated and packaged in nonsafety containers are accessible to children.[10]

Two common household cleaners, ammonia (ammonium hydroxide) and bleach (sodium hypochlorite), appear to result in problems usually only if aspirated or ingested intentionally in large amounts. In a total of 57 cases of household ammonia ingestion, the only significant complications were reported with large or intentional ingestions.[1,8,11-16] These complications were described as severe esophageal and laryngotracheal burns with resultant acquired respiratory distress syndrome (ARDS),[11] gastric necrosis, esophageal perforation, and duodenal and jejunal strictures,[12] airway obstruction due to supraglottic edema resulting in a tracheostomy,[8] and death.[1] Daly et al.[17] reported ulcerative esophagitis in 38 of 59 patients who ingested ammonia. However, the volume and concentration of the ammonia preparations and the severity of the esoph-

Liquid preparations are more likely than solid preparations to produce deep, circumferential esophageal burns and serious gastric and small intestinal lesions.

Ammonia and bleach result in problems usually only if aspirated or ingested intentionally in large amounts.

ageal lesions were not reported. Ingestion of bleach has been reported in 829 patients.[8,13–15,17–20] The only injuries resulting in clinically significant sequelae occurred in two patients who were reexposed to the bleach when they vomited.[21] Both patients required subsequent surgical repair for esophageal lesions. Usually, however, ingestions of household sodium hypochlorite preparations in small amounts either do not produce injury or result in mild esophageal burns without permanent sequelae.[8,13,14,18–20]

TOXICOPATHOLOGY

Factors that influence the extent and severity of gastrointestinal tract burns include the amount, form (liquid or solid), concentration, pH, and viscosity of the alkali ingested; the duration of contact with tissues, transit time, and presence or absence of food in the gut; presence of esophageal reflux after the ingestion; the underlying condition of the gastrointestinal mucosa; and the titratable acid/alkaline reserve.[9,22–25] In general, the larger the quantity of caustic material ingested, the greater the incidence of severe burns.[9,18] Experimentally, volume overdistention of the esophagus with a 10% NaOH solution resulted in an increased rate of esophageal perforation.[24] Titratable acid/alkaline reserve (TAR), the amount of a standard acid or alkali solution needed to titrate, respectively, an alkali or acid to pH 8.0 (approximating normal esophageal mucosal pH), may be a more important measure of caustic potential than pH.[23] For example, lemon juice has a low pH (2.9) and a low TAR value and is well tolerated by the gastrointestinal (GI) tract, whereas soldering flux, which has a near-neutral pH (6.8) and a high TAR value, produces significant mucosal injury. An *in vitro* study of the effects of various alkali and acid preparations on canine esophageal mucosa demonstrated that the incidence and degree of corrosive injury correlated better with the calculated TAR than the pH.[23]

Contact of GI mucosa with caustic alkali compounds results in liquefaction necrosis, a process comprised of protein and collagen destruction, fat saponification, tissue dehydration, and blood vessel thrombosis.[9] This process continues as penetration extends beyond the mucosa for a minimum of several minutes after initial contact.[26] The extent of this continued process depends on the factors enumerated above. Acute effects on the GI mucosa can include erythema, superficial and deep ulcerations, mucosal necrosis and perforation, depending upon the severity of the burn. Endoscopists[27,28] categorize the injuries,

Titratable acid/alkaline reserve (TAR), the amount of a standard acid or alkali solution needed to titrate, respectively, an alkali or acid to pH 8.0 may be a more important measure of caustic potential than pH.

or burns, to the esophageal mucosa into three degrees of severity.

First-degree burn: erythema and edema.

Second-degree burn: erythema, blistering, superficial ulceration, fibrinous exudate.

Third-degree burn: erythema, deep ulceration, friability, eschar formation, perforation.

Esophageal dilation and atony with edema and narrowing at the burn site have been documented within 24 hours of ingestion.[29]

The feline esophagus has significant similarity to that of a child. Experimental *in vivo* NaOH burns in cats have revealed three stages of esophagitis.

Stage 1: Ulceration is complete by 24 hours with a constant narrowing of the burn site noted by 48–72 hours.

Stage 2: Granulation tissue develops by 8–10 days.

Stage 3: Contraction and stricture formation of the wound begins by week 3.[30]

Esophageal perforation may occur immediately or develop within the first few days in cases of severe injury. An experimental canine model has shown that the esophagus is weakest during the second week of the healing process[31] and may be prone to perforation during this time.

It is commonly assumed that alkali caustic ingestions affect the esophagus and, if aspiration occurs, the tracheobronchial tree structures, with a relative sparing of the stomach and small intestine. Many of the studies leading to the development of these beliefs occurred in the pediatric population where ingestions were usually unintentional and involved small amounts. However, deliberate ingestions of larger amounts of alkali caustic substances can result in hemorrhage and perforation of both the stomach and small intestine.[27,29,32–34]

Deliberate ingestions of larger amounts of alkali caustic substances can result in hemorrhage and perforation of both the stomach and small intestine.

CLINICAL PRESENTATION

Initial signs and symptoms vary according to the site and extent of injury and include dysphagia; odynophagia; drooling; vomiting; hematemesis; oropharyngeal, substernal, and abdominal pain; and abdominal rigidity and auscultatory findings of mediastinal air.[9,14,29,33,35] Stridor and respiratory difficulty can result from aspiration of caustic material. Edema and swelling of the larynx, vocal cords, or trachea have been observed; in a child these clinical manifestations can mimic epiglottitis.[3,8,36] Stridor may predict a significant esophageal lesion.[36,37]

When using presenting signs and symptoms to determine the need for diagnostic endoscopy, the clinician should consider the following three points.

1. The presence or absence of oropharyngeal burns does not correlate well with the presence or absence of esophageal lesions (see Table 1) and should not be used in determining the need for further evaluation of the GI tract.

2. In the pediatric population, the presence or absence of drooling, vomiting, or stridor may assist the clinician in determining the need for endoscopy. Two studies examined initial signs and symptoms as possible predictors of esophageal injury in children. Gaudreault et al.[38] retrospectively studied 378 patients for the incidence of vomiting, dysphagia, excessive salivation, abdominal pain, refusal to drink, and oropharyngeal burns. In this study, the majority of patients with these signs or symptoms had mild to no esophageal burns, leading to the conclusion that the occurrence or severity of esopha-

The presence or absence of oropharyngeal burns does not correlate well with the presence or absence of esophageal lesions and should not be used in determining the need for further evaluation of the GI tract.

TABLE 1   Presence or Absence of Oropharyngeal Burns Associated With the Presence or Absence of Esophageal Burns in Alkali and Acid Ingestions

Human Studies		Oropharyngeal Burns Present		Oropharyngeal Burns Absent	
Author	n	Esophageal Burns Present	Esophageal Burns Absent	Esophageal Burns Present	Esophageal Burns Absent
Viscomi et al.[39]	76	16	48	1	11
Wijburg et al.[32]	197	54	31	39	73
Middlekamp et al.[27]*	96	32	54	—	—
Middlekamp et al.[49]	47	21	26	—	—
Anderson et al.[52]	131	60	57	0	14
Chen et al.[29]	5	5	0	—	—
Hawkins et al.[8]	118	35	49	2	32
DiConstanza et al.[18]	94	30	2	46	16
Gaudreault et al.[38]	378	51	228	14	85
Crain et al.[37]	79	6	63	1	9
Cello et al.[14]	17	15	0	2	0
Yarrington et al.[51]	26	12	8	3	3
Bikhazi et al.[15]	105	45	35	6	19
Zarger et al.[43]	41	24	4	7	6
Total	1410	406	605	121	268

* Only 86 patients underwent endoscopy.

geal lesions cannot be predicted from clinical presentation. Using data collected on a standardized form, Crain et al.[37] retrospectively evaluated 79 patients for 3 signs: drooling, vomiting, and stridor. In this study, the presence of two or more signs predicted all the patients with moderate to severe esophageal burns. Of the 65 patients with 0 or 1 sign, 0 had a positive endoscopy. In comparing these findings with those of Gaudreault, Crain et al. noted that if they had included oropharyngeal burns as a serious sign, no statistically significant association between these signs and serious esophageal burns would have been found. The findings of Crain's study may be used as general guidelines when evaluating a child for endoscopy but should be tempered by the clinician's index of suspicion for serious esophageal involvement.

3. In the adult population, presenting signs and symptoms may not help the clinician in determining the need for endoscopy. No studies similar to those of Gaudreault and Crain have been made in the adult population, many of whom have psychiatric impairment and/or suicidal intent and may minimize their symptoms. Here too, larger amounts of caustic material are typically ingested and would be expected to result in injury. In general, the physician should endoscope psychiatrically impaired and/or suicidal patients with a history of caustic ingestion and should strongly consider endoscopy for other adult patients, regardless of symptoms. Wijburg et al.[32] found patients with few or no symptoms who had severe esophageal lesions, and they recommend endoscopy for all patients suspected of caustic ingestion.

In the adult population, presenting signs and symptoms may not help the clinician in determining the need for endoscopy.

DIAGNOSIS

The evaluation of GI tract injury is dependent upon meticulous endoscopy, with occasional use of water-soluble contrast radiographic studies if endoscopy cannot be performed.

The evaluation of GI tract injury is dependent upon meticulous endoscopy, with occasional use of water-soluble contrast radiographic studies if endoscopy cannot be performed. Water-soluble radiographic contrast material should be used if GI tract perforation is suspected because it is less toxic than barium if spillage occurs into the mediastinum or the peritoneum. If the patient's airway is compromised and aspiration may occur, radiographic contrast studies should not be performed since water-soluble contrast materials cause pulmonary irritation leading to ventilatory compromise and pulmonary edema.

Patients should be endoscoped within the first 12–24

hours. Lesions can be visualized by that time, allowing for appropriate treatment or hospital discharge for the patient.[16,28,32] Prior to endoscopy, a careful assessment of airway function should be made. Respiratory compromise may mandate immediate airway management, as described below. An otorhinolaryngeal examination should precede endoscopy in all patients to determine the extent of airway and upper esophageal burns.[9,18] If severe hypopharyngeal burns are observed, perforation may occur with endoscopy. In these cases, diagnostic strategies include limiting the examination and performing radiographic studies with water-soluble contrast material as a substitute for direct visualization.[8] In all of these patients with severe hypopharyngeal burns, prophylactic airway protection is required because of the high risk of aspiration. In the opinion of Wijburg et al.,[32] the technique of inserting a rigid endoscope through which a flexible scope is passed for evaluation may be used when hypopharyngeal burns prevent normal endoscopic examination.

Traditionally, the endoscopist terminates the procedure at the level of the first deep, penetrating, and/or circumferential esophageal burn to avoid perforation.[9,28,39] With the recognition that alkali-induced gastric and small intestinal injuries may be unpredictable from the clinical examination,[13,18,27,29,34] some physicians now advocate flexible endoscopy to include the stomach and duodenum (panendoscopy), regardless of the presence of second-degree or nonperforating third-degree esophageal burns. The flexible endoscope is more pliant than the rigid instrument and, in the hands of an experienced endoscopist, requires minimal air insufflation for passage, thus lessening air-induced distention of damaged tissues. Use of a pediatric fiberoptic endoscope may further minimize the risk of perforation.[13,14] Of a reported total of 135 patients who underwent flexible endoscopy to include gastroscopy, it can be inferred that 32 patients had either a second- or third-degree esophageal burn. Of these 32, 1 patient sustained a perforation during the procedure but recovered. Of a reported 19 patients[8,9,12,14,25,33,34] who suffered gastric necrosis secondary to alkali caustic ingestion, 5 presented with severe epigastric pain, hematemesis, or signs of perforation that led to immediate surgery. Aggressive panendoscopy would not have influenced the clinical outcome in these patients. The remaining 14 patients with gastric necrosis either underwent delayed surgery for perforation or life-threatening GI hemorrhage or were managed conservatively. Nine of these patients died from complications of their gastric necrosis. It is possible that early diagnosis of the gastric necrosis by panendoscopy followed by sur-

Patients should be endoscoped within the first 12–24 hours.

With the recognition that alkali-induced gastric and small intestinal injuries may be unpredictable from the clinical examination, some physicians now advocate flexible endoscopy to include the stomach and duodenum (panendoscopy), regardless of the presence of second-degree or nonperforating third-degree esophageal burns.

Panendoscopy with a fiberoptic endoscope is therefore recommended in all patients with a history of alkali caustic ingestion.

gical resection of the gangrenous GI tract would have improved the mortality rate of this group. Panendoscopy with a fiberoptic endoscope is therefore recommended in all patients with a history of alkali caustic ingestion. The skill of the endoscopist should determine whether the endoscope is passed beyond a deep, penetrating, and/or circumferential esophageal burn in order to examine the stomach and, if possible, the duodenum.

If gastric mucosal damage is suspected and endoscopic examination cannot be performed, two alternative methods for evaluation of gastric and small intestinal injury have been proposed. The first utilizes early radiographic studies with water-soluble contrast.[8] These studies are most useful for documenting a suspected perforation and for evaluation of the presence or absence of mucosal damage. However, determination of burn severity often cannot be made. The second calls for direct visualization of the stomach, via exploratory laporatomy, in any patient with endoscopically documented second- or third-degree esophageal lesions or in any patient with a history of liquid alkali ingestion and a persistent alkaline gastric pH.[6] This approach allows for aggressive surgical management of observed burns (described below).[9,40,41] While laporoscopy may provide a safe and rapid alternative to the two alternatives described above, this technique has not been evaluated in caustic ingestions and therefore cannot be recommended at this time.

MANAGEMENT

Immediate attention to the maintenance of a patent airway is of primary importance. Life-threatening respiratory compromise should be managed initially with orotracheal intubation, cricothyroidotomy, or tracheostomy if massive pharyngeal or laryngeal burns or edema are present. Nasotracheal intubation may be performed using a fiberoptic laryngoscope for direct visualization of the airway followed by insertion of the endotracheal tube over the fiberoptic scope. Stridor indicates hypopharyngeal burns and the need for immediate otorhinolaryngeal assessment of the airway. Most reported cases of airway burns are managed initially or secondarily with tracheotomy.[27,36] Corticosteroids may be useful in decreasing laryngeal edema in patients with airway burns.[18]

Stridor indicates hypopharyngeal burns and the need for immediate otorhinolaryngeal assessment of the airway.

Evacuation of the stomach either by induced emesis or by orogastric tube lavage is contraindicated. Repeat exposure to the alkali will increase esophageal damage. Dilution of the ingested alkali probably offers no benefit as the burn occurs almost immediately with mucosal contact and addition of fluid may induce vomiting. An *in vitro* study demonstrated little change in pH when water was added to NaOH.[42] Also contraindicated is administration of a weak acid, such as vinegar, to "neutralize" the alkali. This therapy may generate an exothermic reaction with subsequent thermal damage to the mucosa, produce gas that can distend and further damage tissues, and provoke vomiting.

Patients should be kept NPO initially and given parenteral analgesics until pain is relieved. Caution must be exercised not to overmedicate to the point where the physical examination is obscured. Opioids are the ideal agents for pain control because of their potent analgesia and easy reversibility. After otorhinolaryngeal examination and diagnostic endoscopy, patients with first-degree burns may be discharged if they are able to take fluids orally. All patients with second-degree burns should be admitted to a regular hospital bed; all patients with third-degree burns should be admitted to an intensive care unit. Patients with diagnosed gastric necrosis, as discussed in the section headed *Diagnosis*, should undergo laparotomy with resection of necrotic GI tract. Uncomplicated patients with second-degree burns should receive total parenteral nutrition (TPN) initially to reverse the hypercatabolism associated with the acute phase.[18] These patients can be started on oral fluids by the end of the first week[30] and advanced to solids as tolerated. In patients with third-degree burns, TPN[18] or a feeding jejunostomy[43,44] should be used until the GI tract has healed. Although H_2-blocker drugs may be used to decrease gastric acidity, their effectiveness has not been studied.

Should corticosteroids be used in these patients to decrease esophageal stricture formation? This indication for corticosteroids remains controversial. In 1950, Spain et al.[45] showed that immediate cortisone therapy decreased fibroblastic activity while allowing epithelialization in murine NaOH-induced wounds. Subsequently, corticosteroid therapy has been examined for its potential to decrease stricture formation in dogs, cats, and rabbits with experimentally induced NaOH esophageal burns. Initial studies indicated a decline in stricture formation when corticosteroids were administered.[24,30,46–48] Some of these studies also employed antibiotics to decrease the potential for infectious complications,[30,46,47] and this therapy was extended to human treatment regimens to protect against secondary bacterial invasion of the esophageal burn, as well as pulmonary and mediastinal infections.[30,40]

A comparison of available human studies in the literature to ascertain the efficacy of corticosteroids is hampered by the lack of or variability in burn classifications when categorizing patients into treatment groups, the difficulty in properly differentiating second-degree from third-degree burns with endoscopy,[39] and the use of varying corticosteroid regimens, with or without antibiotics, and with or without adjunctive esophageal dilation therapy. Early reported corticosteroid successes were noted in studies that did not classify the burns according to severity,[39,50,51] a significant problem since nearly all first-degree and most second-degree burns heal without sequelae, regardless of the therapy (see Table 2). A number of studies were conducted using comparable burn classification systems.[8,27,28,49] These studies concluded that corticosteroids did diminish stricture formation although a reappraisal of this data does not support this judgment (see Table 2). The majority of second-degree burns improve, but the majority of third-degree burns develop strictures regardless of therapy. The most rigorous study thus far is that of Anderson et al.[52] who studied 131 children over an 18-year period. All underwent rigid endoscopy within 24 hours and, if the esophagus was burned, were randomized to treatment either with or without a 5–6 week course of corticosteroids. The findings of this study are listed in Table 2. They concluded that the use of corticosteroids did not alter the rate of stricture formation, which correlated better with the severity of the burn at the time of presentation. This conclusion is hampered by the fact that the power of the study allowed only an 80% chance of finding a 30% difference in the outcomes of the treatment regimens in the study population. Also, due to the small number of untreated patients with second-degree burns, the study did not definitively prove that corticosteroids were ineffective in this group.[53] Nevertheless, at this time, corticosteroids have not been proven to alter the rate of esophageal stricture formation.

Corticosteroids may decrease the need for eventual surgical repair of esophageal strictures if used in conjunction with esophageal dilation. Middelkamp et al.[27] prospectively studied 96 cases of caustic ingestion treated with corticosteroids and antibiotics and found that, of 7 patients with third-degree burns, 3 required surgical replacement and 3 required feeding gastrostomies. One patient died. However, 2 other studies added esophageal dilation to the therapeutic regimen and reported that of 14 patients who developed strictures, 0 required surgical repair.[3,30] Anderson et al.,[52] who used dilation for all strictures, noted a trend toward less surgical replacement of the esophagus in the patients treated with steroids (4 of 10 compared with 7 of 11 nontreated patients), but this did not achieve sta-

At this time, corticosteroids have not been proven to alter the rate of esophageal stricture formation. Corticosteroids may decrease the need for eventual surgical repair of esophageal strictures if used in conjunction with esophageal dilation.

TABLE 2 Effects of Corticosteroid Therapy in the Management of Alkali Injury to the Esophagus

| | Esophageal Lesions Treated With Steroids | | | | | | Esophageal Lesions Treated Without Steroids | | | | | |
| | First Degree | | Second Degree | | Third Degree | | First Degree | | Second Degree | | Third Degree | |
Human Studies*	Total Burns	Strictures	Total Burns	Strictures	Total Burns	Strictures	Total Burns	Strictures	Total Burns	Strictures	Total Burns	Strictures
Webb et al.[28]	4	0	18	5	6	6	9	0	3	0	2	2
Middlekamp et al.[49]	13	0	5	0	3	3	—	—	—	—	—	—
Middlekamp et al.[27]	19	0	6	1	7	7	—	—	—	—	—	—
Hawkins et al.[8]§	—	—	9	2	2†	2†	—	—	11	4	2‡	2‡
Anderson et al.[52]	6	0	15	1	10	9	13	0	5	0	11	11
Total	42	0	53	9	26	25	22	0	19	4	13	13

* Includes only those studies with data acceptable for comparison.
† One patient had early perforation and one had early death; therefore neither is included in the totals.
‡ Both patients died and are therefore not included in the totals.
§ Includes only the prospective portion of the study.

Given the unanswered questions regarding corticosteroids, they should be used only in patients with second- or third-degree esophageal burns in whom esophageal dilation will be used as adjunctive therapy if strictures develop.

tistical significance. Further study is needed to determine if corticosteroid therapy decreases the need for reparative surgery, perhaps by rendering the strictures easier to dilate.

Given the unanswered questions regarding corticosteroids, they should be used only in patients with second- or third-degree esophageal burns in whom esophageal dilation will be used as adjunctive therapy if strictures develop. Corticosteroids may be given to adults as methylprednisolone 40 mg intravenously every 8 hours[54] and to children as prednisolone 2 mg/kg/day intravenously[52] until oral intake is resumed, when equivalent doses of oral prednisone can be substituted. After 3 weeks of full-dose therapy, the corticosteroids are tapered over the subsequent 3–6 weeks, depending on the severity of the injury.[28,52] If corticosteroids are administered, patients should also be given antibiotics to prevent bacterial invasion of the burn sites,[46,47] which may play a significant role in the pathogenesis of the caustic burn and stricture.[55] Ampicillin in doses of 50 mg/kg/day to a maximum of 8 to 12 g/day for adults intravenously (initially) or orally in divided doses (after oral feedings are resumed) is recommended for the duration of the corticosteroid therapy.[5,52] Tetracycline in adults, erythromycin in children, or clindamycin in adults or children can be used in patients who are allergic to penicillin. If corticosteroid therapy is withheld, antibiotic therapy should be used only for documented infectious complications.

Esophageal dilation is used after the second or third week in patients who develop documented strictures.[28,30] Dilation before the end of the second week has been associated with an increased incidence of perforation and stricture formation. The latter may result from repetitive damage with increased scarring.[3,6,24,30] Both anterograde dilations, for mild to moderate burns, and retrograde dilations, for severe burns, have been used.[3,35,52] In patients with severe strictures, retrograde dilation over a guide wire placed via gastrostomy is the preferred method.[56] Dilation is safer when performed over a string or guide wire but may still be complicated by esophageal perforation, especially when performed in the anterograde manner.[56]

Several other management strategies have been used in small numbers of patients. Wijburg et al.[16,32] advocate using a flexible, siliconized nasogastric tube as the sole treatment of caustic esophageal lesions. This tube functions as a stent, keeping the esophagus patent and also allowing for tube feedings at an early stage. Three easily dilated strictures were noted in 43 patients with deep, circumferential burns treated in this manner. A potential complication of nasogastric tube use is the promotion of gastro-esophageal reflux,[26] although this was not reported by Wijburg. Surgery with direct visualization of the esophagus, stomach, and surrounding organs, as described in the section headed *Diagnosis*, allows for accurate staging of third-degree burns, possible prevention of peritoneal caustic contamination, and resection of necrotic tissue with surgical repair and placement of stents or strings for subsequent esophageal dilation.[9,40,41] Regardless of therapeutic philosophy, emergency laparotomy should be performed when signs of perforation, necrosis, or life-threatening hematemesis or hematochezia occur.[33]

Experimental therapies that have been studied in animals include lathyrogens, N-acetylcysteine, and sodium polyacrylate. Lathyrogens, such as β-aminopropionitrile (BAPN), are compounds that prevent covalent cross-linkage in newly formed collagen, decreasing the strength of the scar tissue in esophageal lesions and rendering them more susceptible to dilation. In a canine NaOH esophageal burn study,[57] esophageal patency was compared in control, corticosteroid plus dilation, and BAPN plus dilation animal groups. The treatments were begun at 4 weeks after the burn, after stricture formation had occurred. The BAPN group progressed from a mean esophageal diameter of 7.9 mm at the beginning of therapy to 18.3 mm at the end, compared with changes of 6.5 to 7.7 mm for the control group and 9.0 to 11.0 mm for the corticosteroid group. Another lathyrogen, penicillamine, decreased stricture formation of rats with NaOH esophageal burns (strictures in 2 of 23 rats) compared with the control group (strictures in 18 of 22 rats).[58] N-acetylcysteine (NAC), in a comparison study with corticosteroids and a control group, decreased severity and incidence of stricture formation in rats with experimentally induced esophageal NaOH injury.[59] The rates of reduction of stricture formation were comparable for NAC (48%) and corticosteroids (48%) compared with controls (74%), as was the severity of stenosis (severe stenosis 6% in NAC group, 7% in corticosteroid group, and 30% in control group). Theories for the activity of NAC on newly formed collagen include effects on intermolecular sulfhydryl-sulfhydryl bonds in collagen, disulfide linkages involved in interfibrillar components of collagen, and pro-collagen molecules.[59] Sodium polyacrylate, a viscous, water-soluble synthetic polymer with mucosal protective effects, decreased burn size and prevented weight loss in rats administered 25% NaOH by gastric gavage.[60] No human studies have employed any of these experimental therapies, and BAPN is not currently available for human use.

Emergency laparotomy should be performed when signs of perforation, necrosis, or life-threatening hematemesis or hematochezia occur.

COMPLICATIONS/CLINICAL SEQUELAE

Patients may suffer perforation of the esophagus and/or stomach, gastrointestinal hemorrhage, or chemical pneumonitis that may evolve into ARDS.[27] With few exceptions, perforation and GI hemorrhage occur in the setting of severe, third-degree burns.[8,9,18,33,34,52] These complications have been managed both conservatively, with drainage and antibiotics for esophageal perforation and supportive therapy for GI hemorrhage[34]; and aggressively, with a variety of surgical procedures including total esophagectomy, gastrectomy, or both, and cervical esophagostomy or pharyngostomy and jejunostomy, with subsequent reconstructive surgery.[6,9,49] Duration of healing of the acute esophageal lesions depends upon the burn severity, with first-degree burns healing within 1 week, second-degree burns healing within 20–30 days, and third-degree burns healing within 90 days in survivors.[18] Stricture formation, if it occurs, begins to develop at approximately the second or third week after ingestion,[24,29,32,49] although delays have been reported.[27] Eighty percent of all strictures are manifested within the first 2 months, while 99% are evident by the end of the first year.[28] Strictures that do not respond to dilation and prevent adequate nutritional intake are managed with esophagectomy and colonic interposition.[28,36,49,61,62] Scarring of the pharynx, epiglottis, and gastric pylorus may require pharyngoplasty, resection of the epiglottis or trachea, or partial or total gastrectomy.[36,49,63]

Patients who develop esophageal strictures after caustic ingestions are at risk for the development of esophageal cancer. Patients who develop strictures from caustic ingestion must be monitored for life for the development of malignant disease.

Patients who develop esophageal strictures after caustic ingestions are at risk for the development of esophageal cancer. In a series of 2,414 patients with esophageal carcinoma, Appelqvist et al.[64] reported 63 cases of squamous-cell esophageal carcinoma that developed in patients with a history of alkali ingestion. Hopkins et al.[65] obtained a history of caustic injury in 12 of 846 patients with squamous-cell esophageal carcinoma. The mean ages of the patients at the time of presentation in these series were 48 and 52.8 years, respectively, which is younger than the usual age of 60–62 years for development of esophageal carcinoma. The latency period between ingestion and appearance of the carcinoma ranged from 9 to 71 years, with the average varying from 38.7 to 45.8 years after ingestion.[64,65] The youngest patient reported with esophageal carcinoma was a 15-year-old boy who ingested lye at age 3.[66] The midthoracic region is the most common site of occurrence, and the cancers typically develop at the site of stricture.[64,65,67,68] Patients who develop strictures from caustic ingestion must be monitored for life for the development of malignant disease.

A patient with a normal initial endoscopy does not require routine follow-up evaluation for delayed stricture formation. Of 26 patients with initial negative endoscopies, 8 were reendoscoped 12–18 months later and had normal examinations; none developed delayed strictures.[49] Tewfik et al.[3] performed routine barium swallows at 6 weeks on 68 patients and found 6 esophageal strictures, all occurring in patients who had demonstrated burns on initial esophagoscopy. Stricture formation has not been reported in patients whose initial examinations were negative for upper GI tract burns.

ACID INGESTIONS

Guidelines for the diagnosis and management of acid injuries are less well established than those for alkali ingestions. This is due in large part to the limited number of human cases of acid ingestion, which in the West accounts for only 5% of all reported cases of corrosive ingestions.[43,69] Experimentally, both animal and human studies have concentrated on the more prevalent alkali ingestions. Thus the strategies for treating acid ingestions derive largely from case reports and two larger human series reported from India.[43,69]

Sources and types of acid are numerous and listed in standard reference texts.[4,5] Hydrochloric acid is the most common acid ingested,[43,44,70] followed by sulfuric acid.[44] Acids release hydronium (H^+) ions upon dissociation in water. When ingested, acids produce a coagulation necrosis almost immediately upon contact with the GI mucosa.[69,71] This necrosis may involve destruction of the columnar epithelium, submucosa, and muscularis mucosa, with consolidation of normally loose connective tissue, thrombosis of blood vessels, and hemolysis of erythrocytes forming a coagulum over the burn.[72,73] Whereas alkali-induced liquefaction necrosis may continue to penetrate deeper tissues, the acid-induced coagulum hinders further acid penetration into the tissues and may protect the deeper muscular layers.[9,22] However, full thickness burns with perforation can occur with severe injuries.[71] Acids tend to damage the stomach more than the esophagus, although esophageal burns with subsequent stricture formation can occur.[43,73] In a series of 34 patients ingesting acids, 17 sustained a superficial second-degree esophageal burn or worse.[8] Acids demonstrate a predilection for the distal two-thirds of the stomach. Factors contributing to

Acids tend to damage the stomach more than the esophagus, although esophageal burns with subsequent stricture formation can occur.

this predilection include a pathway along the lesser curvature that facilitates rapid transition of liquids from the esophagus to the pylorus, known as the "magenstrasse"; acid-induced pyloric spasm with subsequent pooling of acid distally, which prolongs mucosal contact time; food in the stomach that shields the greater curvature; and protection of the fundus by air.[74-76] The duodenum is relatively spared,[44] possibly secondary to protection afforded by pyloric spasm.[43]

CLINICAL PRESENTATION

In a large prospective study, oropharyngeal pain (73%) and dysphagia (56%) were the two most frequent presenting complaints.

In a large prospective study of 41 patients with acid ingestion,[43] oropharyngeal pain (73%) and dysphagia (56%) were the two most frequent presenting complaints, followed by salivation (37%), odynophagia (34%), and vomiting (34%). Dysphagia and odynophagia were closely associated with esophagitis, occurring in 96% of patients. Signs and symptoms referable to gastric lesions were less reliably associated, with epigastric pain, tenderness, or both occurring in only 49% of patients with gastric burns.

Oropharyngeal examination may reveal whitish mucosa with a swollen or necrotic uvula.[69,77] As with alkali ingestions, the presence or absence of oropharyngeal burns does not predict the condition of the esophageal or gastric mucosa. One study found no oropharyngeal burns in 20% of patients with moderate to severe esophageal and/or gastric lesions,[43] while in another series, 54% of patients with a normal oropharynx had injury to the upper GI tract.[44] Aspiration of the acid can produce stridor, rales, and rhonchi, and ARDS can develop rapidly.[75,77] Gastrointestinal hemorrhage and signs and symptoms of upper GI tract perforation may be present.[8,43,77] Severe systemic effects, such as metabolic acidosis, disseminated intravascular hemolysis, hyponatremia and hypotension, have been reported.[69,72,77-79] Signs and symptoms referable to these conditions should be sought.

Upper GI tract endoscopy should be performed as soon as possible in any patient confirmed or suspected of ingesting an acid since presenting signs and symptoms often do not predict serious GI tract injury.

DIAGNOSIS

Upper GI tract endoscopy should be performed as soon as possible in any patient confirmed or suspected of ingesting an acid since presenting signs and symptoms often do not predict serious GI tract injury.[43,44] Esophagus, stomach and, if possible, duodenum should be examined. Flexible endoscopy to include stomach and duodenum has been reported without complication in 49 of 56 patients, 51–86% of whom had moderate to severe esophageal lesions.[43,44] Of the remaining seven patients, two were not endoscoped initially past the cardioesophageal junction due to severe injuries of the cardia; repeat endoscopies were successfully completed 2 days later. Five patients with evidence of perforation were not endoscoped. Examination of the GI tract distal to the esophagus is critically important in acid ingestions to assess both the severity of gastric injury and the need for emergent surgery. In a total of 107 patients reported in the literature, death occurred in 16 patients, 14 of whom had severe gastric necrosis and/or perforation. One death occurred from esophageal perforation alone, and one death resulted from pulmonary complications secondary to aspiration of hydrochloric acid.[8,18,43,44,69,72,75,77,80,81] Knowledge of the extent of gastric damage is important in gauging the severity of injury to the patient.

Zargar et al.[43] have defined a burn classification system for acid-induced injury to the esophagus and stomach using five grades.

Examination of the GI tract distal to the esophagus is critically important in acid ingestions to assess both the severity of gastric injury and the need for emergent surgery.

Grade 0: normal examination.

Grade 1: edema, hyperemia of mucosa.

Grade 2a: superficial, localized ulcerations, friability, blisters.

Grade 2b: grade 2a findings plus circumferential ulceration.

Grade 3: multiple, deep ulcerations, areas of extensive necrosis.

On endoscopic examination, the more severe injuries can be expected in the lower two-thirds of the esophagus and in the distal body and antrum of the stomach. Radiologic studies with water-soluble contrast material performed acutely may reveal changes consistent with esophagitis or gastritis but are inadequate to assess severity of injury other than perforation.[43]

MANAGEMENT

The airway should be managed to assure adequate ventilatory support in a manner similar to that for alkali injuries. A nasogastric tube should be placed immediately and suction applied to remove any remaining acid that may be pooled in the stomach due to pyloric spasm. This will decrease gastric contact time with the remaining acid and is a safer procedure than when used in alkali ingestions due to the coagulum-limited penetration of the burn.[69,71] Theoretically, this will also decrease some of the systemic complications associated with acid absorption. Penner[74] re-

A nasogastric tube should be placed immediately and suction applied to remove any remaining acid that may be pooled in the stomach due to pyloric spasm.

viewed 13 cases that reportedly underwent early gastric tube placement without complication. Dilution with water, antacids, or other diluents is relatively contraindicated due to exothermic reactions generating heat (dilution of 91.6% sulfuric acid with an equal volume of water raises the temperature of the resultant 61% sulfuric acid by 79°C).[74] Increasing gastric volume could also precipitate emesis.

Patients should be kept NPO and given intravenous fluids and sufficient parenteral analgesics to relieve pain. Routine laboratory blood studies, including coagulation parameters and blood type and cross-match for transfusion, and chest and abdominal radiographs to evaluate for perforation and chemical pneumonitis should be performed. All patients with a grade 1 or 2a burn should be admitted to a regular hospital bed; those with grade 2b or 3 should be monitored in an intensive care unit. Total parenteral nutrition should be administered to these patients until oral feedings resume.

Corticosteroids should not be administered.

Corticosteroids should not be administered. The efficacy of this therapy remains unexamined and unproven. Additionally, corticosteroids may mask signs of peritonitis, thus delaying necessary surgery.[69] Antibiotics should be used only in cases of documented infection.

The necessity and timing of surgical intervention remains the most controversial aspect of management. In the two series reported from India, surgery was performed only for GI tract perforation, which occurred solely in patients with grade 3 lesions.[43,44] The outcome of these patients was poor. Seven deaths occurred in nine patients who developed either esophageal (1 death) or gastric (6 deaths) perforations, for a mortality rate of 78%. Two patients survived after operative closure. Of the remaining 31 patients who developed either esophageal or gastric strictures, 14 ultimately required surgical repair. The other 17 patients either refused surgery, developed only mild symptoms, or were lost to follow-up evaluation. Chodak et al.[69] identified 25 cases of acid or non-alkali caustic ingestions in a review of the literature from 1960–1977. They noted that 23 of these 25 patients required surgery at some point, 8 emergently for peritonitis or perforation (3 deaths) and 15 electively at a later date for pyloric stenosis or suspected cancer. In the latter elective cases, the surgery was technically difficult secondary to adhesions.

Given the high mortality rate in cases of acid-induced upper GI tract perforation and the ultimate requirement for surgery in the majority of patients reported, an aggressive surgical approach is recommended.

Given the high mortality rate in cases of acid-induced upper GI tract perforation and the ultimate requirement for surgery in the majority of patients reported, an aggressive surgical approach is recommended in the following situations:

1. When endoscopy reveals evidence of grade 3 burns with full-thickness necrosis (blackened, ulcerated mucosa) of the stomach or esophagus.

2. If signs or symptoms of GI tract perforation are manifest on initial presentation.

Again, while the potential utility of laparoscopy is exciting, it remains undocumented in these cases.

The optimal time for surgery is before perforation occurs. Exploratory laparotomy permits direct identification and resection of necrotic GI mucosa, examination of adjacent organs for damage caused by acid soilage of the peritoneal cavity, and peritoneal lavage to remove the acid contaminating the peritoneal cavity. A variety of reparative surgical procedures have been used acutely, including partial gastrectomy with a Billroth I or II anastomosis; total gastrectomy with tube duodenostomy, closure of the distal esophagus and a double-barreled esophagostomy; pancreatoduodenectomy; splenectomy; and resection of gangrenous small bowel.[69,75,82] Feeding jejunostomy and gastrostomy can be performed with string placement for subsequent retrograde dilation. A second-look operation has been advocated to evaluate for further necrosis.[69] Early aggressive surgical resection of gangrenous tissue is advocated to avoid perforation with spillage of acid into the thoracic or peritoneal cavities.

The optimal time for surgery is before perforation occurs.

A second-look operation has been advocated to evaluate for further necrosis.

COMPLICATIONS/CLINICAL SEQUELAE

Many of the complications that occur with severe alkali injuries, such as GI tract perforation, GI hemorrhage, aspiration pneumonitis, and ARDS, can also occur with grade 3 acid-induced injuries.[8,18,43,44] Additionally, metabolic acidosis, disseminated intravascular coagulation, and hypotension may complicate the clinical course.[72,77] Tracheoesophageal fistulae have also been reported.[83]

As with alkali injuries, the time necessary to heal the GI tract depends upon the severity of injury. Endoscopic examination reveals healing in patients with grades 1 and 2a injuries in 21–28 days, in those with grade 2b injuries in 24–40 days, and in survivors with grade 3 burns in 32–54 days.[43] Stricture formation can occur at the sites of grades 2b or 3 upper GI tract burns. Zargar et al.[43] reported stricture formation in 14 of 21 patients with esophageal burns, 16 of 25 patients with gastric lesions, and in the only patient with a duodenal burn. The time to stricture formation is less well established than for alkali injuries, but strictures can be expected to develop as healing progresses. Esophageal strictures may lead to dysphagia, weight loss, and vomiting. Pyloric, antral, or duodenal stenosis can produce gastric outlet obstruction with progressive symptoms of anorexia, weight loss, epigastric fullness, and vomiting.[69,82,84,85] These strictures may respond to dilation or require surgical repair, including esophagectomy with colonic interposition, pyloroplasty, gastrojejunostomy, antrectomy with a Billroth I anastomosis, and subtotal gastrectomy with a Billroth I or II anastomosis.[43,85] Adenocarcinomas arising in the site of acid-induced esophageal and gastric strictures have been reported.[71,86,87] Due to the possible risk of malignancy, some physicians advocate resection rather than dilation or repair of gastric strictures.[71,84] Although the incidence of malignant transformation of acid-induced strictures remains unknown, the risk mandates monitoring these patients for life.

Although the incidence of malignant transformation of acid-induced strictures remains unknown, the risk mandates monitoring these patients for life.

Two problems that have not been reported in alkali-injured patients may arise in those who have ingested acid and sustained severe gastric burns: (1) healing may result in a small, scarred, immobile stomach and frequent small feedings may be needed to avoid a dumping syndrome, and (2) achlorhydria and diminished or absent intrinsic factor may also develop. Patients should be monitored periodically for these conditions. Gastric emptying and motility can be evaluated with contrast radiographic studies. Vitamin B_{12} therapy may be necessary to avoid an acquired pernicious anemia.[72]

SUMMARY

Alkali and acid injuries to the GI tract pose several diagnostic and therapeutic dilemmas for the clinician. Endoscopy should be performed within the first 12–24 hours in alkali-injured patients and immediately in those with a history of acid ingestion. Patients with alkali injuries should be panendoscoped if possible and then treated with nutritional support, analgesics, and antibiotics for documented infections. Corticosteroid therapy remains controversial; its use may decrease the need for surgical repair of the esophagus when used in conjunction with dilation therapy for strictures. Patients with acid injuries should be panendoscoped, and similar treatment with potent analgesics and nutritional support is required. Those with grade 3 burns should undergo immediate laparotomy with resection of necrotic tissue and surgical repair to avoid perforation with acid soilage of the peritoneum. Both types of injury can result in stricture formation in the GI tract that may necessitate long-term dilation therapy or surgical repair. The increased risk of malignancy mandates life-time monitoring in those patients developing strictures. Prevention of these injuries remains the best cure.

References

1. Litovitz TL, Schmitz BF, Bailey KM: 1989 annual report of the American Association of Poison Control Centers national data collection system. Am J Emerg Med 8:394, 1990

2. Grenga TE: A new risk of lye ingestion by children (Letter). N Engl J Med 308:156, 1983

3. Tewfik TL, Schloss MD: Ingestion of lye and other corrosive agents: a study of 86 infant and child cases. J Otolaryngol 9:72, 1980

4. Wason S: Alkaline corrosives. In: Poisondex. Vol. 68. Micromedex, Denver, 1991

5. Hoffman RS, Goldfrank LR, Howland MA: Caustics and batteries. p. 769. In Goldfrank LR, Flomenbaum NE, Lewin NA, et al. (eds): Goldfrank's toxicologic emergencies. 4th ed. Appleton & Lange, Norwalk, 1990

6. Kirsh MM, Peterson A, Brown JW et al: Treatment of caustic injuries of the esophagus: a ten year experience. Ann Surg 188:675, 1978

7. Cleveland WW, Thornton N, Chesney JG et al: The effect of prednisone in the prevention of esophageal stricture following the ingestion of lye. South Med J 51:861, 1958

8. Hawkins DB, Demeter MJ, Barnett TE: Caustic ingestion: controversies in management: a review of 214 cases. Laryngoscope 90:98, 1980

9. Estrera A, Taylor W, Mills LJ et al: Corrosive burns of the esophagus and stomach: a recommendation for an aggressive surgical approach. Ann Thorac Surg 41:276, 1986

10. Edmonson MB: Caustic alkali ingestions by farm children. Pediatrics 79:413, 1987

11. Klein J, Olson KR, McKinney HE: Caustic injury from household ammonia. Am J Emerg Med 3:320, 1985

12. Ernst RW, Leventhal M, Luna R et al: Total esophagogastric replacement after ingestion of household ammonia. N Engl J Med 268:815, 1963

13. Sugawa C, Lucas CE: Caustic injury of the upper gastrointestinal tract in adults: a clinical and endoscopic study. Surgery 106:802, 1989

14. Cello JP, Fogel RP, Boland IR: Liquid caustic ingestion. Arch Intern Med 140:501, 1980

15. Bikhazi HB, Thompson ER, Shumrick DA. Caustic ingestion: current status. a report of 105 cases. Arch Otolaryngol 89:112, 1969

16. Wijburg FA, Heymans HSA, Urbanus NAM: Caustic esophageal lesions in childhood: prevention of stricture formation. J Pediatr Surg 24:171, 1989

17. Daly JF, Cardona JC: Acute corrosive esophagitis. Arch Otolaryngol 74:41, 1961

18. Di Costanzo J, Noirclerc M, Jouglard J et al: New therapeutic approach to corrosive burns of the upper gastrointestinal tract. Gut 21:370, 1980

19. Pike DG, Peabody JW, Davis EW et al: A re-evaluation of the dangers of Clorox ingestion. J Pediatr 63:303, 1963

20. Landau GD, Saunders WH: The effect of chlorine bleach on the esophagus. Arch Otolaryngol 80:174, 1964

21. French RJ, Tabb HG, Rutledge LJ: Esophageal stenosis produced by ingestion of bleach: report of two cases. South Med J 63:1140, 1970

22. Tucker JA, Silberman HD, Turtz ML et al: Tucker retrograde esophageal dilatation 1924–1974: a historical review. Ann Otol Rhinol Laryngol Suppl 16:3, 1974

23. Hoffman RS, Howland MA, Kamerow HN et al: Comparison of titratable acid/alkaline reserve and pH in potentially caustic household products. J Toxicol Clin Toxicol 27:241, 1989

24. Knox WG, Scott JR, Zintel HA et al: Bouginage and steroids used singly or in combination in experimental corrosive esophagitis. Ann Surg 166:930, 1967

25. Ritter FN, Newman MH, Newman DE: A clinical and experimental study of corrosive burns of the stomach. Ann Otol Rhinol Laryngol 77:830, 1968

26. Cotton R, Fearon B: Esophageal strictures in infants and children. Can J Otolaryngol 1:224, 1972

27. Middelkamp JN, Ferguson TB, Roper CL et al: The management and problems of caustic burns in children. J Thorac Cardiovasc Surg 57:341, 1969

28. Webb WR, Koutras P, Ecker RR et al: An evaluation of steroids and antibiotics in caustic burns of the esophagus. Ann Thorac Surg 9:95, 1970

29. Chen YM, Ott DJ, Thompson JN et al: Progressive roentgenographic appearance of caustic esophagitis. South Med J 81:724, 1988

30. Haller JA, Bachman K: The comparative effect of current therapy on experimental caustic burns of the esophagus. Pediatrics 34:236, 1964

31. Johnson EE: A study of corrosive esophagitis. Laryngoscope 73:1651, 1963

32. Wijburg FA, Beukers MM, Heymans HS et al: Nasogastric intubation as sole treatment of caustic esophageal lesions. Ann Otol Rhinol Laryngol 94:337, 1985

33. Allen RE, Thoshinsky MJ, Stallone RJ et al: Corrosive injuries of the stomach. Arch Surg 100:409, 1970

34. Welsh JJ, Welsh LW: Endoscopic examination of corrosive injuries of the upper gastrointestinal tract. Laryngoscope 88:1300, 1978

35. Haller JA, Andrews HG, White JJ et al: Pathophysiology and management of acute corrosive burns of the esophagus: results of treatment in 285 children. J Pediatr Surg 6:578, 1971

36. Ferguson MK, Migliore M, Staszak VM et al: Early evaluation and therapy for caustic esophageal injury. Am J Surg 157:116, 1989

37. Crain EF, Gershel JC, Mezey AP: Caustic ingestions: symptoms as predictors of esophageal injury. Am J Dis Child 138:863, 1984

38. Gaudreault P, Parent M, McGuigan MA et al: Predictability of esophageal injury from signs and symptoms: a study of caustic ingestion in 378 children. Pediatrics 71:767, 1983

39. Viscomi GJ, Beekhuis GJ, Whitten CF: An evaluation of early esophagoscopy and corticosteroid therapy in the management of corrosive injury of the esophagus. J Pediatr 59:356, 1961

40. Ray JF, Myers WO, Lawton BR et al: The natural history of liquid lye ingestion: rationale for aggressive surgical approach. Arch Surg 109:436, 1974

41. Meredith JW, Kon ND, Thompson JN: Management of injuries from liquid lye ingestion. J Trauma 28:1173, 1988

42. Maull KI, Osmand AP, Maull CD: Liquid caustic ingestions: an *in vitro* study of the effects of buffer, neutralization, and dilution. Ann Emerg Med 14:1160, 1985

43. Zargar SA, Kochhar R, Nagi B et al: Ingestion of corrosive acids: spectrum of injury to upper gastrointestinal tract and natural history. Gastroenterology 97:702, 1989

44. Dilawari JB, Singh S, Rao PN et al: Corrosive acid ingestion in man: a clinical and endoscopic study. Gut 25:183, 1984

45. Spain DM, Molomut N, Haber A: The effect of cortisone on the formation of granulation tissue in mice. Am J Pathol 26:710, 1950

46. Rosenberg N, Kunderman PJ, Vroman L et al: Prevention of experimental lye strictures of the esophagus by cortisone. Arch Surg 63:147, 1951

47. Rosenberg N, Kunderman PJ, Vroman L et al: Prevention of experimental esophageal stricture by cortisone. II. Control of suppurative complications by penicillin. Arch Surg 66:593, 1953

48. Weisskopf A: Effects of cortisone on experimental lye burn of the esophagus. Ann Otol Rhinol Laryngol 61:681, 1952

49. Middelkamp JN, Cone AJ, Ogura JH et al: Endoscopic diagnosis and steroid and antibiotic therapy of acute lye burns of the esophagus. Laryngoscope 71:1354, 1961

50. Borja AR, Ransdell HT, Thomas TV et al: Lye injuries of the esophagus: analysis of ninety cases of lye ingestion. J Thorac Cardiovasc Surg 57:533, 1969

51. Yarington CT, Heatly CA: Steroids, antibiotics, and early esophagoscopy in caustic esophageal trauma. N Y State J Med 63:2960, 1963

52. Anderson KD, Rouse TM, Randolph JG: A controlled trial of corticosteroids in children with corrosive injury of the esophagus. N Engl J Med 323:637, 1990

53. Lovejoy FH Jr: Corrosive injury of the esophagus in children: failure of corticosteroid treatment reemphasizes prevention (Editorial). N Engl J Med 323:668, 1990

54. Howell JM: Alkaline ingestions. Ann Emerg Med 15:820, 1986

55. Bosher LH, Burford TH, Ackerman L: The pathology of experimentally produced lye burns and strictures of the esophagus. J Thorac Surg 21:483, 1951

56. Hawkins DB: Dilation of esophageal strictures: comparative morbidity of antegrade and retrograde methods. Ann Otol Rhinol Laryngol 97:460, 1988

57. Madden JW, Davis WM, Butler C et al: Experimental esophageal lye burns. II. Correcting established strictures with beta-aminopropionitrile and bougienage. Ann Surg 178:277, 1973

58. Gehanno P, Guedon C: Inhibition of experimental esophageal lye strictures by penicillamine. Arch Otolaryngol 107:145, 1981

59. Liu AJ, Richardson MA: Effects of N-acetylcysteine on experimentally induced esophageal lye injury. Ann Otol Rhinol Laryngol 94:477, 1985

60. Ehrenpreis ED, Leikin JB: Use of oral sodium polyacrylate in rat gastrointestinal alkali burns. Vet Hum Toxicol 30:135, 1988

61. West KW, Vane DW, Grosfeld JL: Esophageal replacement in children: experience with thirty-one cases. Surgery 100:751, 1986

62. Gossot D, Sarfati E, Celerier M: Early blunt esophagectomy in severe caustic burns of the upper digestive tract: report of 29 cases. J Thorac Cardiovasc Surg 94:188, 1987

63. Leape LL, Ashcraft KW, Mann CM: Tracheal resection for lye stricture. Surgery 72:357, 1972

64. Appelqvist P, Salmo M: Lye corrosion carcinoma of the esophagus: a review of 63 cases. Cancer 45:2655, 1980

65. Hopkins RA, Postlethwait RW: Caustic burns and carcinoma of the esophagus. Ann Surg 194:146, 1981

66. Kinnman J, Shin HI, Wetteland P: Carcinoma of the oesophagus after lye corrosion: report of a case in a 15 year old Korean male. Acta Chir Scand 134:489, 1968

67. Benedict EB: Carcinoma of the esophagus developing in benign stricture. N Engl J Med 224:408, 1941

68. Kiviranta UK: Corrosion carcinoma of the esophagus: 381 cases of corrosion and nine cases of corrosion carcinoma. Acta Otolaryngol (Stockh) 42:89, 1952

69. Chodak GW, Passaro E: Acid ingestion: need for gastric resection. JAMA 239:225, 1978

70. Muhletaler CA, Gerlock AJ, de Soto L et al: Acid corrosive esophagitis: radiographic findings. AJR 134:1137, 1980

71. Fisher RA, Eckhauser ML, Radivoyevitch M: Acid ingestion in an experimental model. Surg Gynecol Obstet 161:91, 1985

72. Jelenko C III, Story J, Ellison RG Jr: Ingestion of mineral acid. South Med J 65:868, 1972

73. Gray HK, Holmes CL: Pyloric stenosis caused by ingestion of corrosive substances: report of case. Surg Clin North Am 28:1041, 1948

74. Penner GE: Acid ingestion: toxicology and treatment. Ann Emerg Med 9:374, 1980

75. Nicosia JF, Thornton JP, Folk FA et al: Surgical management of corrosive gastric injuries. Ann Surg 180:139, 1974

76. Testa GF: Contrileta radiologica e sperimentale alla studio dell lesione esofagee e gastriche nelle causticazioni da alcali. Radiol Med (Torino) 25:17, 1938

77. Greif F, Kaplan O: Acid ingestion: another cause of disseminated intravascular coagulopathy. Crit Care Med 14:990, 1986

78. Linden CH, Berner JM, Kulig K et al: Acid ingestion: toxicity following systemic absorption (Abstr). Vet Hum Toxicol 25:282, 1983

79. Brinklov AMM, Andersen PK, Nielsen PS et al: Dissemineret intravaskulaer koagulation ved saltsyreforgiftning. Ugeskr Laeger 141:2606, 1979

80. Gimmon (Goldschmidt) Z, Durst AL: Acid corrosive gastritis: a plea for delayed surgical approach. Am J Surg 141:381, 1981

81. Lowe JE, Graham DY, Boisaubin EV Jr et al: Corrosive injury to the stomach: the natural history and role of fiberoptic endoscopy. Am J Surg 137:803, 1979

82. Maull KI, Scher LA, Greenfield LJ: Surgical implications of acid ingestion. Surg Gynecol Obstet 148:895, 1979

83. Pense SC, Wood WJ, Zwemer FL et al: Tracheoesophageal fistula secondary to muriatic acid ingestion. Burns 14:35, 1988

84. Scher LA, Maull KI: Emergency management and sequelae of acid ingestion. JACEP 7:206, 1978

85. Chong GC, Beahrs OH, Payne WS: Management of corrosive gastritis due to ingested acid. Mayo Clin Proc 49:861, 1974

86. O'Donnell CH, Abbott WE, Hirshfeld JW: Surgical treatment of corrosive gastritis. Am J Surg 78:251, 1949

87. Eaton H, Tennekoon GE: Squamous carcinoma of the stomach following corrosive acid burns. Br J Surg 59:382, 1972

INDEX

Page numbers followed by the letter *f* refer to figures; those followed by *t* refer to tables.

Liquefaction necrosis, 227
Lithium
   overdose, extracorporeal removal for, 70
   volume of distribution, 29–30
Liver disease. *See* Hepatic entries

MDAC. *See* Activated charcoal, multiple-
      dose therapy
Methanol poisoning
   extracorporeal removal for, 69
   forced diuresis and urine alkalinization
      for, 67–68
   sodium bicarbonate for, 97–99
Methemoglobinemia, from nitrogen oxide
      inhalation, 207–208
   diagnosis and treatment, 219–220
Methylene blue, for methemoglobinemia,
      219–220
Mini-Mental State examination, 150
Monoamine oxidase inhibitors
   hypertension from, 194–195
   toxicity onset, 5
Mushroom poisoning, extracorporeal
      removal for, 71t, 71–72
Myocardial depression, toxins associated
      with, 183, 183t

Naloxone, for delirium, 161–162
Nitrites, and tissue binding, 32
Nitrogen oxide inhalation, 204t, 207–208

Opioid overdose, naloxone for, 161–162
Organic brain syndrome; *see also* Delirium
   defined, 147–148
Organophosphate poisoning, 5–6, 193
Oxygen, hyperbaric. *See* Hyperbaric oxygen

Paraldehyde, for ethanol withdrawal, 167
Paraquat poisoning, extracorporeal removal
      for, 71t, 73
Pentobarbital overdose, sodium bicarbonate
      for, 95–96
Peritoneal dialysis, 66
pH, and drug distribution, 26–27
Pharmacokinetics. *See* Toxicokinetics
Phencyclidine poisoning, activated charcoal
      for, 160–161
Phenobarbital overdose
   extracorporeal removal for, 71t, 72–73
   MDAC for, 53–54

sodium bicarbonate for, 94–96
Phenothiazines, for delirium, 163, 167
Phenytoin
   for digoxin, poisoning, 119
   poisoning, 15
Phosgene inhalation, 204t, 208
Phyencyclidine poisoning, psychosis from,
      153
Physostigmine, for anticholinergic
      poisoning, 196–197
Plant toxins, and fluid loss, 180–181, 181t
Post-distribution plasma concentration, 28
Procainamide/NAPA poisoning,
      extracorporeal removal for, 71t, 74
Protein binding
   and distribution, 30–32
   and extracorporeal toxin removal
      efficiency, 62t, 63
   and sodium bicarbonate efficacy, in TCA
      overdose, 86
Psychosis, drug-related, 152–154
Pulmonary edema, from phosgene
      inhalation, 205, 208

Quinidine poisoning, sodium lactate for, 83

Renal failure
   and clearance, 36
   drugs associated with, 34t
Rhabdomyolysis, sodium bicarbonate for,
      100–101

Salicylate
   absorption, and activated charcoal, 24–25
   distribution, 26
   poisoning
      and cardiovascular compromise, 185
      extracorporeal removal for, 68t, 68–69
      MDAC for, 54
      sodium bicarbonate for, 89–94
Scorpion sting envenomation, 138–139, 140t,
      141
Secobarbital overdose, sodium bicarbonate
      for, 95–96
Sedative-hypnotic agents; *see also individual*
      agents
   cross-tolerance, and delirium tremens
      treatment, 167–168
   for ethanol withdrawal, 167–168
   tolerance, 164–165, 166
   withdrawal from, and delirium, 164–169